Eating Right for Two

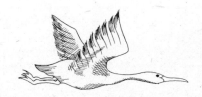

Eating

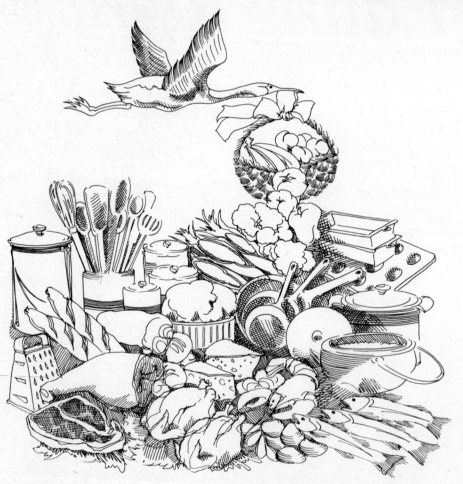

Recipes by

Right for Two

THE COMPLETE NUTRITION GUIDE AND COOKBOOK FOR A HEALTHY PREGNANCY

Text by Diane Klein
Rosalyn T. Badalamenti

ILLUSTRATIONS BY
LAUREN JARRETT

Ballantine Books • New York

To every woman's unborn child

And to my husband, Elliott, and our children, Beverly and Carolyn.

D.K.

To Dot and Marian, good sisters and mothers, both.

R.T.B.

Contents

FOREWORD

Over the past decade, great technological advances have been made in the fields of perinatology and neonatology (the medical specialties devoted to the care of the unborn fetus and the newborn infant, respectively). Obstetricians, using such tools as ultrasound, amniocentesis, and electronic fetal monitoring, can diagnose a wide variety of fetal disorders and, in many cases, effectively treat their unborn and unseen little patients.

In addition, neonatologists have developed elaborate neonatal intensive-care units, where infants weighing as little as one-and-a-half pounds can now be kept alive with the use of specially designed infant respirators, sophisticated monitoring equipment, intravenous feedings, new antibiotics, and expert nursing care.

The cost of premature and other sick infants is staggering, both in terms of the billions of dollars spent each year throughout the United States and in terms of the large numbers of physicians, nurses, and other medical personnel committed to the care of these babies. Furthermore, the enormous cost in emotional stress to the families of such sick children cannot be measured. How much better it would be if more infants were born in good health and fewer required long and expensive medical treatment!

As Diane Klein so vividly points out in *Eating Right for Two*, there are many reasons why a mother may deliver a premature, underweight, or imperfectly developed infant. But, unfortunately, medical science has not yet come up with all of the answers.

For example, we do not know why certain babies are born with severe abnormalities nor why some pregnancies end in miscarriage or in premature labor. On the other hand, through the use of widespread immunization we have been able to prevent German Measles during pregnancy and therefore eliminate the disease's devastating effects on the fetus. We have also made great strides in the care of diabetic women who are pregnant. In the past, many infants of diabetic mothers would be stillborn, grossly overweight, or sickly. As a result of recent advances in our knowledge, most infants of diabetic mothers are now born healthy and of normal birth weight—if the mother has had excellent obstetrical care, beginning early in pregnancy.

While the birth of a normal infant can never be guaranteed, there are a number of steps that should be taken to increase its likelihood. Avoidance of unnecessary drugs, alcohol, tobacco, and environmental pollutants, both before and during pregnancy, is vital to increasing the odds that a baby will be born healthy.

Moreover, the importance of high quality nutrition in improving the outcome of pregnancy cannot be stressed enough. This is very clearly and carefully spelled out here. And as Diane Klein points out, good eating habits should not merely begin at the time of conception or end after delivery or following the end of breastfeeding. Eating well must be a way of life and should become a family affair. The husband of the woman who is either pregnant or planning to have a baby must not only be supportive of his wife's good dietary habits but should also eat well himself.

Few parents realize that their newly born infant will one day be a father or mother, too. It is their duty, therefore, to assure their child a healthy future by providing a nutritious and well-balanced diet and by setting a good example themselves. *Eating Right for Two* can help them achieve this goal: it is a highly useful and informative book—not only for the mother-to-be, but also for the entire family.

To all prospective mothers and fathers—I wish you a hearty appetite and a healthy pregnancy.

—Leonard Glass, M.D.
Professor of Pediatrics and Obstetrics and Gynecology
State University of New York
Downstate Medical Center

Acknowledgments

I would like to thank my literary agent, Barbara Bova, whose idea lit the spark for this book.

I am particularly grateful to both Dr. Arline Cohn, Associate Professor of Biology at York College, City University of New York and to Dr. Burton Sherman, Associate Professor of Anatomy, at the State University of New York, Downstate Medical Center, who jointly reviewed the entire manuscript for technical accuracy and clarity.

And to the following medical experts who so graciously shared their valuable knowledge and time with me. They are: Dr. David E. Barrett, Child Psychologist at Harvard Medical School and the Child Development Unit of Boston Children's Medical Center; Dr. Nathan Dor, Chief of Fetal and Maternal Medicine, Maimonides Medical Center, Brooklyn, New York; Dr. Leonard Glass, Professor of Pediatrics, Obstetrics, and Gynecology at Downstate Medical Center; Dr. Richard H. Schwarz, Professor and Chairman of the Department of Obstetrics and Gynecology at Downstate Medical Center; and Dr. Paul Swyer, Director of Perinatal Medicine at The Hospital for Sick Children, Toronto, Canada and Professor in the Department of Pediatrics at the University of Toronto.

In addition, I am indebted to Dr. Swyer for his kindness in giving me a personal tour of the outstanding facilities at The Hospital for Sick Children, where the smallest and sickest of babies are cared for with love and enormous skill.

Special thanks go to Dr. Alvin H. Kane, Pediatrician and good friend for his patience and expertise in answering my countless questions.

I would also like to thank the Nassau County Chapter of La Leche League International for their cooperation in giving me valuable information on breast feeding.

—D.K.

There are many people who helped me with this book, either offering suggestions for recipes or clerical or tasting assistance, and to them I owe a vote of thanks: Mrs. Dorothy Lyons let me adapt her recipes for Savory Mince (page 255) and Shepherd's Pie (page 256); my sister, Marian Modersohn, gave me her recipe for the excellent Coleslaw on page 210; Margaret Merolla offered me the ideas for what became my Chili Beans with Tofu (page 290) and Eggplant Patties (page 288); Eve Metz gave me the idea for the Zucchini Soup on page 203; and, last but not least, Lina Morielli contributed the Cinnamon-Cheese Toast on page 221.

My sister, Dorothy Summa, helped me with the calorie counts for the recipes and generally bolstered my spirits on the long road to the completion of the manuscript by putting the sections together as they were finished and making cup after cup of tea.

As for the people who lent me their palates and gave me really accurate feedback on the dishes they were asked to taste, I can only say thank you very much to Hank Ginorio, who ate, without complaint, whatever I put in front of him; Pam Lyons, Margery Weinblatt Schwartz, and Kathy Vought, who not only took home little foil-wrapped packages to be warmed up but who faithfully completed their review forms; Lina Morielli and her husband Larry Rosenberg, who never refused to taste-test a dish; Linda MacNeill and her husband Vinny Conzo, who also took whatever I offered and warmed it up. And then there are my niece, Terry Ann Summa, who was interested in whatever I cooked, and my nephew, Nicholas Summa, who said of some of the dishes in the recipe section: "This is the best stuff I've ever eaten!"

To all these generous friends, my thanks.

—R.T.B.

To The Reader

This book is written for the woman of today who wants to give birth to the child of tomorrow. It is a guide to optimal nutrition before, during, and after pregnancy—to help you to bear children who will be able to live successfully in the twenty-first century.

Within the next twenty years, we will see many crucial changes taking place. As the world becomes increasingly crowded, competition for education, housing, and comfortable living in the year 2000 will become even more intense. The growing complexity of our society will require highly intelligent people to run its economic machinery. The news is already filled with pictures of young people, all over the world, clamoring for better housing and decent jobs.

However, there is something you can do, now, to protect your child's future. You can take steps to insure that your baby starts out in life with the maximum physical and mental potential necessary to survive in this future world. For good health is directly tied to higher intelligence, more energy, and a longer, more satisfying life.

What's more, your baby's well-being starts long before birth. In fact, it starts before conception with healthy, well-nourished parents. Some fertility problems are even derived from poor eating habits. But only recently has the full significance of maternal nutrition in pregnancy been recognized.

According to numerous up-to-date scientific studies, there is a smaller incidence of stillbirths, neonatal deaths, premature babies, low birthweight babies and physical and mental retardation among infants whose mothers have had optimal diets before pregnancy and during the growth of the fetus. The intelligence and emotional stability of a school-age child can also, often, be traced to the quality of nutrition in fetal development. Yet about one out of every seven American babies is born too tiny, too weak, or too deformed to survive on its own. And the problem of low birthweight continues to be a growing national concern.

Unfortunately, though much has been learned about maternal nutrition and pregnancy within the past two decades, this knowledge has not always been applied either by doctors or their patients. It is, therefore, the goal of the author to bring to you the latest, well researched information available on your own role in helping to produce a strong, healthy baby.

I have based my conclusions on personal interviews and correspondence with outstanding scientific experts in the field, as well as an extensive and detailed study of the most recent research data available.

This book will show you what you should eat and why before conception, during the nine months of pregnancy (on a month-by-month basis) and after delivery. It will explain the miraculous process of growth taking place inside of you and the special needs of the tiny embryo and developing fetus for specific nutrients.

Although it's true you must eat well throughout pregnancy, certain vitamins, minerals, etc. are especially important at various stages of your baby's development. For example, you are more likely to develop anemia in late pregnancy as the growing fetus makes greater demands upon you for iron. What's more, if the baby receives an insufficient supply of iron during the last three months of pregnancy, it's more likely to also become anemic during the first year of life.

Eating Right For Two will tell you which foods contain the nutrients you need and provide you with easy-to-make tasty recipes, by Rosalyn Badalamenti, for month-by-month menus designed for the whole family to enjoy. The menus are based upon the guidelines for pregnant women that have been set by the March of Dimes Birth Defects Foundation.

Finally, with our increased scientific knowledge, parents can do more than hope and pray they will have a healthy baby. They can try their best to do something about it. Now mothers can make the effort to attempt to give their unborn child the most precious gift of all—a healthy life.

Sadly, I have personally known the sorrow that comes with giving birth to a beautiful baby girl who died in infancy of serious birth defects. If by reading this book, one mother will be spared the pain of such a tragedy, I shall consider my efforts worthwhile.

Diane Klein

Good Nutrition: You Are What You Eat

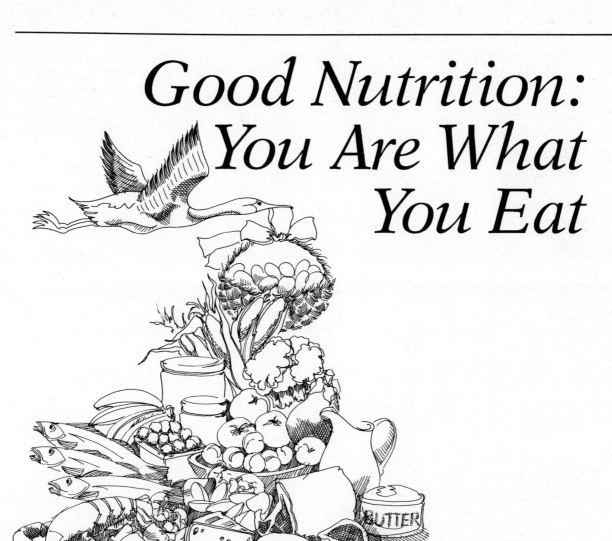

GOOD NUTRITION: YOU ARE WHAT YOU EAT

A mother who eats right is more likely to have a comfortable pregnancy, deliver a healthy baby and be ready with a good supply of milk if she chooses to breast feed.

The March of Dimes Birth Defects Foundation

My Baby, My Body
The Basic Food Groups
How Much Should I Eat?
Daily Requirements

Recommended Dietary Allowances
Recipe for a Healthy Baby
The Pregnant "Gourmet"

My Baby, My Body

Your nutritional needs are at an all-time high when you're expecting a baby. Not only does your body have to take care of its own requirements, but it also has to provide for the "building" of a new human life. Although it's not necessary that you eat a great deal of additional food when you're pregnant (an additional 300 to 400 calories a day is usually sufficient), the *quality of your diet* is crucial.

It's easy to understand this concept if you imagine putting a few quarts of chicken soup into your car's tank when you run out of gas. "Don't be ridiculous," you're probably thinking. "My car needs to run on a good grade of gasoline." Like your car, your body needs to run on high quality fuel suited for its special needs—not on junk foods or a poorly balanced diet. An ample supply of proteins, vitamins, minerals, fats, and carbohydrates in your daily diet is vital for good health.

And you can't expect your body to function well with a lopsided combination of these nutrients. If your body is getting the wrong mixture or an excessive amount of "fuel," you may develop signs of nutritional deficiency or overload. For instance, you may experience a lack of energy from eating foods that contain insufficient iron; you may develop one of a number of deficiency diseases due to an inadequate vitamin intake; and if you eat an excessive amount of food, you will become obese—not a healthy way to enter your pregnancy. (More on this in Chapter 2.)

Just as your car's engine demands a smooth, steady supply of gas, your body also requires a regular supply of fuel. You can't fill it to "overflow" with food for a day or two and then expect it to function properly at "empty" on a starvation diet a week later. Nutrients need to be replenished regularly in your body. Certain vitamins, in fact, like thiamin, niacin, and riboflavin, need to be replenished every day.

Protein Foods: Meat, seafood, poultry, eggs, dried peas, beans, lentils, nuts, and peanut butter.

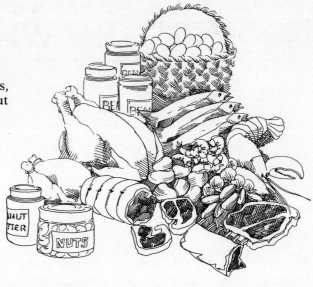

The Basic

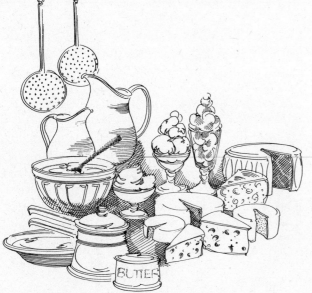

Milk and Milk Products: Whole or skim milk, buttermilk, evaporated milk, hard and soft cheese, yogurt, ice milk, and ice cream.

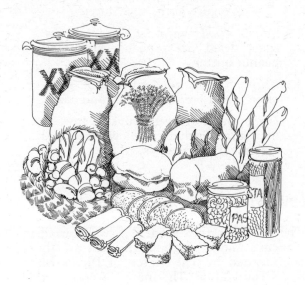

Grain Products: Preferably whole grain or enriched breads, cereals, and pasta.

Food Groups

Fruits and Vegetables: Cooked, raw, or their juices; including yellow, green, and green leafy vegetables.

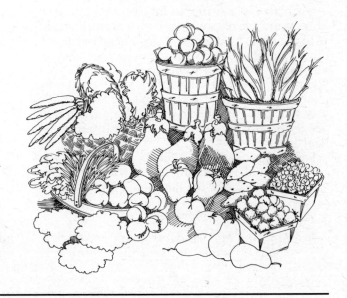

For food to be best digested and absorbed it also should be evenly supplied throughout the day. This is why it's important not to skip meals, especially breakfast. Some of us are accustomed to eating one big meal, generally at dinnertime, and "coasting along" on a scant food supply the rest of the day. But such an irregular eating pattern during pregnancy may deprive the fetus of nutrients for too many hours—and result in irreversible damage to your baby.

During pregnancy the food you eat is truly the "food of life." What better time to brush up on nutrition basics, improve your own diet—and perhaps improve the whole family's diet, too!

The Basic Food Groups

If you're like most of us, you may have some vague memories from your bubble-gum days of a teacher vainly trying to interest you in nutrition. At the age of twelve, the idea of eating right with the basic food groups wasn't nearly as much fun as gobbling down doughnuts, sugared cereals, candy bars, and french fries. But now that you're pregnant it's essential that you know about the basic food groups in order to provide yourself and your baby with the nourishment needed to promote growth and maintain good health.

For a high-quality diet during pregnancy, you must choose the right number of servings of foods from within each of the basic food groups listed below:

The basic food groups are:

1. *Milk and Milk Products:* dairy products such as whole or skim milk, butter-milk, evaporated milk, hard and soft cheese, yogurt, ice milk, and ice cream.

2. *Protein Foods:* meat, seafood, poultry, eggs, dried peas, beans, nuts, and peanut butter.

3. *Grain Products:* preferably whole grain or enriched breads, cereals, and pasta.

4. *Fruits and Vegetables:* cooked, raw, or their juices, including yellow, green, and green leafy vegetables.

How Much Should I Eat?

The daily servings guidelines we've used in the menus and throughout the text are those recommended by The March of Dimes Birth Defects Foundation. The main purpose of this highly respected organization is to help as many women as possible give birth to strong healthy infants.

During the last three months of pregnancy, however, we've given you five servings of protein a day for an extra margin of safety. Some doctors believe this may be helpful to certain mothers at a time when fetal growth is at its maximum.

Recommended Dietary Allowances (The RDAs)

The diets we supply are also based upon information from the latest edition (1980) of the Recommended Dietary Allowances of the Food and Nutrition Board. You'll see frequent mention of the RDAs throughout the text.

Daily Requirements

(March of Dimes Birth Defects Foundation)

Milk and Milk Products

4 servings/Pregnant Woman
5 Servings/Breast-feeding Woman

Grain Products

3 Servings/Pregnant Woman
3 Servings/Breast-feeding Woman

Protein Foods

4 Servings/Pregnant Woman
4 Servings/Breast-feeding Woman

Fruits and Vegetables

4 Servings/Pregnant Woman
4 Servings/Breast-feeding Woman

But what are they? Recommended Dietary Allowances are the levels of nutrients considered "on the basis of available scientific knowledge to be adequate to meet the known nutritional needs of practically all *healthy* persons." They are, simply, recommendations for the average daily amounts of nutrients people should eat over a period of time. Standards have been set for pregnant and breastfeeding women, as well.

The scientists and nutrition experts who make up the Committee on Dietary Allowances of the Food and Nutrition Board make their recommendations every five years based upon the latest available information. Changes and revisions of standards are made after a careful study of new scientific research. But the advice from this panel of experts isn't permanent; changes and revisions of standards are made as soon as additional scientific information becomes available.

Next time you buy a box of cereal or a can of tuna fish, look at the label. You'll probably see a listing of the nutrients and the food value the product gives you according to the RDAs. Unfortunately, governmental regulations don't require that manufacturers of all packaged or canned goods provide you with this important information.

Recipe for a Healthy Baby

There are specific RDAs for the following nutrients during pregnancy: protein, vitamins A, D, E and C, thiamine, riboflavin, niacin, vitamin B_6, folacin, vitamin B_{12}, calcium, phosphorus, magnesium, iron, zinc, and iodine. Suggested intake levels for sodium, potassium, chloride, vitamin K, biotin, and pantothenic acid have also been given. And suggested intakes have been made for the additional trace elements copper, selenium, molybdenum, manganese, fluoride, and chromium.

All of these nutrients and their functions will be discussed at various months during pregnancy, so that you'll readily understand why a lack of even a single nutrient can be devastating to your baby's well-being. Though specific nutrients will be mentioned for their special importance during certain months of pregnancy, they are essential throughout your pregnancy. *All* of the nutrients known to be necessary for the optimum growth and development of your baby will be provided in the menus *every month*.

The Pregnant "Gourmet"

Before we go any further, let's understand that eating properly is *not* going to be a grim prospect but rather a delightful experience for you and your family. In addition, you may gain a sense of well-being and radiant good health you haven't felt for a long time. What's more, I'm sure you'll enjoy using some of the recipes we provide long after your pregnancy is over, since the menus combine interesting ideas for making foods that taste good and look appealing.

Because few women have the time to spend long hours in the kitchen, we'll stick to easy-to-make recipes. If your previous eating habits have been fairly good, meals will be simply somewhat expanded to give you extra calories and additional nutrients. Food faddists, junk-food enthusiasts, constant dieters, and breakfast skippers, however, will find they need to make greater changes in their eating habits.

You will notice that we have reduced sugars and fats in your diet along with the consumption of "empty calories." Some foods provide you with little but calories. We will show you how to replace these foods with quality nourishment that gives you proteins, vitamins, and minerals, in addition to good flavor.

We also stress a variety of foods so that all of the necessary food groups are covered on a daily basis. We don't yet know the precise requirements for all of the necessary trace elements, for example. But if you eat a wide selection of foods, your chances of obtaining all of these elements are good.

Finally, the menus are meant to be flexible; once you understand the principles of good nutrition during pregnancy, you can make up your own menus or alter the ones we have provided. Suppose, for instance, you don't like bluefish and Day 3 has a bluefish recipe for dinner. You can easily substitute another of the seafood dishes, like Sautéed Scallops or Salmon Patties. And if a fruit or vegetable such as melon or asparagus is not in season or is too expensive to buy, you may substitute a different fruit or vegetable. Simply try to exchange one green vegetable for another, or an orange vegetable like sweet potatoes for another orange vegetable like carrots. The principle here is to provide a similar food substitution from the same food group.

The menus will start you on the road to better eating habits. But don't worry. Many of the foods will be familiar, though enriched with high-quality ingredients. Your diet will be well balanced, varied and delicious. For we will show you good nutrition does not have to be either boring or expensive.

PREPARING FOR PREGNANCY

Half of the U.S. population is malnourished.

Dr. Myron Winick

For a long time it was widely believed the baby was a perfect parasite, able to draw from the mother all of its dietary needs, regardless of the mother's nutritional status. What's more, this harmful myth led to relatively little interest in the pregnant woman's diet and how it affected fetal development. And there are still some doctors who continue to see the fetus as "an arrogant bastard," taking whatever it needs from the mother's body.

Fortunately, scientists began to suspect the falseness of this assumption as a result of two so-called natural experiments that took place during World War II. At the siege of Leningrad in 1942 the people were subjected to near starvation, as the Nazis desperately tried to destroy the Russian resistance. Afterward, it was found there was a significant decline in fertility during this period, a dramatic reduction in the survival rate of newborns, and considerable increases in stunted, low birth-weight babies.

In occupied Holland there was also a six-month period of near famine in the 1940s. Even though the Dutch women had fairly ample diets prior to the occupation, they too gave birth to smaller babies with a greater incidence of stillbirths and congenital malformations.

However, in Great Britain during the war years, pregnant women were supplied with special priority ration cards for better nutrition. Despite the difficult wartime conditions—and without any improvement in prenatal care—the death rate of newborn babies in Britain actually declined between 1940 and 1945.

More recent studies have also confirmed the importance of a well-balanced diet during pregnancy. A healthy, well-formed baby will rarely develop without every link in the nutritional chain of life: all the amino acids, carbohydrates, fats, vitamins, and minerals needed for the building and nourishment of billions of brand-new cells. Otherwise, cell functions break down and the normal process of growth cannot occur. The effects of breaks in the nutritional chain of life may be devastating to the fetus, especially when its cells are undergoing rapid division. And dietary deprivation does not have to be severe to affect fetal growth and development.

Admittedly, we cannot blame all birth defects upon faulty nutrition. Maternal infections, genetics, alcohol, drugs, uncontrolled hypertension, and even severe emotional stress can damage your unborn baby. But becoming a well-nourished mother is a crucial factor over which *you* can exert control.

Unfortunately, many American adults eat poorly. In fact, according to an eminent nutrition expert, Dr. Myron Winick, head of Columbia University Medical School's Institute of Human Nutrition, half of all American adults eat too much or not enough. Among younger women the number is probably even greater. In a country of great affluence, why are so many of us poorly prepared for motherhood?

The Slenderella Complex

There has never been a period when so many Americans have spent so much time, money, and emotional energy on trying to lose weight—thereby enriching those people who write countless books on how to do it! Just take a look at the *New York Times* Best Sellers list every week and you'll see at least two or three diet books, each promising to magically turn you into a carbon copy of Bo Derek.

The only problem is that many of the popular diets are nutritionally unbalanced, if not downright unhealthy. For example, the "Beverly Hills Diet," according to an editorial written by Drs. Susan and Orland Wooley in the *International Journal of Eating Disorders*, produces bodily purges through diarrhea caused by the excessive eating of large quantities of fruit.

Yet this extraordinary preoccupation with weight, which author Kim Chernin describes as "the tyranny of slenderness," seems to have affected women far more than men. It's incredible to realize that with more than half the people of the world going to bed hungry, there are American women so obsessed with their weight that they literally attempt to starve themselves to death. This eating disorder is known as anorexia nervosa, and more than 90 percent of those suffering from it are young, middle- and upper-class women in their late teens and twenties.

As if that isn't enough, we now have a new eating disorder to cope with, reports Jane E. Brody, the well-known medical writer. She states that psychotherapists at eating disorder clinics all over the country warn of a new eating practice called bulimia. Apparently, a fair number of young women threaten their health and their lives by continually eating huge amounts of food and then vomiting or taking laxatives to prevent themselves from gaining weight. "The typical bulimia victim is a single white woman (only about 5% are men) from the middle and upper classes who has some college education. Most are of normal weight ..." Jane Brody points out. This amazing eating pattern, which is kept secret by the victims, starts with a stringent diet to lose weight.

Thin, Thinner, Thinnest

> Mirror, mirror, on the wall,
> Who's the thinnest of them all?

The desire to be "fashionable," which in our culture, generally means being very thin and childlike, is continually being promoted in the pages of every magazine devoted to women. The models are young, many of them slim-hipped and boyish looking, without an extra ounce of fat to be found anywhere. Even prestigious high-fashion magazines like *Harper's Bazaar* and *Vogue* have been using twelve- and thirteen-year-old girls as role models of feminine beauty.

Is it any wonder so many women want to be as thin as possible at any price? Or as the late Babe Paley (who was considered a great beauty in society circles) was fond of saying, "You can never be too thin or too rich." Obviously, lots of women have taken such advice seriously. And too many try to maintain a weight that is, as Dr. Orland Wooley puts it, "below their normal set point."

Pregnancy in the Underweight Woman

Why are we making such a fuss about being too thin before pregnancy? It seems doctors have become increasingly aware of the medical problems and complications for both mother and baby when the mother-to-be is 10 percent or more *below* the standard weight for her height and age, *before* pregnancy.

A study by Dr. L. E. Edwards and his colleagues, published in the *American Journal of Obstetrics and Gynecology* in 1979, shows that underweight women tend to have premature infants. In addition, these babies, even at one year of age, show inadequate growth and evidence of delayed neurological development. What's more, underweight women have a higher rate of anemia and premature rupture of the amniotic membranes.

Dr. Roy M. Pitkin, a well-respected authority in the field of fetal nutrition, believes the greatest danger the underweight woman faces in pregnancy is giving birth to a low birth-weight baby, for such tiny babies have a lower rate of survival during the first year of life.

Furthermore, Drs. J. Churchill, J. Neff, and D. Caldwell studied the relationship between birth weight and intelligence. They reported observations on two groups of school children in Detroit with widely different IQs. Although none of the youngsters was a premature baby, those

Ideal Weight Chart for Women

Height (with shoes)	Small	Medium	Large
	(with 3 pounds of clothing)		
4'10"	102-111	109-121	118-131
4'11"	103-113	111-123	120-134
5' 0"	104-115	113-126	122-137
5' 1"	106-118	115-129	125-140
5' 2"	108-121	118-132	128-143
5' 3"	111-124	121-135	131-147
5' 4"	114-127	124-138	134-151
5' 5"	117-130	127-141	137-155
5' 6"	120-133	130-144	140-159
5'-7"	123-136	133-147	143-163
5' 8"	126-139	136-150	146-167
5' 9"	129-142	139-153	149-170
5'10"	132-145	142-156	152-173
5'11"	135-148	145-159	155-176
6' 0"	138-151	148-162	158-179

(Source: Metropolitan Life Insurance Company, 1983)

children who had weighed more at birth (an average of 8.3 pounds for boys and 7.3 pounds for girls) had superior IQs, above 120.

While being model-thin with hollow cheekbones may be ideal for the pages of *Vogue*, it's clearly no good for the optimum growth and development of your baby. The infant's good health will strongly depend upon your nutritional state before and during pregnancy.

Obesity and Pregnancy: Is Overweight Harmful?

Let's define what we mean by "overweight." Dr. Roy M. Pitkin states that such a woman is 20 percent or more *above* ideal weight for her height and age. He points out the overweight woman, like the underweight woman, is at increased risk of complications when pregnant. But the problems are different. Dr. Pitkin has observed a higher rate of chronic hypertensive vascular disease and diabetes in heavy mothers-to-be. Both of these ailments can possibly have damaging affects on the growing fetus. Delivery may also be more difficult for an obese woman.

So, if you're markedly overweight, try to reduce *before* becoming pregnant. *Successful Dieting Tips* by Bruce Lansky is a good book that may be a help in teaching you how to slim down—and stay that way.

However, you should be back eating normally the month *before* you conceive, warns Dr. Charles Mahan of the University of Florida College of Medicine. Pregnant women should *not* be dieting.

Yet not too many years ago doctors used to place overweight women on a reducing diet during pregnancy. A woman wouldn't show any change in weight as a result of a strenuous diet, and after pregnancy she was twenty pounds lighter. But medical experts today realize this can be a dangerous practice, because the fetus may be deprived of vital nutrients.

The Junk-Food Junkie

Too many of us have been conditioned from early childhood, especially by TV advertising, to eat poorly. We've been taught to enjoy the foods best suited for rapid turnover in the supermarket, "fun" food made by mass production with the goal of higher profits for big business.

Highly salted or sugared snacks are a substantial part of the junk-food lover's diet. Cookies, candy bars, sweetened cold cereals, pretzels, cup cakes, sodas, and fruit drinks with only 10 percent fruit juice are pushed relentlessly through the persuasive power of advertising. Everything is made to appeal to your jaded taste buds and keep you coming back for more. Incidentally, have you ever seen *anyone* stop after eating a single potato chip?

Food products for people are rarely advertised on TV as being "good for you." But just for the fun of it, concentrate on some of the commercials for dog food. You may be surprised to discover your dog is eating better than you are! "Buy Blah Blah dog food for your pet. It has all the necessary protein, vitamins, and minerals your dog needs to grow strong bones and teeth and maintain a healthy coat." Can you say the same for the artificially colored and flavored chocolate "Pudgie Bars" you may eat?

Unfortunately, according to the Food and

Nutrition Board of the National Research Council, "Many persons in the U.S. derive a large part (30% or more) of their energy from foods of low nutrient concentration that provide almost no vitamins and minerals, or at best only a narrow spectrum of nutrients."

So maybe you've been able to get along by eating a lot of junk food in the past, but if you're planning to become pregnant, now's the time to kick the habit. Your baby's entire future may depend upon it.

Foods for Fertility

With all of the talk we hear about contraceptives and the raging controversy over who should use birth control pills, are IUDs safe, and how about going back to the diaphragm, we forget the couples who are desperately trying to have a baby. Drs. Richard Amelar, Lawrence Dubin, and Patrick Walsh estimate in a recent book, *Male Infertility*, that 15 percent of married couples in the United States are in this unhappy predicament. And another 10 percent have fewer children than they would like to have. In about 30 percent of these infertile couples the husband has been found to play an important role in the woman's inability to become pregnant; in an additional 20 percent he contributes to the infertility problem.

What's more, medical authorities predict we will see a further rise in infertility problems as more and more women postpone having their babies until they're past thirty. There is a sharp increase in the chances that you or your husband may discover you are infertile in your thirties. Yet during the past eight years, the number of women having their first baby after the age of thirty has almost doubled, from 58,000 to more than 100,000.

Although some couples can be helped to achieve their dream of having a baby through medication or surgical procedures, others, sadly, cannot. Unfortunately, medical experts simply don't have all of the answers to what causes male or female infertility.

Zinc Supplementation

One of the most recent advances in nutritional research is the discovery that trace elements are essential for human reproduction. A relatively new method of treatment now being tried for certain infertile men is the nutritional supplementation of zinc.

As long ago as 1966, researchers at the University of California demonstrated that female rats raised on a nearly zinc-free diet of soybean protein were unable to reproduce. These females showed severe disruption of their reproductive cycles, and in most cases no mating took place.

The sole missing factor in the animal's diet was this one trace element, zinc. The experimental conditions were controlled and standardized, since a similar control group of female rats received zinc supplement in addition to their regular soybean diet.

In 1980 researchers reported on the results of an experiment, using men volunteers, to test dietary zinc deficiency and its relationship to fertility. Dietary zinc intake was restricted from twenty to forty weeks for five men; a significantly *decreased sperm count* was found in four of these men. The decrease occurred both during zinc restriction and in the early phase of zinc replacement, before the body stores were reestablished. It lasted six to fourteen months.

The low sperm counts, luckily, were reversed after zinc supplementation was restored, but it took six to twelve months for this to happen. As a result of such information, some physicians are attempting to treat men with low sperm counts of unknown origin with zinc sulphate. However, your husband shouldn't self-medicate if there's a fertility problem. He needs to see a urologist who specializes in male infertility.

Although physicians have used zinc tablets in treatment, this mineral is found naturally in meat, especially liver, poultry, eggs, and seafood; true deficiency is rare. Oysters and herring are particularly rich sources of zinc. It's found in lesser amounts in milk and whole grains.

Vitamin Deficiencies

Dr. Bruce Stewart of the Cleveland Clinic Foundation is a sterility expert who has found a relationship between what you eat and drink and your fertility index. He notes that a severe vitamin A deficiency in the male, for example, can cause a decrease in the number of cells that will eventually become mature sperm. Since many millions of sperm cells are required for fertilization to take place, this could be a crucial factor in certain men.

The best dietary sources of vitamin A are liver, eggs, cheese, butter, fortified margarine, and yellow, orange, and dark green vegetables and fruits, like carrots, broccoli, cantaloupes, apricots, peaches, sweet potatoes, winter squash, and spinach.

Dr. Stewart also points out the need for an adequate amount of vitamin C in the diet, since this vitamin is vital for the production of motile sperm. It's known to prevent sperm agglutination (the clumping together of sperm cells). If millions of sperm cells are unable to swim freely after being deposited into the vagina, this markedly cuts down on their ability to enter the cervix successfully and eventually swim up the Fallopian tubes to fertilize the egg cell.

Vitamin C is found in oranges, lemons, grapefruit, melons, strawberries, green peppers, potatoes, tomatoes, and dark green vegetables.

Get your vitamins naturally by eating foods that contain them. And don't stuff yourself with massive doses of vitamin pills. You can do more harm to your body than good. Huge amounts of vitamins, especially of vitamin A, can cause serious health problems.

Alcohol and Babies Make Bad Mixers

Although the ancient Greeks were aware of the dangers of alcohol to pregnant women and forbade them to drink, the subject was not taken seriously by modern-day physicians until recently. In fact, you can still find books written by well-known doctors and published as late as 1973 that will tell you, "There's no logical reason to prohibit the moderate use of alcohol during pregnancy to the patient who enjoys and tolerates it."

However, in 1973 Drs. David W. Smith and Kenneth Jones published a description of eight babies born of alcoholic mothers. The babies were suffering from severe growth deficiencies, heart defects, and malformed facial features. Several subsequent large research studies confirmed the theory. Alcohol was the culprit—even in well-nourished, nonsmoking mothers.

This pattern of serious birth defects became known as the "fetal alcohol syndrome."

Babies of drinking mothers are stunted, and about half of them, according to the March of Dimes Birth Defects Foundation, have heart defects. Their heads are small and their brain size has been affected. Unfortunately, unlike many other small newborns, such babies never catch up to normal growth and often die in infancy.

Other affected youngsters are poorly coordinated, hyperactive, have short attention spans, and are behavioral problems. Their IQs don't improve with age.

Although not every fetal alcohol syndrome baby has all of these defects, there seems to be a correlation between the severity of the physical characteristics and the degree of mental impairment. The most severely retarded children are generally those with the most obvious physical defects.

How Much Alcohol Can Damage My Baby?

No one is sure how little or how much alcohol can harm an unborn baby. But scientists are now attempting to find such answers. It is known, for instance, that alcohol passes rapidly through the placenta, the organ which nourishes the fetus, and that the baby feels a drink almost as fast as you do! In fact, if you drink beer, wine, or a cocktail, your baby has a drink too. And since he's tiny, he may be much more strongly affected than you are.

In addition, alcohol damages the liver and interferes with its ability to store needed vitamins and convert them to their active chemical forms. The use of alcohol also leads to poor absorption of vitamins from foods that you eat, so that you may be actually depriving the growing fetus of essential nutrients despite a fairly good diet.

In July 1981 the Surgeon General's Advisory sent the strongest warning thus far on alcohol and its effect on fetal development, to health professionals all over the United States. It warned, "Sizable and significant increases in spontaneous abortions have been observed among women who drank the equivalent of as little as four cocktails a week during pregnancy." It also warned of reduced birthweight among the infants of women who drank the equivalent of only two cocktails a week during pregnancy.

Moreover, a notice in the July 1981 *Food and Drug Administration Drug Bulletin*, aimed at the *casual drinker*, was sent to over a million doctors and nurses. It said, "The Surgeon General advises women who are pregnant—or *considering pregnancy*, not to drink alcoholic beverages and to be aware of the alcoholic content in foods and drugs." This means staying away even from such foods as Irish coffee, rum and fruit cakes, or eating desserts that are liberally laced with liquor. Cough medicines, too, often contain a fairly high alcohol content.

How Does Alcohol Hurt the Baby?

Besides depriving the fetus of nutrients, scientists theorize alcohol adversely affects the baby's fast-growing cells by killing them or slowing their growth. Furthermore, since the brain develops throughout pregnancy, this organ is affected by the mother's drinking.

No one yet knows how much alcohol is "safe" for the expectant mother to drink. And some women and their babies may have a lower tolerance than others. So in the words of the March of Dimes Birth Defects Foundation, "If you're pregnant, think before you drink." The risks are much too great to take chances on your child's future!

Smoking: Destroying the Baby's Nutritional Environment

It's not fair but it's true. Smoking can be much more damaging to women than it is to men, for men don't give birth to babies. Unfortunately, evidence continues to mount linking smoking during pregnancy with serious problems in the fetuses and the newborns of mothers who smoke.

According to a recent report from the Surgeon General, "Increasing levels of maternal smoking result in a *highly significant increase* of placental abruptions, placenta previa, bleeding early or late in pregnancy, premature and prolonged rupture of the membranes and preterm delivery—all of which carry high risk of perinatal loss."

Sadly, there's little question now about the effects of heavy smoking during pregnancy; we have positive proof that it is strongly tied to miscarriage, low birth-weight babies, birth defects, and early infant death.

Yet cigarette smoking is immensely popular among young women of childbearing age. One study revealed up to 40 percent of working women over the age of twenty now smoke; teenage girls who smoke cigarettes presently outnumber teenage boys. What's even more disturbing is the belief that half of all pregnant women continue to smoke.

"You've come a long way, baby," proclaims the highly successful slogan that entices you to smoke by tagging along on the coattails of the feminist movement. But if you do you're hurting yourself and your unborn baby, while enriching the male-dominated tobacco industry. Is this liberation?

How Can Smoking Damage My Baby?

According to Dr. Leonard Glass, director of Neonatology at Downstate Medical Center in Brooklyn, New York, "Smoking impairs fetal nutrition because it constricts the blood vessels to the placenta and it can interfere with the oxygenation of blood." Since the fetus is totally dependent upon you to receive a steady supply of oxygen and nutrients to support its growth and survival, you're choking off a portion of its lifeline when you smoke.

And the more you smoke during pregnancy, the greater the fetal danger. In addition, the later you continue to smoke, the more devastating the consequences can be to your child. What's more, researcher Patricia Diebel points out that several essential vitamins and minerals have been shown to be inefficiently assimilated by the mother who smokes. The following nutrients may be affected by your smoking habit.

Calcium

Calcium—desperately needed for fetal development—is one of the nutrients affected by smoking. It's believed more rapid calcium metabolism takes place in the smoker. Therefore, calcium is reabsorbed from the bones to maintain the necessary serum calcium level to support other vital functions in the body. But the fetus of a smoking mother may be at risk of not receiving sufficient calcium for its own skeletal development, bone density, and tooth bud formation.

Vitamin B_{12}

Levels of this vitamin, necessary for the formation of red blood cells in the fetus and a coenzyme in protein metabolism, are definitely lower in the woman who smokes; and they are actually related to the number of cigarettes she smokes! British researchers Drs. J. M. McGarry and J. Andrews found reduced levels of vitamin B_{12} in the blood of pregnant women who smoked and suggested that cyanide in the inhaled smoke may be detoxified by a process in the body that depletes vitamin B_{12}.

Vitamin C

A large-scale two-year study by the Canadian government revealed that those people who smoke one and a half packs of cigarettes a day have 30 to 40 percent *less* vitamin C in their blood than nonsmokers. And a U.S. Department of Health, Education, and Welfare survey showed vitamin C levels are quite a bit lower in pregnant women who smoke. In fact, a single cigarette depletes vitamin C levels in your body by 25 milligrams, about the amount of the fresh orange you may have just eaten.

Since this vitamin has a number of vital functions in fetal development, its reduction can definitely affect your baby. For vitamin C is involved in tissue formation and healthy collagen production. (Collagen is the fibrous substance in connective and vascular tissues.) Vitamin C also increases iron absorption and helps insure the integrity of blood vessels.

Amino Acids

Proteins are the essential building materials in the human body; amino acids are vital components of the protein molecule. They provide not only for the formation of body tissues, but also for hormones to regulate body processes and enzymes to control chemical reactions in our bodies.

Protein is indispensable for the growth of the breasts, the placenta, and the uterus during pregnancy; a constant supply of ample amounts of protein is required to insure your baby's normal growth and development. Studies of 182 pregnant women by Dr. Warren Crosby and a team of experts, under a grant from the National Institute of Child Health and Human Development, clearly showed that blood levels of ten amino acids were closely related to fetal growth. On the other hand, cigarette smoking by the mother was correlated with reduced blood levels of amino acids and with reduced fetal growth.

Smoking and Your Baby's Future

The March of Dimes Birth Defects Foundation cautions that pregnant women who smoke heavily tend to have low birth-weight babies. Many of these tiny infants are not merely small but stunted in their physical development. Such a baby often has permanent brain damage, which can be expected to hurt the child's ability to learn throughout life. This may not show up until the youngster enters school and the teacher tells you, "Your child has a learning problem."

Another matter of grave concern, now that so many young women have become smokers, is the possibility that the children of these mothers run a high risk of developing cancer as a result of their unhealthy intrauterine environment. A recent study of the placentas of women who smoke revealed they contain an enzyme that could possibly trigger the growth of cancer cells. This particular enzyme is not found in the placentas of nonsmoking mothers.

Walk Away From Cigarettes

In 1980 about 3.5 million Americans were able to give up cigarettes, according to the National Center for Health Statistics. You can do it too!

Groups like Smokenders have proven successful for many people who want to stop. And *Good Housekeeping* magazine recommends a self-help plan "that's worked for millions of former smokers." It's a little book called *Quit* by Charles F. Wetherall, which contains a clever twenty-five-step program for quitting by eliminating one cigarette a day over a period of ten to thirty days. Soon, your body can be free from cigarette smoke and nicotine juices for longer and longer periods each day. The chain that binds you to dependence on cigarettes will be broken. And you and your baby will both benefit. For if there was ever a time in your life to get rid of the cigarette habit, this is it.

Fathers Who Smoke

A recent study conducted at Cleveland Metropolitan General Hospital/Case Western Reserve University has shown that even when a non-smoking pregnant woman is exposed to the cigarette smoke of *other* people, the fetal blood contains significant tobacco smoke byproducts. Although the effects on the fetus of second-hand exposure to a smoke filled environment are not yet known, it's possible that constantly inhaling your husband's cigarette fumes may harm the fetus.

How Caffeine Affects You

Caffeine readily crosses the placenta, the lifeline between you and your baby, and enters the fetal circulation. The fetus, however, seems to lack the necessary enzymes to metabolize the caffeine properly.

In an analysis of the medical records of eight hundred obstetrical patients at the University of Illinois, researchers identified sixteen mothers who had a high intake of caffeine (six hundred milligrams or more per day) during pregnancy. Only one of these women had an uncomplicated delivery. The other fifteen pregnancies ended in spontaneous abortion, stillbirth, or premature birth. These women were young, in good health, and there was nothing in their medical histories to indicate they might have a problem in pregnancy. In addition, most of them were Mormons who neither drank alcohol nor smoked.

Their caffeine intake was calculated using the values of seventy-five milligrams for a serving of coffee, thirty milligrams for tea and forty-five milligrams per serving of cola. Yet this amount can vary. Brewed coffee, for example, has eighty-three milligrams of caffeine per six-ounce cup, while instant coffee has only sixty milligrams for the same amount. Even cocoa has ten milligrams of caffeine per six ounces, and chocolate also contains caffeine. Decaffeinated coffee contains a much smaller level of caffeine per six-ounce cup (three milligrams) and when women drank large amounts of this, their pregnancies were unaffected in the Illinois study. According to the March of Dimes Birth Defects Foundation, if you must drink coffee during your pregnancy, many doctors suggest you change to decaffeinated coffee.

But since coffee and tea act as diuretics and remove fluid from your body, they must not be the main sources of liquids in your diet. You and the baby are going to need an *increase* in body fluids during pregnancy.

Although the research on caffeine has not been as definitive as that on the harmful effects of alcohol and smoking on your baby, the Food and Drug Administration still advises pregnant women to avoid caffeine. Furthermore, the FDA Drug Bulletin published in November 1980 cautions that many over-the-counter drugs, such as cold and allergy preparations, headache tablets, antacids, and stimulants also contain caffeine and should be avoided during pregnancy.

Is Trouble "Brewing" Among the Experts?

There is no real consensus among the experts about the dangers of caffeine during pregnancy. Researchers at Boston's Brigham and Women's Hospital, who interviewed more than 12,000 women over three years, concluded coffee did not cause birth defects, underweight babies, or stillbirths. Instead they indicated smoking as the culprit in many of the problems blamed on coffee, in a January 1982 article in the *New England Journal of Medicine*. However, the Brigham team did find a small risk of premature rupture of membranes among women who drank four or more cups of coffee a day during the first three months of pregnancy. Dr. Kenneth Ryan, Chief of Obstetrics and Gynecology at Brigham and Women's Hospital, qualified these conclusions by adding it wouldn't hurt for heavy coffee drinkers to cut down on caffeine during pregnancy.

Obviously, more research will be done in the future on the effects of caffeine in pregnancy, in view of the conflicting findings of the experts. In the meantime, you'd be wise to drink coffee, if you choose to, in moderation. Milk, fruit juices, and soups are much better choices.

The Medicine Menace

Even when the organs of the baby's body have already been formed, prescription drugs, over-the-counter medications, and any chemical substances you take into your body may still damage the baby's further development. For the fetus is almost always an unwilling recipient of the medication you absorb.

In fact, most drugs, except those with a large molecular weight, readily cross the placenta. Though not too long ago doctors believed the placenta was an "impenetrable barrier" that protected the growing fetus from harmful substances, we now know this is untrue. And the 10,000 children who were born without limbs because their mothers took thalidomide are a tragic reminder.

Therefore, *never self-medicate* when you are pregnant or planning to become pregnant. Medicines that may be perfectly safe when you are not expecting, can be toxic to the fetus, depending upon its stage of development. For example, the antibiotics—tetracycline, sulfa drugs, and streptomycin—must not be taken near the end of pregnancy. Tetracycline may cause discoloration of the baby's permanent teeth and affect bone growth. Some of the sulfa drugs disturb the baby's liver function. And some tranquilizers are known to increase your risk of having a baby born with a cleft palate. Sleeping pills, pain killers, central nervous system depressants, antinausea medication, and even heavy use of aspirin can cause problems, too.

So check with your doctor *before taking any medicine,* including the so-called harmless over-the-counter stuff. Your doctor has a long list of medications that are potentially harmful to the fetus. And with increasing research, the list keeps growing longer!

The Hazards of "Recreational" Drugs

Few women are unaware of the dangers of heroin addiction to an unborn infant. Most of us know a pregnant user can addict her baby and cause it to suffer withdrawal symptoms after birth. Yet many middle- and upper-class women have become accustomed to pot smoking, the use of amphetamines, and even cocaine usage.

What effects do these drugs have on the fetus's health during pregnancy? Cocaine is known to markedly decrease your appetite, a condition you certainly don't want to happen during pregnancy. And scientists now believe marijuana, which crosses the placenta, may have a toxic effect on the embryo and the fetus. Laboratory

tests have shown female monkeys treated with THC (the mind-altering ingredient of marijuana) are four times more likely to abort or to give birth to dead babies.

Then why haven't these tests been done on women instead of animals, to confirm the results? It would be hard to justify taking such risks with the lives of human mothers and their newborn babies. Nevertheless, some women who have admitted being "heavy" pot smokers, especially in the last trimester of pregnancy, have given birth to babies who were unusually drowsy. And some amphetamine users have hyperactive infants.

No one can be sure of the problems that may develop in your child later on, as a result of your taking drugs in pregnancy. So even if scientists don't have all the answers yet, don't make your baby a medical statistic!

Biological Variability

By now, some of you are surely saying to yourselves, "I have a friend who smoked when she was pregnant and her little girl turned out okay." Or, "My sister-in-law used to drink before the baby was born and nothing bad happened to her."

And it's true. *Every* woman who smokes during pregnancy isn't going to give birth to a defective newborn nor is *every* woman who drinks destined to produce a damaged baby. There are definite subtle differences in genetic hardiness between people that are still poorly understood by medical experts.

Dr. Richard Schwarz, director of Obstetrics and Gynecology at Downstate Medical Center in Brooklyn, explained it this way: "Two fetuses can be exposed to the same damaging substance and you'll get different results, even at the identical time in gestation. Apparently, there's something in the genetic makeup of a particular fetus and, perhaps, even of the mother, that allows a lethal agent to cause its full-blown manifestation in one baby but not in the other. So, theoretically, if we were able to line up a group of ten fetuses and expose them to the same nutritional deprivation or toxic agent, most of them would die—yet for some unknown reason, one or two might live."

We can see this principle of biological variability operating in adults as well. Most of us know someone who's smoked two packs of cigarettes daily since he was a teenager and, now is a hearty eighty-five year old and still going strong. Nevertheless, these people are the exceptions. Smoking *does* pose great health risks for the average person, and we've got abundant evidence to prove it.

Betting Against the Odds

You're playing Russian roulette with your baby's life if you become pregnant and continue to ignore the known medical hazards. It's far more important to try to *prevent* a birth defect than to have to salvage an abnormal child.

As the March of Dimes Birth Defects Foundation points out, there are currently about fifteen million Americans whose daily lives are drastically affected, in some way, by having been born with birth defects.

Tragically, "Too many babies come into the world deformed in ways that could have been prevented," say Drs. Robert Rugh and Landrum B. Shettles of Columbia University's College of Physicians and Surgeons. "Half of the children in our hospitals are there because their parents did not exercise reasonable care during pregnancy."

Still, you have every reason to look forward to the birth of a beautiful healthy baby. Don't spoil its chances for a full normal life. For at no other time, except during pregnancy, is the well-being of one person so totally dependent upon another.

THE FIRST MONTH

... The future health of mankind depends, to a very large degree, on nutritional foundations laid down during prenatal life.

Dr. Roy M. Pitkin

Let's Start at the Very Beginning ...

When you become a physically mature female, a ripe egg, called an ovum, bulges from the surface of one of your ovaries about once a month, under the powerful influence of a hormone from the pituitary gland. The egg is pushed out of the side of the ovary into the nearby Fallopian tube. The two tubes, each about five inches long, are located on either side of your uterus leading from the abdominal cavity to the interior of the uterus. The Fallopian tubes form the pathway for the upward journey of the sperm cells and the downward travels of the ovum.

If you have sexual relations within seventy-two hours before ovulation or within twenty-four hours afterward, fertilization can take place. Although the exact way the sperm cells find the egg is still not clearly understood, we do know that only a few thousand of the millions of sperm cells ejaculated by the male are able to reach the mid-segment of the Fallopian tube containing the ovum. The rest remain in the vagina, exposed to the hostile environment of its acid secretions and are destroyed.

So the one sperm that unites with the egg has won against gigantic odds. And the baby that will eventually develop, according to the late Dr. Alan Guttmacher, has a far greater chance of becoming president than the sperm had of fathering a baby!

This is the miracle of fertilization, that wondrous moment when a single tiny sperm cell unites with the egg nucleus and their content is combined. The sex and the genetic blueprint of your baby are also assigned simultaneously and cell division begins only a few hours later.

Just think of it: A speck scarcely visible to the human eye will become a seven-and-one-half-pound fully developed infant nine months later—if all goes well. In fact, this period between conception and the birth of the newborn is the most important time span in all human development.

However, fertilization, implantation in the uterus, and early development of the ovum are incredibly complex. According to Dr. Guttmacher, about 30 to 50 percent of fertilizations do not result in babies. Many more eggs are fertilized than babies are ever born. But unless pregnancy had progressed for several weeks, you would not have known the egg had been fertilized. Your menstrual period might just have been a little late.

This is why the preparation of your body *before* pregnancy is vitally important. Wonderful and exciting things will be taking place in your body during the first month of pregnancy. The minute embryo uses your nutritional stores and daily food intake for its growth. And it can be subjected to either a fertile environment that will enhance its development or a hostile one that may destroy its chances for normal growth and survival. All of this—before you know you're pregnant.

Am I Having a Baby?

At first it's not always easy to tell whether or not you're expecting a baby. Even a woman who has had a baby before can be mistaken. To begin with, you may notice your menstrual period is late. But this isn't always a reliable sign, as menstruation can be delayed by emotional upset, illness, dieting, or even a change of climate. And some women have light periods and bleed even though they are already pregnant.

However, if you are expecting a baby, you will probably notice other symptoms. You may feel sleepier than usual or notice a sudden swelling and tenderness of your breasts. Perhaps you need to urinate more often. Many women also feel slightly nauseated in the mornings or when they are hungry.

The signs of pregnancy often appear two or three weeks after fertilization has taken place, the week after a period should have begun. These changes are caused by hormones that your reproductive system is producing. So if your period is about two weeks overdue or you have other early signs of pregnancy, it's important to find out. The doctor will do a pregnancy test and a pelvic examination to estimate how many weeks pregnant you may be.

Preparing for Pregnancy

It's very possible you may not be certain if you're going to have a baby until the end of the first month or even the beginning of the second. But if you have read this book before becoming pregnant and have changed your smoking, drinking, and dietary habits accordingly, you should be in excellent condition to "make" a baby. The prepregnancy diet is rich in proteins, vitamins, and minerals, with sufficient fat, carbohydrates, and liquids to sustain the healthy growth and nutritional needs of the tiny embryo during its first two months.

A final warning! Almost everything you eat or drink gets to your baby through the placenta, the thick wall of tissue in the uterus that nourishes the unborn child. Therefore, though prescription drugs, over-the-counter medications, and all chemical substances you ingest are not, strictly speaking, "foods," nevertheless they can affect the development of your baby.

This is the strongest possible reason for discontinuing their use before you plan to become pregnant, or as soon after as possible.

My Baby's Environment

	Points
1. I don't smoke cigarettes or marijuana.	15
2. I don't drink alcoholic beverages or take cough medicines or foods that contain alcohol.	15
3. I take no medication or pills (except what is absolutely necessary and under my doctor's supervision).	15
4. I don't drink coffee—and if I drink decaffeinated coffee, I have no more than two cups a day.	5
5. I am of normal weight for my height.	10
6. I've given up eating junk foods.	5
7. My diet has enough calories for proper weight gain.	10
8. I eat high-quality foods with sufficient protein, vitamins, minerals, and carbohydrates.	10
9. I am receiving regular prenatal care by a physician or a clinic.	10
10. I am taking an iron supplement.	5
	100

In order to do the best for your baby, your score should add up to 100!

The March of Dimes Birth Defects Foundation cautions that *any type of drug may be especially dangerous to the early developing embryo.* The effect is often greatest during the first three months of pregnancy and you will soon understand why, as we begin to see how your baby grows and receives its nourishment.

The Embryo: Stage 1

After the fertilized egg divides into two cells, it soon becomes four, then eight, doubling the number of cells with each successive division at a dizzying rate of geometric progressions. At the same time, the egg is moving slowly down the Fallopian tube into the uterus. The fertilized egg soon becomes a ball-shaped cluster of rapidly dividing cells. And by the time it's implanted within your uterus, about nine or ten days after fertilization, it's already a hollow ball of as many as one hundred individual cells.

But even before the embryo is formed, certain cells already have fashioned a see-through bubble. Fluid seeps into the bubble from the surrounding maternal tissues, and it becomes the home in which the developing embryo, and later the fetus, will live—snug, warm, and protected. This fluid-filled bubble is known as the amniotic fluid, or the "bag of waters."

A small number of the early cells will develop into the embryo and the rest into the placenta and other membranes. Meanwhile, the cluster of cells continues its division at an astonishing rate, increasing every hour.

During the second week after fertilization, the new cells build a type of "shield" around the embryo, which contains rudimentary tissues for the entire body. But most of its wide top is the brain region, which starts to develop very early. In fact, the nervous system begins to form about eighteen days after fertilization. What's more, by only twenty days after conception the foundation for the fetal brain, spinal cord, and the entire nervous system will have been laid down, as well as the rudiments of its eyes.

By the third week, the embryo is only one-tenth of an inch long but the brain has formed two lobes, and the early spinal cord is visible, with its future vertebrae and muscle segments. The embryo has what looks like the beginning of a tail, an extension of its spinal column. This "tail" is temporarily longer than the rest of the body and will eventually become the tip of the adult spine, the coccyx.

On the twenty-fourth day after fertilization, the tiny embryo has no visible arm buds. Yet suddenly, only forty-eight hours later, the beginning of arm buds miraculously appear and the leg buds make their appearance two days later. It's as if a magician waved his magic wand and chanted, "Now you don't see them; now you do." The primitive heart is beating by the twenty-fifth day after conception, and even certain internal organs can be recognized within the first month of embryonic life. The liver can be seen on the twenty-seventh to the thirtieth day after conception and the thyroid gland, which plays an important role in metabolism, enters its first stage of development at this time.

By the end of the first month the embryo is only one-quarter-inch long and one-third of its length consists of its head. The miniature body has a trunk, arm and leg buds, but no distinguishable face. There are only outlines of the eyes at the sides of the head. Simple kidneys, a digestive tract, and a primitive blood stream are also present. The embryo's heart is large in proportion to its body size at this stage, as is its brain.

Yet the month-old embryo is minute in size. When seen under a high-powered microscope by the untrained eye, it can easily be mistaken for the embryo of an animal or a fish. However, the four weeks after conception are extremely important ones. The embryo shows an amazing rate of growth during this period. It has grown to be 10,000 times larger than it was as a fertilized egg, although it is still no bigger than a grain of rice. In addition, *all* of the major organs of the body have begun to develop.

The Placenta: Your Baby's Lifeline

How does the rapidly developing embryo get its nourishment? When the cluster of cells reaches the uterus, it remains free in the uterine cavity for only about three days before it's implanted into the wall of the uterus. Within a very short time the placenta, a network of tiny blood vessels and tissues, forms in the uterus and attaches itself to the ball of cells by means of a stalk, the umbilical cord.

The placenta is the organ, formed in part by maternal and in part by embryonic tissues, through which the growing embryo obtains its food, water, and oxygen supply. After you eat a meal, your food is digested and absorbed. The breakdown products are then passed into the liver, which releases essential nutrients into your bloodstream. The nutrients pass through the very thin walls of the embryo's capillaries into its circulatory system by means of the placenta (although your blood does not actually mix with the baby's). Waste materials from the embryo, in turn, are carried to the placenta, absorbed into your blood stream and eliminated by your kidneys. It is truly an ingenious system!

Moreover, the normal growth of the placenta is an important factor in the healthy development of your baby. For the human placenta increases its weight during the entire course of pregnancy, tapering off during the last month. When the embryo (which is generally called a fetus after the second month) grows, the placenta normally gets proportionately larger to provide greater nourishment. At birth, a healthy placenta weighs about one and a half to two pounds and is eight inches wide and about an inch thick.

If the placenta is reduced in size, it's incapable of providing the fetus with the necessary nutrition. A small placenta has less surface area and fewer cells available for the transfer of nutrients, and the baby will suffer the consequences. Dr. Pedro Rosso, of the Institute of Human Nutrition at Columbia University's College of Physicians and Surgeons has shown that the mother's food intake *before* and *during* pregnancy is one of the environmental factors that influences placental growth.

What's more, Dr. Aaron Lechtig and his research associates at the Institute of Nutrition in Central America and Panama have concluded that even moderate protein-calorie malnutrition leads to a lower placental weight. "This effect," they say, "may be the mechanism by which maternal malnutrition causes a high prevalence of low birth-weight babies...." And as we discussed earlier, underweight infants have a poorer chance of survival during the first year of life.

The Great Weight Myth

Doctors have always agreed the pregnant woman needs to gain weight to provide for the baby's growth and development. But the question is, how much? Unfortunately, as recently as ten or fifteen years ago, many obstetricians believed pregnant women should gain no more than a total of fifteen or eighteen pounds. However, increasing scientific evidence has proven that restricting the woman to such a small weight gain is unhealthy for the mother and her unborn baby.

Then how did doctors come to accept this false assumption about weight gain in pregnancy? Incredible as it may seem now, the theory was based upon the hypothesis of a German obstetrician, Dr. Ludwig Prochownick. He proclaimed in the early 1900s that "semi-starvation is really a blessing in disguise, because curtailment of food should produce a small lightweight baby" that would be easy to deliver. He therefore advocated a diet low in calories, carbohydrates, and protein and restricted in water and salt. Despite the lack of any scientific data to support Dr. Prochownick's conclusions with regard to the infant's health and well-being, doctors passed down this myth in obstetrical textbooks from one generation of physicians to another!

When I was pregnant with my first child I gained a total of twelve pounds, although I have always been slim. And I remember my doctor's chubby nurse wagging her finger at me, as if I was a naughty child because I had gained three-and-one-half pounds during my sixth month. My pregnant friends then told me their secret. They never ate lunch before their appointment with the obstetrician. But you'll soon realize why such a small weight gain during pregnancy is woefully inadequate.

First, let's consider the large bodily changes you must undergo in order to supply the fetus with the necessary calories and nutrients it will need for growth, and to meet your own requirements during pregnancy. In a sense, making a baby probably causes the greatest bodily stress to which any woman is subjected during her lifetime.

According to Dr. Sue Rodwell Williams, co-author with Drs. Bonnie Worthington and Joyce Vermeersch of *Nutrition in Pregnancy and Lactation,* the "average costs" of pregnancy are as follows:

Mother

- Breast tissue weight increase   3 pounds
- Blood volume weight increase   4 pounds
- Maternal fat stores   4 to 8 pounds
- Increase in the size of the uterus   2½ pounds

Baby

- Weight of the fetus   7¼ pounds
- Placenta   1 pound
- Amniotic fluid   2 pounds

Total Increase in Weight   23¾ pounds

As you can see, you will most likely need to gain about twenty-four to twenty-eight pounds just to maintain a pregnancy for a single baby of average weight. Other experts now believe a twenty- to thirty-five-pound gain is within normal limits. Even a high of forty pounds is considered desirable by some doctors, *if* you entered pregnancy underweight.

In the 1960s maternal stores of fat were not considered an important factor in the mother's weight gain. But we have learned recently that additional fat tissue is required for extra energy to sustain rapid fetal growth in the later months, for labor and birth, and for milk production during breast feeding.

Obviously, there is no absolute consensus of medical opinion as to how much you should gain during pregnancy in order to produce the best possible fetal outcome. In addition, many questions regarding maternal nutrition and the fetus still remain unsolved. For instance, Dr. Roy M. Pitkin believes the *pattern* of your weight gain and the *quality* of the foods you eat are as important as how much you gain. For example, you can fulfill your calorie quota for lunch by eating a large piece of chocolate layer cake, a bag of potato chips, and a bottle of soda. Although this would probably give you ample calories, it wouldn't provide you with the high-quality nutrition the fetus needs to build its body tissues.

Weight gain during the first ten weeks should be minimal, because it's due mainly to the expansion of the mother's uterus and a small increase in her blood volume. A weight gain of about two to four pounds at the end of the third month is considered adequate by many experts. After that, however, you should be gaining steadily, about one pound a week until your baby is born. As there is a consensus of opinion that weight gain is one of the indicators of how well a pregnancy is progressing, keep a record of your weight, week by week.

Counting Calories

The latest Recommended Dietary Allowances (1980) for pregnant women from the National Academy of Sciences advises 2,400 calories per day throughout the entire pregnancy. The March of Dimes Birth Defects Foundation suggests 2,100 calories per day during the first trimester of pregnancy and about 2,400 calories for the fourth through the ninth month. The Canadian Dietary Standards call for 2,600 calories per day during pregnancy. So as you can see, there is a difference of opinion among the experts. Yet advising you to eat a certain number of calories per day doesn't take into account how physically active you are, how quickly your body burns up calories, nor your present weight and height.

In general, the best way to judge your dietary needs is to make every calorie count during pregnancy by emphasizing nutrient-filled foods and watching your weekly weight gain. We will provide you with menus for delicious meals for all nine months of pregnancy. The amount you eat, however, will depend upon your individual rate of weight gain.

If you are not gaining sufficiently, add larger portions of food or additional snacks between meals. On the other hand, with a too-rapid weight gain (unless you are expecting more than one baby) decrease the size of the portions you eat, drink skim milk instead of whole milk, or cut back on between-meal eating. The main reason for not gaining an excessive amount of weight is the difficulty you may have in taking it off after the baby is born. Most of us know someone who gained a lot of weight with each pregnancy. After the birth of the baby, such a woman is left with an extra fifteen or twenty pounds. By the time she has had three children, she is often obese.

If You Gain Too Little

There is a direct correlation between your own weight gain during pregnancy and the weight of your baby at birth. And almost all recent major studies of fetal development have clearly documented this relationship. Dr. David Rush of the Institute of Human Nutrition at Columbia University proved this point in a study of 7,000 births. Furthermore, when Dr. Jean-Pierre Habicht and his associates offered supplementary feeding to pregnant women in four Guatemalan villages where chronic mild malnutrition was present, the average birth weight of the babies of women who received the improved nutrition was higher than that of the control group of unsupplemented mothers. Their data suggest the optimum time to begin calorie supplementation is as early as possible in pregnancy, and that supplementation should continue until the baby is born.

Drs. Kenneth Nisander and Esther Jackson analyzed data from nearly 12,000 pregnant women and concluded "... birth weight shows a positive association with maternal weight gain, increasing on the average about nine grams for each pound increase in maternal weight gain."

Strangely enough, the connection between your weight gain in pregnancy and the size of your newborn was not generally accepted by many doctors as recently as ten or fifteen years ago. In fact, there are still some who believe the baby's birth weight is "preordained" solely by heredity. So that if the father is a husky six footer, you can expect an eight-and-one-half-pound "buster," but if the father is a slim, five foot six inches tall, the baby will weigh much less. Nevertheless, we have strong scientific evidence that good nutrition on the mother's part and a sufficient weight gain during pregnancy, result in a *bigger* baby, even with small parents. And this is as true in Texas as it is in India or Guatemala.

Low Birth-Weight Babies

Fortunately, there is today a realization that low birth-weight infants are not always perfect babies "in miniature." For these tiny babies (below five-and-one-half pounds) are at much greater risk than normal weight babies for cerebral palsy, mental retardation, learning disabilities, respiratory distress syndrome, serious infections, and death in early infancy. "About 8 percent of the newborn in the United States," says Dr. Frank Zlatnick, "are of low birth-weight, but this minority is a clear majority of the neonatal deaths."

Of course, not all low birth-weight babies will have problems, but there's little question the chances are much greater than for a normal weight baby, closer to seven-and-one-half pounds.

The U.S. government, in recognition of the importance of good nutrition to pregnant women, has provided a special feeding program (known as WIC, or Women, Infants and Children) to improve the diets of poverty-level women who are known to be at great risk of producing low

birth-weight babies. They receive certificates that entitle them to get free high-nutrient foods at the supermarket: milk or cheese, eggs, iron-fortified cereal, fruit juice, and dry beans or peas. A 1981 study by the Massachusetts Department of Public Health showed a death rate one-third lower for the babies of women who participated in the program, as compared with other low-income pregnant women who had not.

These are compelling reasons for making sure you eat well and sufficiently during fetal development, in order to give birth to the healthiest possible baby. Yet you can be rich and eat poorly; live on a much more modest scale and eat well. Your baby doesn't care if you have a T-bone steak or a can of tuna fish, jumbo shrimp or two slices of pizza. All of these foods give you high-quality protein necessary for healthy fetal development.

Doctors and Diets

Perhaps you're wondering, "Why hasn't my doctor prescribed specific dietary guidelines for me to follow during pregnancy?" For a long time, the study of nutrition was considered a stepchild in the field of medicine. In fact, most medical students graduated from medical school without ever having been exposed to a single course on nutrition! Therefore it's easy to understand why most pregnant women still receive relatively little dietary advice from their obstetricians. As a mother with three young sons told me, "If you're not anorexic or diabetic, you could be living on chocolate cake, milk, and iron tablets and they wouldn't know the difference."

Unfortunately, some physicians aren't very knowledgeable about specific nutritional needs during pregnancy and other doctors don't take the time to sit down and talk about them to expectant mothers. However, as research continues on the importance of the foods we eat—not only during pregnancy but in relation to cancer, heart disease, and even depression—nutrition will take its rightful place both in the medical curriculum and in the doctor's office.

Nutritional Requirements: The First Month

The tiny growing embryo needs warmth, oxygen, available energy, plenty of water and, as biochemist Dr. Roger J. Williams points out, "an environment containing every link in the nutritional chain of life—all the amino acids, minerals, and vitamins that are needed for cell nourishment and for the building of billions of brand new cells."

As we have seen, the single original egg cell multiplies into many different kinds of cells within the first month. These cells are greatly different in size, shape, composition, and biochemical functioning. Nevertheless, the fundamental activity of *all* living cells is metabolism. This is the process by which each cell converts the nutrients it receives into energy and the special materials necessary to perform specific functions in the body. The supply of raw materials to "build" the baby comes from the foods you eat each day, which are digested, absorbed, and circulated in the blood stream and eventually passed through the placenta to the developing embryo.

In addition, certain nutrients may be stored in your body, to be drawn against later in pregnancy, when your needs and those of the fetus will greatly increase. The capacity for storage, however, varies a good deal for different nutrients. Fats, for example, can be stored. Water-soluble vitamins and some minerals need to be continually replenished.

Although the nutritional requirements for the embryo during the first month are very small, the first six weeks of development are critical, because the major body parts and systems are taking shape. What's more, the embryo is highly vulnerable at this time, precisely because of the early formation of the vital organs, such as the heart, the brain, and the spinal cord. Poor nutrition during the early months of pregnancy can affect both the embryo's development and its ability to survive.

Protein

Protein is one of the key nutrients that should be increased in your diet as soon as you know you're expecting a baby. Not only is it an essential part of every living cell, but additional protein is crucial for the building of new tissues during pregnancy. These nine months are the most rapid building period in the entire human life span.

Proteins consist of many units called amino acids, and the protein value of foods depends upon the amounts and the proportions of the amino acids they contain. Foods with complete protein value include lean meat, fish, cheese, eggs, and milk. These foods are not only rich in proteins, but they also contain all of the essential amino acids in the right proportions to build new cells in the body.

Protein-Counter Chart

These are some of the common foods we eat that contain protein.

FOOD	SERVING SIZE	GRAMS PROTEIN	FOOD	SERVING SIZE	GRAMS PROTEIN
Beans, kidney	½ cup cooked	7.2	Macaroni	1 cup cooked	6.5
Beans, lima	½ cup cooked	6.5	Milk, skim or whole	1 cup	9.0
Beans, navy	½ cup cooked	7.4	Noodles, egg	1 cup cooked	6.6
Beef, chuck roast	3 oz. cooked	24.0	Peanut butter	2 tablespoons	8.0
Beef, lean ground	¼ lb. raw	23.4	Peas, green	1 cup	9.0
Bluefish	3 oz.	22.0	Pizza with cheese	5½ in. piece	7.0
Bologna	3 slices (3 oz.)	10.2	Rice, brown	1 cup cooked	4.9
Bulgur	1 cup cooked	8.4	Rice, white	1 cup cooked	4.1
Bread, whole wheat	1 slice	2.6	Salmon, pink, canned	3 oz.	17.0
Bread, white	1 slice	2.4	Scallops	3 oz. sautéed	16.0
Cheese, Cheddar	1 oz.	7.0	Shrimp	3 oz. sautéed	11.6
Cheese, cottage	½ cup	15.0	Soup, cream of mushroom	1 cup with milk	6.9
Cheese, Swiss	1 oz.	8.0	Soup, cream of tomato	1 cup with milk	6.5
Cream cheese	3 oz.	7.0	Soup, split pea	1 cup	9.0
Chicken, broiled	3 oz.	20.0	Soybeans	½ cup cooked	9.9
Eggs	2 medium	11.4	Spaghetti	1 cup cooked	6.5
Flounder	3 oz.	25.5	Spinach	1 cup cooked	5.0
Frankfurter	1 (2 oz.)	7.1	Tuna fish, canned	3 oz. drained	24.4
Ham, boiled	3 slices (3 oz.)	16.2	Turkey	3 oz.	26.8
Hamburger, lean, broiled	3 oz.	23.0	Walnuts	10 large	7.3
Hamburger, regular, broiled	3 oz.	21.0	Wheat, shredded	2 biscuits	5.0
Ice cream or ice milk	1 cup	6.0	Yogurt	1 cup	8.3
Lentils	½ cup cooked	7.8			
Liver, beef	2 oz.	15.0			
Liver, chicken	1 liver	6.6			

(Source: Agriculture Handbook No. 456, U.S. Department of Agriculture)

There are other protein sources; vegetables and grains such as rice, beans, dried peas, and wheat that are called incomplete proteins because they lack some of the essential amino acids or have poorer amino acid proportions. However, they cost less and can be combined with small amounts of some of the complete protein foods to prepare inexpensive high-quality main dishes.

In addition, two vegetable proteins that complement each other's amino acid deficiencies, such as rice with beans or beans with corn, can also be eaten together to make a complete protein. (In fact, many ethnic dishes, like rice and beans, are based upon this scientific principle.) But both types of protein must be eaten *at the same meal* in order to provide proper nourishment. For proteins don't sit around waiting for each other to "catch up" at your next meal, because they aren't stored in your body.

Four servings of protein *each day* during the first month of pregnancy, are considered ample. Although the embryo in the first month contains little protein, it's important that you get enough protein to make up for any possible deficiency you may have had before becoming pregnant. Besides, your own need for protein as well as the baby's will soon expand enormously.

Calcium

Calcium is another important nutrient that you should begin to add to your daily diet as soon as you know you're pregnant. Although calcium is not used for the fetal skeleton until the last three months of pregnancy, some researchers believe some amounts of this mineral are stored in your body, possibly in anticipation of your greatly increased needs and those of the fetus, later in pregnancy. Even though most body calcium is eventually found in the bones and teeth of the fetus, a small amount of it remains in the soft tissues and body fluids, where it regulates nerve and muscle activity and helps in the absorption of iron.

The human body is amazingly complex; we have not yet unraveled many of its nutritional threads. The nutrients we ingest, like protein and calcium, all have complex roles to play in the future health and development of your baby. Unfortunately, we don't yet know all of the specific functions of each nutrient. But we do know a nutritional deficiency can strike anywhere and everywhere in the baby's body.

How to Combine "Incomplete" Proteins to Make "Complete" Proteins

Food	Add
Rice, brown	Milk, meat, fish, soybeans
Whole wheat cereal	Milk
Green leafy vegetables	Meat, eggs
Rice, white	Milk, Meat, Fish Soybeans
Potato	Eggs, cheese
Kidney beans	Beef, eggs, rice
Peanut butter	Milk
Bread	Milk
Macaroni	Cheese
Vegetable	Eggs or Cheese

Therefore, the National Research Council advises you to drink four eight-ounce glasses of milk (or its equivalent) during pregnancy to satisfy your calcium requirements. By this time, however, some of you are surely grumbling to yourself, "I hate milk," or "I haven't drunk milk since I was ten years old!" But you can substitute cheeses, yogurt, custards, milk puddings, cream soups, or ice milk instead. For example, a one-and-one-half-inch piece of hard cheese is the equivalent of a glass of milk; so is one-and-one-half cups of creamed cottage cheese or a cup of yogurt. However, a quart of whole milk will add six hundred calories a day to your diet, so if you're gaining weight too rapidly, switch to skim milk. (You'll save about fifty calories a glass.) And though you may not love the taste of it at first, many women, like myself, learned during pregnancy to prefer skim milk to whole milk, which soon tasted "too rich."

Luckily, dairy products not only contain calcium, but they add to your body's store of proteins and they provide you with vitamins, zinc, magnesium, sodium, potassium, and phosphorus. It's no wonder a glass of milk gives you more good nutrition than an equivalent serving of any other food.

Iron

According to Dr. Pedro Rosso, Professor of Pediatrics at Columbia University's College of Physicians and Surgeons, lack of iron is the most common dietary deficiency affecting pregnant women in the United States. Why does this happen? Some physicians believe menstrual loss each month, previous pregnancies, or lack of iron-rich foods in our diets contribute to the problem.

Yet until recently, doctors believed the fetus was protected from any iron deficiency in the mother. This assumption was based upon studies that showed the hemoglobin concentration, even in the infants of anemic mothers, was normal. But we have become aware these babies are often born with poor iron stores and are more susceptible to being iron deficient themselves during the first year of life.

"In general," says New York Times science writer Jane Brody, "the iron from animal foods is better absorbed than that from vegetable foods. From 15 percent to 30 percent of iron in meats and fish is absorbed, compared to only 5 percent from vegetable sources." She also advocates eating a vitamin C-rich vegetable or fruit along with food containing iron to increase the iron absorption you get from your meals. Possible combinations are meat and potatoes, an iron-enriched cereal with orange juice or a tomato salad with broiled liver and onions. (Try Chicken Livers Florentine with sliced tomatoes.) Good food sources of iron include liver, liver sausage, lean meats, shellfish, egg yolk, dried peas and beans, dried fruit, green leafy vegetables, dark molasses, potatoes, whole-grain and enriched cereals and cereal products.

The demand for iron in pregnancy is so great however, that it may be difficult for you to meet such a high iron requirement (eighteen milligrams per day) solely by your diet. Many doctors routinely prescribe iron supplementation in the form of pills or capsules, in addition to an iron-rich diet. The need for this will become clear as you read on in the text.

Vitamins

Apparently, having a baby increases the need for all vitamins. The Food and Nutrition Board of the National Academy of Sciences advises pregnant women to increase their intake of vitamins A, C, D, and E, thiamin, riboflavin, and niacin, vitamin B_6, and vitamin B_{12}, and folacin (also called folate or folic acid). It's been well documented in hundreds of animal experiments that a dietary deficiency of *any* of these vitamins can wreak havoc not only with the process of reproduction, but also in the development of the offspring.

For instance, Dr. Roger Williams points out in his fascinating book, *Nutrition Against Disease*, that when high-grade breeding sows were deliberately fed a diet deficient in vitamin A early in pregnancy, many serious abnormalities were found in the baby pigs. Yet there were no defects whatever in the litters in which the mothers received plenty of vitamin A. And if folacin is omitted from the diet of female rats nine days after fertilization, the rat fetuses cease to develop. If the pregnant rats are deprived of folacin on the eleventh day after conception, young are produced but 95 percent of the baby rats are abnormal. When human mothers were given drugs that destroyed this vitamin during the first three months of pregnancy, some of their babies developed severe congenital problems and most died soon after birth.

But not even the experts know precisely what vitamins the embryo requires during its first four weeks of development, nor in what specific proportions. We will, therefore, provide menus varied enough to contain all of the necessary vitamins from the latest Recommended Dietary Allowances.

Fortunately, just as each nutrient serves different functions in your baby's development, certain foods contain many nutrients. So your job of eating well is made much easier. For example, a single large egg has a high amount of protein and vitamin A, iron in the yolk, plus calcium, phosphorus, some of the B vitamins, and vitamin E.

Iodine

The thyroid gland, which regulates the rate at which our bodies use energy, enters its first stage of development during the first month of pregnancy. The mineral iodine affects the thyroid gland and is an important part of the thyroid hormone, thyroxine. If the fetus doesn't get enough iodine, it will fail to develop normally.

In certain parts of the world, iodine deficiency is common due to the poor iodine content of the soil, as good sources of iodine include vegetables grown in iodine-rich soil. Northwestern sections of the United States and the Great Lakes Basin area, in particular, have iodine-poor soil. The best sources of iodine, however, are seafood and iodized salt. To make sure you're getting the iodine you and the baby need, use iodized salt to taste both on the table and in cooking, and be sure to eat seafood regularly.

Zinc

Zinc is another mineral that is particularly important early in prenancy. It plays an active role in the metabolism of protein, so it's essential for the growth of all tissues. In addition, Dr. Joyce Vermeersch indicates the nervous system is highly susceptible to zinc deficiency. The foundation for the entire nervous system is, in fact, laid down by only twenty days after conception.

You will need additional amounts of zinc every

day during pregnancy. A deficiency of this mineral is harmful, for although the mother may not suffer from this deficiency, her baby will. The best sources for zinc are oysters and herring but other high zinc foods are meats (especially liver) and fish, milk, eggs, nuts, and legumes. The daily menus contain ample amounts of zinc, because they're based on foods rich in milk and animal proteins.

Sodium (Salt)

In the past, many physicians placed all women who were expecting a baby on salt-restricted diets. They believed damage might be done to both the mother and child by the use of salt in the diet during pregnancy. Yet researchers have proven this is a myth and that salt is necessary for fetal growth and development.

Nevertheless, there are still certain doctors who were trained in the old school and who continue to restrict the salt intake of their patients. According to the Food and Nutrition Board of the National Research Council, however, "It's difficult to justify dietary restriction of sodium in healthy women during pregnancy on the basis of either experimental work in animals or clinical evidence in humans."

Therefore, you'd be wise to salt your food to taste. However, if you are already a heavy salt user (and studies have shown that many Americans eat twenty times the salt they need), you may need to cut back somewhat on your salt intake. For pregancy, please read "The Salt Controversy" and "Salt and Toxemia," discussed under the third and fourth months.

THE SECOND MONTH

If we cannot yet control nature, we do, nevertheless, have means to control nurture. It is potentially within our grasp to eliminate vast numbers of defective births.

Dr. Roger Williams

The Embryo: Stage II

During the first three weeks of the second month the tiny embryo growing peacefully inside you is still *less than an inch long*, smaller than a paper clip. It weighs only about one-thirtieth of an ounce and is lighter than an aspirin tablet. Nevertheless, it is changing miraculously, day by day.

The head continues to grow rapidly and is large and top-heavy in proportion to the miniscule body. The brain is now composed of a series of five cavities and, remarkably, already has begun to send impulses to coordinate the functioning of the other organs.

The delicate creature begins to develop a more human-looking face during this month, with eyes, ears, nose, lips, tongue, and even milk-teeth buds in the gums. The jaws are well formed, and there is an actual neck.

On the thirty-third day after fertilization the pigment has just formed in the retina of the eyes, and they look dark for the first time. The eyelids are beginning to appear around the ridges of the eyes. And within a week the eyelids have grown so that they cover almost all of the eyeball. On the thirty-seventh day the nose is fully formed with two separate nasal passages. The ears take shape in the fifth and sixth weeks after conception, forming out of two folds of tissue. Although this description may make the two-month-old embryo sound rather attractive, it is not, yet, very appealing in appearance.

The arms and legs are beginning to form as protruding buds, and soon the hands and feet are visible, looking quite human. The arms, however, are unbelievably tiny and delicate, no longer than a one-quarter inch eraser on the top of your pencil. The slower-growing legs soon have recognizable knees, ankles, and toes.

The internal organs are starting to grow, too. Simple kidneys are taking uric acid from the blood during the second month. The stomach and the esophagus are beginning to form. And the stomach produces some digestive juices. The intestines are also growing. Blood starts to form in the spleen soon and has begun forming in the liver.

But as you can see, the embryo does not progress evenly. It seems to grow in a topsy-turvy way: now here, now there. Muscles begin to make their appearance in the pelvic region and the muscles throughout the body are lengthening. The internal hearing mechanism of the ear is nearing completion.

By the sixth week after conception, the little embryo has a complete skeleton made of cartilage. It is not yet composed of bone. But by the forty-sixth to forty-eighth day, the first bone cells appear to replace the cartilage in the bones of the upper arm. The appearance of the first bone cells is said to mark the end of the embryonic period. From now on, the embryo will be called a fetus.

By the end of this second month, the fetus is about one and a quarter inches long and resembles a tiny plastic doll, with a big wobbly head and arms and legs thinner than matchsticks!

Under the skillful baton of its genetic conductor, the developing embryo has emerged day by day. Its timetable for development is orchestrated so perfectly during the first forty-eight days of life, that any embryologist could observe the little creature and tell its exact age from the body formation!

"The development during the first two months is crucial. Once the fetus weathers this successfully, the odds are in its favor," say Dr. Landrum Shettles and Dr. Robert Rugh, co-authors of *From Conception to Birth*. But remember, all this incredible growth is taking place quietly, within the sheltering warmth and darkness of your womb, before you see or feel anything within your body. The foundation for the physical structure of your unborn baby is essentially complete by the end of the second month.

Nature versus Nurture

There are two extremely important factors that contribute to the growth and development of your baby. One is the genetic heritage the infant receives at the precise moment of fertilization. This determines, for example, whether your child will be a boy or a girl, blue-eyed or brown-eyed, tall or short, and whether it will resemble you, your husband, or even Grandpa Joe. These are "harmless" inherited physical characteristics.

There are a very small percentage of babies, however, who, at the moment of conception, inherit genes that are dangerous, either to the baby's survival or to its normal physical or mental development. For instance, in about one in every one thousand births, a baby inherits a so-called fragile X chromosome. Almost all male children with a fragile X chromosome are mentally retarded, and the genetic defect also affects a small number of girl babies. Fortunately, only about 20 percent of all birth defects are solely genetic in origin.

Nurture refers to the environment that *you* provide for the baby's development during its nine-month stay in your uterus. Alcohol, smoking, drugs, pills, dieting, and poor eating habits can all help to destroy a fetus that has inherited perfectly normal genes.

Obviously, both the baby's genetic heritage and its environment will determine your child's future. If either of these factors goes wrong, the baby will suffer the consequences. If you're planning to become pregnant or if pregnancy comes as a delightful surprise, make the necessary changes in your life-style.

Fetal Neural Tube Defects

Not only do the twin factors of nature and nurture contribute to the baby's growth and development, but doctors are beginning to realize there is also a relationship between certain genetic disorders and how they interact with the environment. In other words, the quality of nurture can actually affect nature. This is a very exciting idea because it enables us to try to do something to improve the baby's growth *despite* a genetic problem.

For example, there have been a number of British research studies that have explored the origin of fetal neural tube defects in babies. These abnormalities are serious and often crippling, because they involve malformations in the central nervous system such as faulty development of the spine or the brain. The defects originate early in pregnancy; as we have learned, the foundations for the brain and the spinal cord begin to develop within the first couple of weeks and continue into the second month.

Some experts believe that genetic predisposition plus certain intrauterine factors combine to do this terrible damage. And though there are still missing pieces to the puzzle of neural tube defects, some medical experts strongly suspect the mother's inadequate nutrition, before and during early pregnancy, plays a vital role in susceptible babies.

In a recent large-scale British study of 174 mothers who had already given birth to children with neural tube defects, many of these mothers received dietary counseling before their next pregnancy. There were *no* recurrences of such defective babies in the mothers who were given counseling and therefore improved their diets, despite the fact that there is a higher incidence in families where one child already has the disease. But there were eight recurrences of infants born with central nervous system damage to the forty-five women eating poor diets without counseling, and a number of miscarriages in these women as well.

What were the mothers who were considered to be on a poor diet eating? They had a deficient intake of high-quality protein, ate few fruits and vegetables, and enjoyed excessive amounts of potatoes and potato products (although potatoes are good for you, they must be part of a nutritionally well-balanced diet), refined cereals, sweets, chocolates, and soft drinks.

Another study at the University of Leeds in England showed that mothers who gave birth to infants with neural tube defects had lower levels of vitamin C and folacin in their bodies during the first trimester of pregnancy than mothers who later delivered normal babies.

At present it is widely accepted that defects of the central nervous system, which are among the most serious of congenital disorders, cannot be attributed to a single cause, either genetic or environmental. But if *one* relevant factor, poor nutrition, is eliminated, this may be enough to affect the genetic balance. Perhaps, with optimum nutrition, mothers-to-be may be able to compensate for nature's inborn errors.

This is why we stress the importance of an excellent diet so early in pregnancy. The first two months are critical! Even though the tiny embryo does not use a large amount of nutrients, all of the essential vitamins, amino acids, minerals, and trace elements must be present in the mother for the normal development of the baby's vital organs.

To Supplement or Not to Supplement

Iron

Somewhere during the second month most women suspect they are pregnant. At this time you should definitely begin to see an obstetrician or attend a clinic *regularly* for prenatal care. When your doctor verifies that you are expecting a baby, you'll probably be advised to start taking an iron supplement. And you may very well ask, "Why do I need iron pills if I'm eating such a good diet?"

It is very difficult to plan a pregnancy diet sufficiently rich in iron, because iron needs increase greatly during pregnancy, as iron is used for the manufacture of hemoglobin for you and the baby. You would have to eat liver twice a day for all nine months in order to provide enough iron for your pregnancy needs—and who would be willing to do that! (Besides your diet would lack variety.)

The usual American diet, in fact, contains only about ten to fifteen milligrams of iron per day, though the requirement when you're having a baby is eighteen milligrams per day. And only 10 to 20 percent of the iron you take in is actually absorbed by the body. Dr. Roy Pitkin points out that iron from foods usually provides only slightly more than the amount lost through stool, urine, and perspiration. In addition, most women have little iron stores available in the bone marrow.

Many doctors want you to start taking thirty to sixty milligrams of iron a day in the second month of pregnancy. Others wait until the beginning of the fourth month to prescribe supplementation, when the hemoglobin needs of the mother and the fetus are much higher.

Certain women have trouble tolerating some of the iron preparations. So if what you're taking doesn't agree with your stomach, ask your doctor to suggest another brand.

Folacin (Folic Acid)

There is little medical controversy over giving all women iron supplements during pregnancy. But routine supplementation of one of the B vitamins, folacin, is controversial. Some doctors want their pregnant patients to take it; others don't.

Yet, according to Dr. Pedro Rosso, "After iron deficiency, the inadequate intake of folate (folacin) represents the most common deficiency found in pregnant women in the U.S." This is important because folacin is needed for the development of every part of the human body. The requirement for it increases markedly during pregnancy, although the reasons for this are not completely understood.

Nevertheless, it's believed folacin plays an important role in the growth processes of pregnancy. For instance, it's involved in the production of blood and in the formation of all new cells. And because our bodies don't store this vitamin, we need daily supplements of it.

Lack of this vitamin is particularly a problem for women who have been taking birth control pills until shortly before conceiving. For some reason, this seems to deplete folic acid levels. In addition, the Food and Nutrition Board of the National Research Council, which sets the U.S. Recommended Dietary Allowances, advises oral supplementation of folacin for *all* women during pregnancy.

Folacin is present in a wide variety of foods, such as liver, nuts (especially peanuts), wheat germ, dried beans and peas, whole-grain cereals, oranges, and orange juice. It's also found in asparagus, broccoli, cauliflower, endive, and dark green leafy vegetables.

Other Vitamins

Nutrition expert Dr. Roy Pitkin believes additional vitamin supplementation is unnecessary during pregnancy. He would much prefer to see expectant mothers on a quality diet instead, because he believes that such supplementation is costly and gives a false sense of security about the mother's nutritional status. Even doctors who do advise vitamin pills during pregnancy admit they are no substitute for a balanced diet. We do not yet know *all* of the specific requirements in pregnancy, and the chances of getting a wide range of the essential nutrients is greater from eating a high-quality varied diet, than from taking vitamin pills and continuing to eat poorly.

Never take vitamins without asking your doctor and *never above* the dosages he recommends. An overdose of vitamin A or vitamin D supplement is known to be toxic and can produce abnormalities in your unborn baby. But it's practically impossible to overdose on these vitamins by eating natural foods. You would have to eat nothing but bushels of carrots like Bugs Bunny to cause a significant problem!

Nutritional Requirements: The Second Month

Calcium

You should be continuing to increase your calcium intake. Four eight-ounce cups of milk, or the equivalent, are recommended during the second month of pregnancy.

By the second month, there are milk-teeth buds already in the gums, and calcium is a definite requirement in the building of strong teeth. What's more, the first bone cells have also appeared this month and calcium is necessary for adequate future bone growth. In fact, your deficient calcium intake during pregnancy could eventually result in poor skeletal development in your newborn.

According to Dr. Joyce Vermeersch, about 40 percent of the calcium in your foods is absorbed. In addition to milk and milk products, she suggests cabbage, turnip greens, nuts, legumes, and dried fruits as calcium sources that are absorbed well by the body.

Phosphorus

Calcium and phosphorus are thought of together, since they coexist in a specific ratio in the blood, like a finely matched duet. Together they lend rigidity to bones and teeth. Phosphorus, in addition, has more functions than any other mineral in the body. It is found both in the body fluids and in every individual cell. Many of the B vitamins are effective only when combined with phosphate in the body.

The early formation of your baby's skeleton

and teeth buds in the second month require phosphorus and calcium. And the rapid division of huge numbers of new cells demand phosphorus as well.

Fortunately, this mineral is so widely available in foods, a deficiency is rare. It's found in most protein-rich foods, such as meat, fish, chicken, eggs, milk, and cheese. Even snack foods and processed meats contain phosphorus.

The level of phosphorus should be increased during pregnancy, but if you are eating additional foods for your increased protein and calcium needs, you will be getting an ample amount of phosphorus too. In fact, it's possible to get excessive amounts of this mineral. So cut back on processed snacks and sodas, both of which generally contain high amounts of phosphorus but little else of nutritive value. If too much phosphorus is taken in, "It will bind calcium in the gastrointestinal tract and limit the amount of calcium absorbed," says Dr. Joyce Vermeersch. And Dr. Myron Winick makes a similar point in his new book, *Growing Up Healthy: A Parent's Guide to Good Nutrition.*

Folacin (Folic Acid)

As we have discussed, lack of sufficient folacin may contribute to cruel defects of the central nervous system (the brain and the spinal cord) in the growing embryo. It is also essential for the utilization of protein in early pregnancy. And a deficiency of it can lead to impaired cell division in the fetus and the placenta.

Folacin is involved in the production of vital elements in each cell and in the synthesis of DNA, the basic chemical blueprint of life. With the enormous need for making increasing numbers of healthy cells within the second month, any deficiency in cell division can be damaging. "The effects [of a lack of folacin]," warns the National Research Council, "are most noticeable in rapidly growing tissues."

Diverse abnormalities are found in baby animals that have been deliberately deprived of folacin. They develop malformations of the heart, the blood vessels, cataracts of the eyes, and serious skeletal and brain abnormalities. Since the structure of your baby's brain, its skeleton, eyes, and internal organs are forming at this stage, you can understand the crucial role folacin plays.

In addition, blood cells start to form at one and a half months in the liver and at two and a half months in the spleen. A severe lack of this vitamin, especially late in pregnancy, can cause anemia, in which the red cells are stunted and produce immature cells and reduced hemoglobin levels.

But do remember that long storage and overcooking will destroy 50 percent of the folacin in the foods you eat. So when you buy fresh vegetables use them within a day or two. Frozen vegetables should also be eaten quickly after cooking and not lie around in your refrigerator for days. Also, get into the habit of cooking vegetables in a small amount of water or stir-frying them in a little oil, Oriental style, until crisptender. Vegetables never tasted so good!

Protein

The need for increased protein in your diet throughout pregnancy is crucial. You are "building" the baby, month by month, by expanding your own tissue development in the uterus, the breasts, and the placenta as well as the miniscule body of the little fetus. And the rate of new tissue growth begins to accelerate in the second month.

As you may remember, protein forms the structural basis of *all* cells in your tissues and those of the fetus. In fact, according to Dr. Kamran Moghissi, a research expert in fetal nutrition at Wayne State University School of Medicine, proteins seem to exert the greatest impact on the growth and development of your baby.

Therefore, during the second month of pregnancy, your protein intake should be thirty grams a day above nonpregnant levels. Four servings of protein each day, plus occasional "booster snacks" containing protein, like peanut butter and crackers with a glass of milk or a chunk of cheese, should be ample during the second month.

Fortunately, good-quality protein does not mean you have to buy expensive cuts of meat. In fact, there is more protein in three ounces of drained canned tuna than there is in three ounces of lean ground beef and slightly more than in three ounces of a beef chuck roast!

Calories

Your change in expenditure of calories is still minimal by the end of the second month, because the fetus is only about one and a quarter inches long and has gained little weight despite its remarkable growth and development. But by this time you should have begun to gain a pound or two. If you have had no weight gain at all, slightly increase the portions of food you are eating, or eat more frequent snacks of good quality. (Please see the daily menus for easy and nutritious snack suggestions.)

Manganese

One of the more recent advances in nutritional research, is the discovery that other minerals, called trace elements, are essential for human reproduction, growth, and good health. Manganese is one of these that we're beginning to learn more about. It is, apparently, necessary for the healthy development of baby animals and for reproduction in mature animals. A deficiency of manganese in chickens, rodents, or swine causes congenital defects in the offspring, such as abnormalities in the inner ear. This results in poor balance or a lack of equilibrium. Some research experts also believe that manganese is involved in the skeletal development of the human embryo and the little fetus.

Since the embryo in the second month has a complete skeleton made of cartilage (the first bone cells begin to appear between the sixth and seventh weeks), manganese is thought to be a necessary element in early human development. The internal hearing mechanism of the ear is nearing completion as well during this month, and manganese has a definite relationship to the growth of the labyrinth of the inner ear in many different animals, according to researchers Drs. Kamran Moghissi and Roger Williams.

The National Research Council suggests a safe and adequate manganese intake for adults should be in the range of 2.5 to 5 milligrams per day. It should not be difficult to maintain this level, since nuts and unrefined grains are rich sources of manganese; vegetables and fruits contain moderate amounts; and dairy products, meats, and seafoods have small quantities of manganese.

Vitamin D

This vitamin plays an important role in your baby's bone development, as it's responsible for regulating the metabolism of calcium and phosphorus. It promotes the intestinal absorption of these two minerals; it is also believed to directly influence the mineralization of bone tissues and tooth buds, which begin their early development now. Your need for vitamin D doubles during pregnancy.

This nutrient is found in canned salmon, sardines, eggs, butter, fortified margarine, and you guessed it—liver. A quart of vitamin D fortified skim or regular milk each day will supply you with enough vitamin D. But milk is a poor source of vitamin D unless it's vitamin D enriched. So read the labels. The milk you buy should say "vitamin D milk" or list the amount of added vitamin D in the nutritional information.

Women nineteen to twenty-two years of age should have even greater amounts of vitamin D (the equivalent of five glasses of milk a day or one quart of milk plus other food sources of the vitamin). But don't overdo it: too much vitamin D, like too much of any vitamin, serves no useful purpose and potentially can be harmful.

Amazingly enough, vitamin D can also be formed by the action of sunlight upon your skin. But it's unwise to depend upon this source during the colder months of the year. Besides, the pigment of your skin is another variable that affects the amount of vitamin D you receive from the sun.

Perhaps you have noticed by now the marvel-

ous interrelationship between the various nutrients. For example, while protein affects the growth of the fetal skeleton, so do calcium, phosphorus, manganese, and vitamin D. When you provide the body with all of its needs, the nutrients generally work together harmoniously with amazing precision, like musicians in a well-rehearsed orchestra.

Therefore, despite the fact we are mentioning only specific nutrients each month that particularly affect your baby's growth and development, we are including in the monthly menus *all* of the vitamins, minerals, and nutrients presently known to be needed during pregnancy.

Why Should I Read Food Labels?

Early in pregnancy is the perfect time to learn about nutrition. And it's a habit that will benefit you and your family for a lifetime. Although we have included high-quality foods in the menu sections, it's important for you to know what nutrients you are eating and why. Because more than half of the foods Americans eat come in packages or cans, it's necessary to read and understand food labels in order to improve your diet.

So when you have a little free time, play the label game. Go to your grocery cabinets and refrigerator and pull out five or six cans, jars, or boxes. Then, sit down at the kitchen table and begin to read the labels. I think you will be as surprised as I was when I did this for the first time! In fact, I found that most often, I knew very little about what I was eating.

Unfortunately, the issue of product labeling is

still in a state of legislative chaos. Although some foods do list the ingredients they contain, there may be no information about food values. One popular hot cocoa mix, for example, has the ingredients on the box but no information about the amount of fat, protein, calories, vitamins, or minerals the product contains. The clue is, however, that according to government regulations, ingredients have to be listed in order of their prominence, by weight. Therefore, as the first ingredient labeled on the box is sugar, we know that in terms of weight this cocoa mix contains more sugar than any other ingredient.

Now, let's get back to the labels from your pantry. First, if possible, try to find two similar items to compare. I took two containers of cheese,

one a pot-style cheese and the other a whipped cream cheese.

For the same amount of calories, you can see the pot cheese is a better nutritional buy than the cream cheese. In order to get a similar amount of protein from the whipped cream cheese, you would need to eat about seven-and-one-half ounces and consume 750 calories instead of the 100 calories for the pot cheese.

I then looked at an expensive box of "gourmet" crackers I had purchased. The label said "baked with wheat flour, corn starch, whole milk powder, sugar and salt." It sounded good—whole-wheat flour and only 32 calories for two crisp four-and-one-half by two-inch crackers. But in terms of the U.S. Recommended Dietary Allowances the two crackers provide only 2 percent of the daily requirement for protein, calcium, and iron. And they contain little else of food value!

Yet a seven-ounce can of white meat tuna, (packed in water) has an amazing amount of good nutrition.

POT CHEESE	WHIPPED CREAM CHEESE
Serving Size 4 ounce = 100 calories	Serving Size 1 ounce = 100 calories

Percentages of U.S. Recommended Daily Allowances (per serving)

Protein	30%	Protein	4%
Riboflavin	10%	Riboflavin	2%
Calcium	6%	Calcium	2%
Vitamin B_6	8%	Vitamin A	8%
Phosphorus	15%	Fat	9 grams
Vitamin B_{12}	10%		
Fat	2 grams		

Percentages of U.S. Recommended Dietary Allowance
Canned Tuna Fish
Serving Size 7 ounce

Protein	110%	Vitamin B_6	45%
Thiamine	6%	Vitamin B_{12}	60%
Riboflavin	8%	Phosphorus	40%
Niacin	130%	Magnesium	15%
Iron	4%		

It's easy to understand the importance of becoming conscious of labels in order to get the best food value for your money and your baby.

Help! I Feel Nauseated!

Sometime during the second month of pregnancy, or even as early as the first, you may begin to feel mildly nauseated or even sick enough to vomit. This feeling seems to be worse, generally, in the mornings. But so-called morning sickness can make you feel uncomfortable at other times too, and it doesn't affect all women who are expecting a baby. What's more, each pregnancy may be different. I felt sick with my first child, yet nausea didn't bother me at all when I was pregnant with the other two babies.

Doctors aren't really sure why certain women feel nauseated early in pregnancy. The current theory is that the higher level of estrogen produced during pregnancy accumulates even in the cells of the stomach. As acids build up this causes irritation and then that awful queasy feeling begins. Nausea can also be made worse by stress, anxiety, and poor dietary habits.

Luckily, it doesn't last long in the majority of women, and within a few weeks you will feel fine again. "That's great," you're probably saying, "but what do I do now?" So here are some suggestions to minimize that uncomfortable feeling.

1. Don't let yourself get really hungry.
2. Carry crackers or a small nutritious snack in your pocket or purse.
3. Leave dry crackers or saltines at your bedside.
4. Eat a cracker or two *before* getting up in the morning, and then rest a little before getting out of bed.
5. Eat lightly throughout the day.
6. Smaller, more frequent meals are better than three big ones.
7. Avoid greasy or spicy foods.
8. Drink liquids between meals rather than with your food.
9. Remember that "morning sickness" rarely lasts long.
10. Think positive!

Severe, persistent vomiting during pregnancy is quite rare. If it should be a problem, call your doctor. The treatment is usually brief hospitalization with intravenous feeding to prevent dehydration or any complications.

THE THIRD MONTH

Animals do not need to consume flagrantly bad diets in order to produce malformed young.

Dr. Roger Williams

How Big Is the Baby?

By the ninth week, the fetus is still very tiny, about one and a half inches long and approximately one-seventh of an ounce in weight. It could comfortably fit into a jumbo hen's egg, with a little room to spare. The large head is perched precariously atop its puny little body.

Yet within the third month one of the marvels of human development takes place. The organs, the muscles, the brain, and the spinal cord start becoming interconnected. This advancement is made possible because of an increase in nerve-muscle connections that takes place during the ninth and tenth weeks of your baby's development.

Now, when the brain signals, the fetus can respond by kicking its fragile legs, curling its toes, turning its head, and opening its mouth. Its arms can bend at the wrists and the elbows and the hands may even form tiny fists. And films taken by researchers show the three-month-old fetus is capable of making facial expressions. It can squint, frown, and purse its lips —despite its miniature size! But the eyes, which move closer to the bridge of the nose, are still sealed tight, like a newborn puppy's.

It's unlikely that you will feel the baby kicking and moving around, doing its "sitting-up exercises" at this early stage of development, for it's still too small and its newly formed muscles are very weak.

Nevertheless, the third month of pregnancy is a time of amazing fetal growth and change. The skeleton and all of the muscles are rapidly forming; the ribs and the vertebrae turn to hard bone. And bones are forming in many places throughout the tiny body, even in the fingers and toes.

Tooth formation is continuing as well. It's believed enamel and dentine are starting to develop for all twenty baby teeth and sockets (for the teeth also grow in the jawbone). What's more, the upper part of the mouth forms at ten weeks. Two bony plates come together to form the palate. If this does not happen properly the baby will be born with a cleft lip or cleft palate, which generally requires surgery.

Little by little the fetus grows. Nerve cells fill the tubular cord along which the spinal cord is forming. The nail beds form on the fingertips.

The kidneys begin to spill out small amounts of urine in the amniotic fluid.

During the tenth week the delicate fetus gets a little heavier, though it still weighs only one-quarter of an ounce, or about as much as a teaspoon and a half of sugar. Yet some of the internal organs, like the thyroid gland, the gall bladder, and the pancreas, are already complete. In fact, insulin begins to develop in the pancreas at this time. The vocal cords of the larynx also are beginning to form. The head, however, does not grow quite as rapidly as the body this week.

By the eleventh week the fetus is two and one-half inches long and may weigh one-third of an ounce. By the end of the month the fetus is forming its own digestive system and has working digestive glands. The female is starting to form the urinary bladder.

Changes in the reproductive system start to take place, too. The testes and the prostate gland start forming in the male fetus, which now has an external penis. The female fetus is beginning to develop the uterus and the vagina. The reproductive organs not only become well formed but they already contain some primitive egg and sperm cells. Yet just one month earlier it would have been difficult to tell, by observation, whether the fetus would become a baby girl or boy, as the sexual organs were similar in appearance and poorly defined.

In the twelfth week of fetal development, even more bits and pieces of the little body's growth become apparent. The salivary glands form; the tiny creature can bend its thumb and forefinger to meet. The three-month-old fetus may even practice expanding and contracting its primitive lungs, as though rehearsing for the future. And researchers have observed it swallowing amniotic fluid. By the end of the third month, despite its minute size, the fetus has developed all of its major systems. Within the next three months no new organs will begin to form.

What is even more remarkable is that the fetus, at this stage, is beginning to show its individual behavior patterns! Some fetuses are content and placid. Others busily move about in their watery chamber. The actual muscle structure also varies from one baby to another. The inherited differences in the genetic blueprint of your baby are beginning to reveal themselves.

It's easy to understand why the first three months of pregnancy are so vital to your baby's eventual good health. This period is the most rapid in terms of fetal growth and development of the major systems and organs. And if your baby has had a good start from the first trimester, she's on the way to becoming a strong, lusty infant.

Nutritional Requirements: The Third Month

Vitamin A

An increased amount of vitamin A is essential throughout pregnancy, but it's especially important during the third month of your baby's development. This vitamin is vital for cell development, and great numbers of new cells are being produced now as many different parts of the fetus form. Some of the internal organs, like the thyroid gland, the gallbladder, and the pancreas, are, in fact, completely formed but will continue to grow larger. There is also continued development of the reproductive organs and the digestive system. Vitamin A is also necessary for the linings of the internal organs, such as the gastrointestinal tract, and for the growth of enamel-forming cells in gum tissue. It also contributes to bone growth—and as you know, the skeleton is forming rapidly in the third month.

According to Dr. Myron Winick, a vitamin A deficiency in rats not only slows fetal growth but reduces the number of cells in the placenta.

The National Research Council advises a 25 percent increase in intake of vitamin A during pregnancy to meet your needs and the needs of the fetus. Good sources of vitamin A include organ meats, such as liver; dark green vegetables, such as broccoli, green peas, and turnip greens; and deep yellow or orange vegetables and fruits, such as apricots, peaches, papayas, bananas, oranges, sweet potatoes, carrots, and cantaloupe (a particularly rich source). Vitamin A is also found in butter and fortified margarine.

Zinc

It's important to continue with increased zinc levels this month, as this mineral helps with the maintenance of vitamin A levels in your body by releasing stores of vitamin A in the liver. Here, again, we find an example of the complex and wonderful relationship that exists between the various nutrients as they work together to help the body function.

Iodine

By the end of the third month the thyroid gland, which is located in the neck, is already complete. This small gland takes up iodine from the blood, combines it with other chemicals, and forms thyroxine, an important hormone.

Although the fetus gets its iodine requirements and stores from you, it must begin to make thyroxine on its own. In the cells, thyroxine is changed into several more active hormones that regulate the rate at which the cells change glucose through oxidation into heat and energy. The thyroid hormones are vitally important not only for body growth but for your baby's mental development.

If there is insufficient iodine in your diet, the little fetus fails to develop normally. In fact, in extreme cases the baby will be born both physically and mentally retarded. So continue to eat seafood regularly and use iodized salt to taste in your foods.

Magnesium

This mineral, found in living cells and involved in cell metabolism and tissue growth, is thought to be a coenzyme in protein and energy metabolism and is necessary for the building of your baby's bones. According to the National Research Council, magnesium is also essential for nerve and muscle membranes. Since there is a considerable rise in nerve-muscle connections during the ninth and tenth weeks of your baby's development, magnesium appears to be particularly important at this time.

In animal experiments, researcher Dr. Lucille Hurley found that when magnesium deprivation occurred throughout pregnancy, all of the rat fetuses were malformed and there was damage to almost every organ system. However, the role of magnesium deficiency in humans is not too clear, as yet, although it's known a deficiency can lead to neuromuscular problems with tremors and convulsions.

The Recommended Dietary Allowances for

1980 advises a 50 percent increase in this mineral during pregnancy. Magnesium is plentiful in salad greens, nuts, soybeans, and whole grains.

Calcium

Your calcium intake continues to be important for your baby's development in the third month because of the accelerated skeletal growth and rapid bone and tooth formation of the fetus. In addition, calcium is known to regulate nerve and muscle activity, which is also increasing now.

Calories

Even though the fetus weighs only about one-third of an ounce at the end of the third month of pregnancy, you should begin to lay down fat stores. This extra fat will provide you with the energy reserves needed to sustain fetal growth in the latter part of pregnancy.

By this time your weight gain should be between two to four pounds for the first trimester. If you have not gained this much by the time you have completed the third month, decrease your physical activity and rest more. Eat larger amounts of high-quality food at mealtime or frequent snacks, even if you have to carry them with you. Cheese and crackers, nuts and raisins, milk, a banana, or a sandwich are good between-meal choices.

Remember, if you gain properly, so will your baby.

Protein

Good-quality protein must be an important part of your diet throughout pregnancy. Foods rich in protein, such as meat, fish, eggs, cheese, and milk are vital for the new tissue growth that is accelerating during the third month. It's best to divide your protein allowance, as we have done in the menus, rather than to eat most of it at any one meal. The monthly menus will provide you with ample protein.

Vitamin B_6

This is another of the vitamins that should be increased during pregnancy as it's necessary for the metabolism of the additional protein in your diet. In fact, newborn babies who were accidentally subjected to a deficiency of vitamin B_6 developed convulsions and grossly abnormal electroencephalograms (brain wave tracings). The infants were "miraculously" cured by the restoration of vitamin B_6 to their diet.

Cereals and grains are good sources of this vitamin but according to Dr. Joyce Vermeersch, up to 75 percent of it is removed in food processing and is not restored by "enrichment." B_6 is also found in wheat germ, meat (especially liver), peanuts, corn, bananas, sunflower seeds, and soybeans.

Animal Experiments: Are They Valid?

A great deal of the information we have learned about nutrition in pregnancy has come from carefully controlled animal experiments. In the chapter devoted to the second month, for example, we mentioned that depriving pregnant animals of manganese causes certain congenital defects in animal babies. You will see this kind of research study cited throughout the book.

You may think, "But I'm not a rat, a chicken,

a guinea pig, or a pregnant chimp!'' Why don't we have more information on human mothers and the effects of specific nutrients on *their* babies? Restricting human mothers from any of the known essential nutrients could cruelly hurt their babies. For ethical reasons it's impossible to carry out such experiments.

As we have seen, most of the information we do have on pregnant women, we have learned as a result of natural disasters—war, famine, or accidents. However, during the 1950s an English physician, Dr. Margaret Robinson, restricted the salt intake of certain pregnant women in a large-scale controlled study. Dr. Robinson divided the women (similar in age and in the number of children they had) into two groups. The 1,019 women in one group were advised to take more salt during pregnancy, by eating salted fish, salted nuts, bacon, and salted butter. The other group of 1,000 women, were told to use as little salt as possible in cooking, to refrain from adding salt at the table, and to eat no salty foods. Otherwise, the diets, advice, and prenatal care were exactly the same for both groups.

The study lasted for three years. Sadly, there were twenty-two more babies who died in the group of salt-restricted mothers than in the group that used salt during pregnancy. This tragic study was too high a price to pay for scientific knowledge. But it clearly demonstrates why these kinds of experiments must be done on animals and not on human subjects.

The Rat and I: How Different Are We?

There are both differences and similarities between human mothers and pregnant animals. The rate of fetal growth is much faster in animals than in humans, and the animal mothers bear a number of babies with each pregnancy. There is also a proportionate difference between the weight of the mother and the weight of the babies at birth. None of us will ever give birth to a baby that weighs half of what we do. Yet with some animals, the total weight of the newborn babies may be nearly half the mother's weight.

But there are important similarities. The animal fetus, like the human fetus, is totally dependent upon the mother's nutritional status for its growth and survival. And there is an increase in fetal requirements as pregnancy advances. What's more, both animal and human fetal growth is retarded when the mother's diet is restricted!

Does the nutritional research done on experimental animals hold true for human babies, despite our differences? Thus far, we are finding there are striking similarities in the effects of nutritional deprivation. For instance, research scientists have shown that experimentally induced folacin deficiency in pregnant rats leads to fetal death or birth defects.

In addition, a zinc deficiency in pregnant rats was found to be especially harmful to the rat babies, 90 percent of whom were born with gross malformations. And as we have noted, doctors now realize the importance of zinc to you and your developing baby.

Scientists have recently come upon an even more amazing discovery. Young animals and young children who were nutritionally deprived prenatally and early in life show somewhat similar behavior patterns! According to fetal nutrition expert Dr. Pedro Rosso, the young of protein-restricted animal mothers reveal behavioral abnormalities and learning disabilities. These young rats reacted to other animals with what Dr. Rosso describes as "antigroup" attitudes. They also showed an increased lack of attention span and a reduced ability to learn when confronted by maze tests.

Moreover, Dr. David Barrett, a psychologist at Harvard Medical School, and his coauthors, Dr. Marian Radke-Yarrow, of the National Institute of Mental Health, and Dr. Robert Klein, of the Institute of Nutrition in Central America and Panama, have just completed a fascinating study on the effects of mild caloric deficiencies in the diet of infants and pregnant women.

Their findings, carried out over a period of five years both in Central America and San Diego, California, show that even mild early dietary deficiencies can disrupt a child's emotional stability by the time he or she reaches school age. The youngsters whose mothers were mildly malnourished during pregnancy and who did not receive a high-calorie supplement the first two years of life were more passive and dependent upon adults, showed a lack of interest in the environment, and were sadder and unfriendlier at six and eight years of age. Yet children who had better-nourished mothers during pregnancy and who received nutritional supplements in early life were more active and helpful, less anxious, and friendlier.

Moreover, these scientists point out, the subtle alterations in the development of the central nervous system coupled with a poor home environment often result in stunting the child's emotional growth. Admittedly, this probably doesn't happen with rat babies. Nevertheless, the results of the two studies are intriguing. We may not be that different from animals in some respects, after all.

Common Nutritional Complaints

Constipation

Some women have a problem moving their bowels during pregnancy. Doctors believe that in the early months this is caused by greater amounts of the hormone progesterone, which slows down the smooth muscles of the gastrointestinal tract. Later on, constipation may be made worse by the crowding of the enlarging uterus and its pressure upon the lower portion of the intestine.

How do you deal with it? Most of the time, simple dietary changes are enough to "get the machinery working again."

Here are some suggestions to help with this common problem.

1. Eat more raw vegetables and fruit to add additional roughage to your diet.

2. Dried fruits like apricots, raisins, prunes, and figs are especially helpful.

3. Drink more liquids. Prune juice is great if you like it.

4. Eat whole-grain "natural laxative foods," such as bran muffins or bran flakes.

5. Frequent small meals rather than three big ones may solve the problem.

6. Avoid rice and chocolate, both of which tend to be binding.

7. You don't *have to* have a bowel movement every day to feel well or be

"normal." So don't get uptight about
it.

8. *Don't medicate yourself with laxatives!*
(Diarrhea can result in a loss of
potassium.)

If you're still having trouble despite the
changes in your diet, check with your doctor.
Some iron tablets can cause constipation, and
your doctor may want you to switch to another
brand.

Heartburn

Occasionally during pregnancy you may be
troubled by an unpleasant burning sensation in
your chest or throat after eating. This is
commonly known as "heartburn" and results
from stomach acid being pushed up into the
esophagus. Some women never experience this
sensation, but others are frequently bothered by
it.

To minimize your discomfort, don't lie down
after eating or go to sleep soon after dinner. Eat
smaller meals to help you avoid heartburn and
that "full feeling" a lot of women complain about,
even in the third month of pregnancy. Finally,
stay away from such greasy foods as deep-fried
doughnuts, sausages, fatty hamburgers, under-
cooked bacon, and soggy French fries.

THE FOURTH MONTH

A good and proper diet of the pregnant woman can alter drastically the baby's health during its first six months.

Dr. Landrum B. Shettles
Dr. Robert Rugh

Jack and the Beanstalk

During the fourth month, the fetus shoots up like a seedling planted in fertile soil. It grows about six inches until it is up to eight to ten inches long. This is about half the length of many babies at birth. However, despite its amazing growth, the fetus is a fragile creature, weighing a mere six ounces at the end of the month. Even though the fetus is growing more rapidly no new organs or body systems develop during the fourth month.

However, the bony skeleton continues to develop, and the fetus looks more erect and less "curled up." The body grows larger in relation to the oversized head, which is no longer one-half of the total length of the fetus. Now the head is only one-third of the length of the delicate body. And the neck muscles have formed.

Other developments are occurring as well. The female fetus is beginning to catch up to the male in the development of its sexual organs. The tiny fetal heart is already recirculating twenty-five quarts or so of blood each day through the body. The features of the face are becoming clearer. Tiny lips appear on the mouth. The groove between the upper lip is developing. The permanent teeth, which are to replace the baby teeth, begin to develop within the jawbone in the fourth month of pregnancy. But the fetus is still not terribly appealing, as its skin is thin, loose, and wrinked.

Toward the end of this month (or early in the fifth) some women will feel a slight fluttering in the abdomen, as if butterflies were moving about. This is an exciting moment for most of us! And it usually comes from the kicking of the little matchstick legs of the fetus.

The Growing Placental Lifeline

The placenta is now a little more than three inches in diameter. Its role in your baby's development is crucial, as the fetus takes food, oxygen, and water through the placenta to sustain its remarkable growth.

During this month the placenta normally increases in size to provide greater nourishment. Moreover, it will continue to grow, at least until the baby weighs about seven and one-half pounds.

However, if you are eating poorly or not gaining sufficiently, the placenta will be smaller, and weigh less. A placenta of reduced size is unable to provide your baby with the necessary food and oxygen it requires for optimal growth and development. Research has shown that the placentas from infants who are small and stunted at birth, are not only lighter in weight but they have fewer cells than that of normal infants.

Placental Problems (or Abruption of the Placenta)

Occasionally, the placenta may separate prematurely from the wall of the uterus (placental abruption). It can occur as a result of an unfortunate accident, from toxemia of pregnancy, or, more commonly as a result of the mother's heavy smoking or poor nutrition. Sometimes, there is no known cause.

This tragic condition is seen more often in malnourished women, and it can spell disaster for the infant. Toxic wastes rapidly build up in the tissues of the fetus, and the brain survives for only about eight minutes without oxygen. The baby often dies even before the mother can be rushed to the hospital.

Yet according to Dr. Thomas Brewer and his wife, science writer Gail Brewer, "Nontraumatic abruptions (of the placenta) do not occur in well-nourished women. Good nutrition early in pregnancy fosters secure implantation of the placenta on the uterine wall. Continued good nutrition assures that the placenta will grow to meet the demands of the developing baby."

A Final Reminder

If you are still smoking cigarettes, this is your last chance to stop before possibly doing serious permanent damage to your unborn baby. From now on, the fetus needs increasing amounts of food, water, and oxygen to sustain its rapid growth. Each cigarette you smoke chokes off the supplies available to the infant. And the more you smoke, the more danger to your baby!

High Blood Pressure in Pregnancy

Hypertension, the medical term for high blood pressure, is a fairly common problem in women who are expecting a baby. According to Drs. Jan Drayer and Michael Weber of the University of California Medical Center, high blood pressure affects 10 to 15 percent of all pregnancies. The authors of *Our Bodies, Ourselves*, a fine book about women by the Boston Women's Health Collective, believe the increased rate of hypertension in certain young pregnant women may be related to their use of birth control pills.

Why should you be concerned about your elevated blood pressure during pregnancy? You will notice your doctor will be checking it regularly, each time you come to the office. Unfortunately, an increase in blood pressure can result in reduced placental blood flow to the fetus, and a decreased supply of oxygen and nutrients can seriously damage your baby. What's more, as the blood pressure of hypertensive mothers rises, there's a gradual but dramatic increase in the death rate of their infants.

Some women have what doctors refer to as "essential hypertension," the name given to the majority of cases of high blood pressure that are not caused by specific glandular or hormonal abnormalities. This is usually present in early pregnancy, less than twenty weeks. Others have hypertension complicated by kidney problems. And certain women develop "gestational high blood pressure" during pregnancy, generally after the twentieth week. In these women, blood pressure may remain higher for the first two or three weeks after the baby is born, and then it gradually returns to normal six to eight weeks after birth.

Luckily, not every mother with hypertension during pregnancy will develop complications. If they receive excellent prenatal care, many women with this problem go through pregnancy and deliver normal babies of average weight.

Treating Hypertension

If you have mild to moderate high blood pressure, usually you will be asked to limit your activities and rest frequently. Although being inactive may be "a pain in the neck," it's a very good way to reduce your blood pressure. In addition, your doctor will probably go over your diet with you to make sure you are eating properly—without restricting your salt intake. (We're talking about "regular" salt, sodium chloride, and not any other salt, such as potassium salt.

Products like Morton Lite Salt and potassium chloride should not be used during pregnancy.)

The Salt Controversy

Allowing women to eat a normal salt content diet even if they are hypertensive, has been a startling idea for many older physicians. Restricting salt in pregnancy was first suggested in 1906 as a means of preventing toxemia, a dreaded complication of pregnancy. And even twelve to fifteen years ago, most doctors believed in limiting salt intake for *all* pregnant women for fear of this problem. How well I remember being afraid to eat even a bite of a sour pickle when I was expecting a baby. However, the theory has since been proven to be without any scientific validity. Therefore, salt your food to taste but *do not use salt tablets.*

You may be aware that patients with hypertension are generally told to stay on a low-salt diet. But nutritional needs of pregnant women vary from those of women who are not pregnant. According to Dr. Harold Kaminetsky, writing in the *Journal of Obstetrics and Gynecology* in April 1978, "... It is now known that pregnant women actually have difficulty retaining all of the sodium (salt) necessary to carry out the normal physiology of pregnancy. There is no evidence that the abnormal handling of sodium may produce toxemia."

Dr. Kaminetsky further points out that you must retain a great deal of sodim in your body in order to retain sufficient water. For during the second trimester of pregnancy, beginning in the fourth month, your breast tissue should increase, as well as the size of uterus, the amount of amniotic fluid, the weight of the placenta, and the size of the fetus. And about 60 percent of all new tissue is composed of water.

Pregnant women with hypertension, in fact, do better with a normal salt intake, because it maintains the blood volume of the mother and that of the developing infant. Moreover, it has been seen that hypertension causes increased resistance in the blood vessels and a diminished blood volume, both of which are dangerous for the well-being of the fetus.

Ways to Halt Hypertension

According to researcher Dr. Lionel Schewitz, of the University of Illinois College of Medicine, the majority of pregnant women with high blood pressure will respond to bed rest and an improved diet, with an adequate amount of salt, fluid, and protein. Of course, *your doctor should be checking you frequently, monitoring your blood pressure and taking blood and urine tests*.

"But what happens if my pressure *still* doesn't go down enough?" you ask. You will, most probably, be admitted to the hospital, where your activity can be controlled further. Antihypertensive drugs, most of which are diuretics, may be used.

Although diuretics do a good job in lowering blood pressure, there are disadvantages to using them, because they reduce the blood plasma volume. Further, according to Drs. Jan Drayer and Michael Weber, "Only a few of the antihypertensive agents available in this country have been proven safe and effective in the treatment of gestational hypertension, although preferably *none* of these drugs should be given before the sixteenth week of pregnancy." If a diuretic must be used, Aldomet is one they consider safe during pregnancy.

The Increase in Blood Volume

As pregnancy progresses, the placenta needs much more blood flowing through it to work at an optimal level. Despite its small size, the fetal heart recirculates about twenty-five quarts of blood during the fourth month. The mother's blood volume, therefore, must increase at a relatively rapid rate to meet this need. Towards the end of the third month, the plasma volume (the fluid component of blood) starts to expand. By thirty-four weeks, according to Dr. Joyce Vermeersch, it's about 50 percent greater than it was at conception.

Researchers have shown that the increase in blood plasma volume is directly related to the outcome of pregnancy. In fact, women who have a small increase, by comparison to the average, have a greater number of stillbirths, abortions, and low birth weight babies.

How can you be sure that your blood volume is increasing adequately? Since salt causes the body to retain fluid, which is then kept by the bloodstream, restricting salt in pregnant women will limit the expansion of blood volume. A lowered blood volume will then result in either a slower-growing placenta or one with areas of dead tissue that cannot transfer all of the nutrients for the growing fetus. Therefore, salt your food to taste.

It's also imporant for you to drink more liquids at this time to help increase the blood volume in your body. Aim for seven or eight glasses a day, including milk, fruit juices, water, and soup.

Tea and coffee, however, are diuretics. They cannot really be considered as part of your fluid intake, since they don't retain fluid, but will cause you to lose fluid by urination.

Nutritional Requirements: The Fourth Month

Carbohydrates

In the fourth month your energy needs begin to increase because of the rapid fetal growth. The monthly menus that we provide will give you ample amounts of carbohydrates, the sugars and starches in your diet that should supply you with your main source of energy.

Nearly all of the carbohydrates we eat originally come from plants. Grains, fruits, and vegetables are common examples of the "natural" carbohydrates we eat. These foods are important because they provide fuel and contain a wide variety of vitamins, and essential minerals.

But many of us are accustomed to getting a large amount of carbohydrates from refined sugars and products made from them. For instance, cookies, cakes, and pies contain a great deal of refined sugar in addition to flour, which gives you calories for energy but little nutritive value.

Why do we need to eat carbohydrates? Why can't we use the protein and fats in our diet for all of our energy needs? When your body has a steady supply of calories from carbohydrates, the protein you eat can be used for making new tissue for you and your unborn baby. It's especially vital during pregnancy that protein be "spared" and not used up for your energy needs. Carbohydrates are then burned for energy instead. Carbohydrates are also needed to digest protein and some of them supply dietary fiber. This fiber gives you roughage to keep your digestive system running well and regularly eliminating waste products.

Fats also require the presence of carbohydrates in order to burn properly. When no carbohydrates are being metabolized, it's possible your blood may become polluted with ketones (the waste products of fat). They are toxic and can accumulate in the body and damage the fetal brain.

Fats

As we have seen, if your body had to depend solely upon stored fat for energy during pregnancy, serious problems could develop. However, a daily amount of fat in your diet is both necessary and desirable. Fats "carry" certain fat-soluble vitamins into your body through the walls of the digestive tract. And without some fat in your diet, you wouldn't be able to absorb vitamins A, D, E, and K, because they don't mix with water.

Polyunsaturated fats, such as corn, peanut, soybean, and safflower oils are also a source of linoleic acid, an essential fatty acid needed for many functions including growth. In addition, fats are a concentrated source of energy. They supply nine calories per gram, more than twice the energy supplied by the same amount of protein and carbohydrates. But they're an easy way to gain too many calories. To put it simply, you can get fat quickly from eating too much fat.

Protein sources such as meat, fish, cheese, milk,

and peanut butter will supply sufficient fat in your diet. Other foods that are high in fat content are ice cream, sour cream, mayonnaise, olives, nuts, margarine, butter, and pastries.

Protein

During the fourth month, your need for protein begins to increase sharply and will remain high until that wonderful day when your baby is born! (If you are planning to breast feed, of course, additional protein will still be necessary.)

For the next three months, however, the extra protein will be used mainly to take care of your own needs. Your circulating blood volume will gradually expand. The growth of tissues in your breasts and uterus also require protein. In addition, the placenta will develop further—and the mature placenta stores protein. What's more, so does the amniotic fluid, which surrounds the fetus like a large, protective, clear balloon.

Calories

By the beginning of the fourth month you should be gaining about three-quarters to one pound a week, a rate of gain that should continue until the baby is born. Most of the weight gain in pregnancy should take place after the third month. According to researcher Dr. Kamran Moghissi, a good average weight gain in a normal pregnancy is twenty-four to twenty-eight pounds. But twenty to thirty-five pounds is still within a "practical range," he feels. And if you were underweight before conception, even forty pounds is okay.

Vitamin B_{12}

We know that a slightly increased supply of this vitamin is necessary in pregnancy, but experts are not sure of the exact amount. B_{12} is involved in the formation of red blood cells, which begin to assume increased importance during the fourth month, due to the expansion in fetal blood circulation. It's also needed for protein metabolism, the process by which cells convert nutrients into special materials necessary to make new cells. A vitamin B_{12} deficiency can produce anemia.

Fortunately, this vitamin is present in all food of animal origin. So that, probably, only prolonged eating of a vegetarian diet might cause a lack of B_{12}. However, Dr. Myron Winick cautions that women who have been on birth control pills for several months or more prior to pregnancy may have depleted their supply of vitamin B_{12}. He therefore believes that you should have a blood test if you have been on the pill, and if you are lacking B_{12}, take a supplement containing this vitamin.

Vitamin B_6

Like vitamin B_{12}, this vitamin is involved in protein metabolism and is important for your baby's increased growth in the coming months. According to Dr. Winick, vitamin B_6 affects the developing brain in both humans and experimental animals. But, "The exact biochemical alterations in the brain are unknown at this time."

B_6 is another of the vitamins that may have been depleted if you have recently been on the pill. According to the National Research Council's Food and Nutrition Board, we don't yet know exactly how much increased vitamin B_6 is necessary during pregnancy. But numerous research studies within the past twenty-five years suggest there's a need for an increased amount of this vitamin when you're expecting a baby. The monthly menus include additional vitamin B_6. Wheat germ, whole grain cereals and breads, avocados, green beans, green leafy vegetables, bananas, fish, poultry, potatoes, and certain meats like liver supply vitamin B_6 in fairly high amounts.

Biotin

This vitamin plays an important role in the metabolism of fat and carbohydrates, helping both in the formation of fatty acids in the body and in the release of energy from carbohydrates. Good sources include *cooked* eggs, liver, dark-green vegetables, dried peas and beans, chocolate, cauliflower, and mushrooms.

Unfortunately some babies inherit a rare metabolic disorder in which the fetus requires very large amounts of biotin in order to stimulate defective enzymes to carry out normal body-chemistry processes. In a recent medical breakthrough, a March of Dimes researcher, Dr. Mitchell Globus, used amniocentesis to discover a mother was going to bear a second child with "biotin dependency." Essential enzyme activities in the unborn baby's cells were found to be abnormal. From the time this mother was twenty-three and one half weeks pregnant, she received daily biotin injections. The additional vitamin given to the mother was absorbed by the fetus and the baby was diagnosed and treated successfully *before* birth!

This is another remarkable example of how genetic disorders interact with the environment. In this case, scientists were able to change the fetal environment despite a genetic problem. But if the fetus had not been diagnosed and given continual doses of biotin through the mother, an inherited birth defect could have killed the child.

THE FIFTH MONTH

His [the physician's] knowledge of nutrition, in general, is deficient; formal instruction in nutritional principles is notably absent from medical school curricula and graduate programs.

Dr. Roy M. Pitkin

Stunts and Somersaults
Nutritional Requirements:
*   The Fifth Month*

Toxemia: A Serious Complication

Stunts and Somersaults

During the fifth month the fetus grows another two inches, until, by the end of the fifth month, it will be almost a foot. However, it is still extremely fragile and weighs only about a pound.

The fetal muscles are becoming stronger, though, and the little creature is a lot more active now, bobbing about in the transparent bubble of amniotic fluid. You can probably feel its faint attempts at gymnastics, because by the end of the fifth month the fetus is capable of doing somersaults, kicking, turning, and even hiccuping. You can awaken it if you wish, by tapping gently on your stomach or making a sudden jarring movement. Obviously, your womb isn't soundproof!

Much of the skeleton is bony hard at present, and the fetal heartbeat is louder. Although the body organs are well developed by this stage, the baby would quickly die if it were exposed outside of the cozy, protected environment of your uterus. Before six months, the lungs, skin, and digestive organs are not sufficiently mature to allow the fetus to survive on its own.

More and more "finishing touches" are beginning to appear now. Very fine hair starts to grow on the eyebrows and on the head. A fringe of delicate eyelashes develops on the eyelids, which are still tightly closed like those of a newborn kitten. Hard nails form on the nail beds of the fingers, and, a bit later, on the toes. In addition, all babies, whether boys or girls, develop pale pink nipples on the chest.

The fetus also grows a soft downy covering, called lanugo, over its entire body; it is especially prevalent on its arms, legs, and back. Luckily, most of it falls out before birth, or the baby would appear quite fuzzy!

Oil glands begin to secrete a fatty substance that mixes with the loosened dead cells on the surface of the skin to form a protective, paste-like covering, called the vernix caseosa. This acts as a buffer for the baby's tender skin, which is constantly being bathed by the mineralized amniotic fluid. The vernix cushions the delicate skin from abrasions.

Nutritional Requirements: The Fifth Month

Potassium

In the fifth month of pregnancy, as we have seen, the muscles of the fetus become stronger and it is much more lively. At this time the mineral potassium, which we have provided in your diet throughout pregnancy, becomes especially important. For potassium, which occurs mainly in the intracellular fluid in the body, helps in the release of energy and other activities in muscle cells. In fact, it influences the contractibility of muscles affecting body movement.

Potassium also aids in regulating the water balance in the body and in the transmission of nerve impulses. Nerve-muscle connections, which started to become interconnected in the third month of pregnancy, are now more developed.

Potassium-rich foods include bananas, oranges and orange juice, dried fruits, nuts, peanut butter, and dried peas and beans. Since laxatives can cause a serious loss of potassium and fluids in the body, they should be avoided as soon as you are expecting a baby. This is also one reason why hypertension should be treated without diuretics, if possible.

Iodine

During the second half of pregnancy, your basic metabolic rate may increase up to 23 percent, says Dr. Benjamin Burton of the National Institutes of Health. This additional metabolism, associated with increased activity of the thyroid gland, makes it necessary for you to be sure your intake of iodine is still ample. Goiter, an enlargement of the thyroid gland, is more likely to develop during pregnancy as a result of iodine deficiency. So please continue to use iodized salt in your diet and eat seafood regularly.

Vitamins

Your baby's need for vitamins as well as all of the other nutrients will increase in the crucial months ahead. These compounds cannot be made by your body and must instead be obtained from your diet. Unfortunately, there is no one food that contains all of the vitamins in sufficient quantity to satisfy human requirements, especially during pregnancy. But a varied diet is the best guarantee that you're getting all the vitamins you need.

The different vitamins vary greatly, not only in their chemical composition but in their functions. Vitamins A, D, E, and K are the so-called fat-soluble vitamins, which normally tend to be stored in the body in moderate amounts. They are absorbed along with dietary fats you eat, but since they can be stored you aren't dependent on their day-by-day supply in your diet.

The water-soluble vitamins include vitamin C, thiamin, niacin, biotin, pantothenic acid, vitamin B_{12}, riboflavin, vitamin B_6, and folic acid. They are not stored in your body, and the excess you don't use immediately is excreted in the urine. You are dependent, therefore, upon a constant dietary supply of these vitamins.

Vitamin C

Vitamin C is believed to be particularly important during the second and third trimesters of pregnancy. When the mother has sufficient vitamin C in her diet at this time, the placenta normally transmits a high amount of the vitamin from you to your baby. Scientists do not completely understand the reason for this as yet.

We do know that vitamin C is involved in tissue formation (and, of course, during the fifth month of pregnancy, not only is the fetus growing larger, but so are your breasts, and the placenta). It is also vital in the production of collagen, a cementlike substance present in connective and vascular tissues.

Vitamin C also helps in greater iron absorption, and is essential for the transfer of iron to the liver for storage.

Good sources for this vitamin are fresh, canned, and frozen citrus fruits and juices, strawberries, tomatoes, potatoes, cantaloupes, green peppers, broccoli, cauliflower, cabbage, brussel sprouts, and turnip greens. But do be careful not to overcook vegetables containing vitamin C, as most of it will be destroyed at prolonged high temperatures. In addition, be careful not to allow a vitamin C-rich vegetable or fruit to sit at room temperature for a prolonged period of time after cutting it, as this reduces its vitamin C content.

Vitamin E

This vitamin is an essential nutrient in the fifth month, since its deficiency can cause fragility of red blood cells and a general weakness in cell walls at a time when plasma blood volume must be built up. Laboratory studies reveal that a lack of vitamin E also results in greater excretion of creatine in the urine, indicating muscle loss. In the fifth month, however, the fetal muscles should normally grow stronger.

The best sources of vitamin E are vegetable oils, and margarine. Wheat germ is also a good source and can be added to a meat loaf, hot cereal, sprinkled over pancakes, or even put in a cookie batter for extra nutrition.

The B-Complex Vitamins

Although scientists believed at first that they had discovered a single vitamin, it was later proven they had actually found a number of vitamins: thiamin (B_1), riboflavin (B_2), niacin (B_3, nicotinic acid), pyridoxine (B_6), pantothenic acid, and cobalamin (B_{12}), plus folic acid, all of which perform vital functions in the body. A lack of any of them can cause serious problems for the little fetus.

Pantothenic Acid

Dr. Roger J. Williams, author of *Nutrition Against Disease*, believes that pantothenic acid plays "an unusually vital role in reproduction" because the body requires relatively large amounts of it to aid in producing strong healthy babies. "Human muscle, for example," he stresses, "contains twice as much pantothenic acid as the muscle of other animals and human milk, which nature provides for human babies, is relatively rich in this vitamin."

The Food and Nutrition Board recommends four to seven milligrams of pantothenic acid per day for adults and that "a higher intake may be needed during pregnancy and lactation (breast feeding)." But no specific amount is mentioned. It is, fortunately, widely distributed in foods and is abundant in meat, whole-grain cereals and breads, and legumes. It's also found in lesser amounts in milk, dark green vegetables, nuts, eggs, and fruits. With the diet provided in this book, you will receive ample pantothenic acid. More research is still being done on the vitamin and its role in pregnancy and breast feeding.

Thiamin, Niacin, and Riboflavin (the B Triplets)

These three water-soluble vitamins are often lumped together, possibly because they are all involved with energy metabolism in the body. However, their functions are distinct. Thiamin helps to release energy from carbohydrates. Riboflavin helps to release energy from proteins and fats as well as carbohydrates. And niacin participates with thiamin and riboflavin in helping to produce energy in cells.

The need for these vitamins, of course, is increased during pregnancy because your calorie consumption is greater, especially by the beginning of the second trimester.

Thiamine, riboflavin, and niacin can be found in whole-grain and enriched breads, pastas, and cereals as well as peas, milk, and eggs. Riboflavin is present in dark green vegetables and mushrooms; niacin can be found in liver and chicken; and liver and pork are good sources of thiamin.

When you read the labels on the packaged breads you buy, see that they are enriched with the B triplets; otherwise, change brands. Two more helpful hints: Don't store milk in a clear glass bottle, as riboflavin is sensitive to light and can be destroyed. Secondly, use very little water when cooking vegetables containing these vitamins, and cover the pot in which you cook them.

Protein

Why do you need it now? Aside from your own bodily needs which increase sharply at this time, Mother Nature is thinking ahead. You need additional protein to enable you to accumulate stored fat, in order to provide energy for labor and birth. In addition, you are building up protein reserves in the fifth month to be able to breast feed the baby after birth.

Calories

According to Dr. Roy M. Pitkin, if you have gained less than 2.2 pounds last month, your weight gain is inadequate. On the other hand, a weight gain of more than 6.6 pounds in any one month is too much.

So check your weight in between doctor's visits. Do this at the same time each day—if possible, in the morning before breakfast. You can easily adjust your own weight gain by eating additional quality snacks, if you're not gaining sufficiently. And chubby mamas should slightly decrease their portions of food to slow down the excess weight. (Unless, of course, you are expecting more than one baby!)

Toxemia: A Serious Complication

Toxemia, a disease of pregnancy that has baffled physicians for centuries, can be a serious problem for some pregnant women. This condition may occur anytime *after* the twentieth to the twenty-fourth week of pregnancy, but it commonly develops late in pregnancy.

Toxemia has several stages; in the first stage, which is called pre-eclampsia, the pregnant woman may have swelling of the body, high blood pressure, a sudden large weight gain, and protein in her urine. In the second stage she may have, in addition, trouble with her vision, terrible headaches, and abdominal pain. In severe *untreated* cases of toxemia, during the eclamptic stage, the expectant mother may have convulsions, lapse into a coma and die—often with the baby still in her uterus.

According to Dr. Bo S. Lindberg, between 4 and 15 percent of all pregnant women are affected. Other experts feel this may be true only in a poverty-stricken, poorly nourished clinic population, but that the rate is much lower among middle- and upper-class women. In fact, Dr. Nathan Dor, chief of Fetal and Maternal Mdicine at Maimonides Medical Center in Brooklyn, feels this disease is very rare in well-nourished middle- or upper-class women who generally have constant prenatal care and supervision.

The Medical Skeptics

Certain doctors continue to believe there's a relationship between a mother's gaining too much weight and toxemia, although within the past ten or fifteen years many researchers have shown there's no scientific evidence to support this theory. Other physicians still feel the causes of toxemia are unknown, and they dismiss the idea that malnutrition could play an important role in the development of toxemia. Nevertheless, there are some interesting facts that do point to a definite relationship between poor-quality nutrition and toxemia.

For example, the rate of incidence of the disorder in the United States reveals a close association, statistically, with low income and poor nutrition. The greatest death rates from toxemia are found in Mississippi and South Carolina, the states with the lowest per capita incomes. While the overall rate of mothers dying of toxemia in the United States is 6.2 per 100,000 live births, the death rate from toxemia in South Carolina is 20.3 deaths per 100,000 live births and a high of 30.2 deaths per 100,000 live births in Mississippi, an even poorer state.

Is this disease related to the black race in some ways as some doctors have proposed? No. Because a high rate of toxemia does not hold true for middle-class blacks. They have a very low rate of the disease, as do middle-class whites. But other poverty-stricken groups, such as the American Indians in Arizona and New Mexico, also suffer from a high rate of toxemia. And they often have had a lifetime of poor dietary habits. It seems obvious that there is some connection between poverty, poor nutrition, and toxemia of pregnancy.

There are, in addition, certain conditions that may also make you more prone to developing toxemia, such as hypertension, diabetes, and chronic kidney disease. Your doctor should be watching you during pregnancy even more carefully if you have any of these problems.

Anemia and Toxemia

Dr. John C. McFee has found an association between lack of iron during pregnancy and the development of toxemia. He cites a recent study done on five hundred pregnant women in India revealing that a much higher percentage of women who were iron deficient early in pregnancy later developed toxemia, compared to those who were not iron deficient.

"Although anemia cannot be said to cause toxemia," says Dr. McFee, "the two frequently coexist." He therefore concludes, "Various attributes of poverty, such as poor nutrition, often result in anemia and are no doubt important in the etiology [cause] of toxemia."

Is Edema a Sign of Toxemia?

According to Dr. Thomas Brewer, a diagnosis of toxemia is automatically made by some obstetricians when a pregnant woman develops edema (swelling of the hands and feet). He believes that many thousands of well-nourished women have been diagnosed as being toxemic and treated for toxemia they didn't have!

Moreover, Dr. Nathan Dor says, "At least 50 percent of normal pregnant women have edema at some time. This is *not* an abnormal condition during pregnancy." The swelling may be related to venous pressure in the legs due to the pressure of your uterus on the pelvic veins. If you're bothered by this, Dr. Dor suggests you just lie down and get off your feet. Frequently this is enough to make your swollen ankles disappear.

Signs and Symptoms

If you have a sudden spurt in weight gain and you haven't been eating well or feeling well, or you have *any unusual symptoms*, such as persistent headaches, abdominal pains, or blurring of vision, *contact your doctor or clinic at once.* Fortunately, according to Drs. Gordon Bourne and David Danforth, "With modern care the risk to the mother [in toxemia] is extremely small in the most severe cases; the risk to the baby is much reduced by skillful care, but if the disease develops early or is severe the baby is definitely jeopardized."

This is another excellent reason for seeing your doctor regularly during pregnancy and becoming an educated patient responsible for your own welfare and that of your unborn baby.

Salt and Toxemia: Savior or Sinner

Since abnormal sodium retention and edema are present in toxemia, salt and toxemia are still strongly linked together in the minds of many physicians. But researchers like Dr. Roy M. Pitkin and Dr. Harold Kaminetsky point out there's no scientific proof that restricting salt in pregnancy helps to prevent toxemia.

What's more, severely restricting sodium, even in a woman who may be developing toxemia, can be dangerous for the baby. Laboratory tests reveal these women have a markedly reduced blood volume and less extracellular fluid. Therefore, depriving them of salt further cuts down the blood volume, which can lead to a reduced placental flow. This, in turn, jeopardizes the baby's oxygen and nutritional supplies.

Treatment of Toxemia

Dr. Nathan Dor prescribes bed rest, an excellent diet with low-level vitamin and mineral supplementation, and close observation as the best method of treating the pregnant woman with mild toxemia. Sometimes, however, if the mother (often a poor teenager) has had little prenatal care and her condition is already serious, a Caesarean section may have to be done immediately. But the best approach to toxemia in pregnancy is its *prevention* through quality prenatal care and good nutrition, including the use of salt.

THE SIXTH MONTH

For reasons as yet unclear, being born to a better-nourished mother is protective to children even after two years of age.

Dr. Beverly Winickoff
Dr. George Brown

Standing Tall
Nutritional Requirements:
  The Sixth Month

Trace Minerals

Standing Tall

The fetus is growing so rapidly during the sixth month that you will need and store more protein at this time than at any other. Furthermore, you should be continuing to gain about three-fourths to one pound a week.

The fetus is getting a little plumper and increases its weight to about one and three-fourths pounds. It also grows two additional inches, to become about fourteen inches long. The body of the fetus is now even more erect than it was in the fourth month. This enables it to make room for the enlarging internal organs, particularly the liver and the heart. Its eyes are structurally complete, and it may open and close them. It is an increasingly lively little creature, well able to tumble about in the "bag of waters" like a tiny weightless astronaut. What's more, the hair is growing long by the sixth month; some babies could use a trip to the "Unisex" Beauty Shop by the time they are born!

Still, the fetus is not very pretty nor cuddly, as it's scrawny, with skin that is reddish and wrinkled.

Although adult bones contain 90 percent calcium, there is as little as 12 percent calcium in the bones of the fetus during the sixth month. It cannot protect itself against cold nor regulate its own body temperature yet, for there are little or no fat deposits beneath the skin. This is why a fetus delivered prematurely in the sixth month has a terrible struggle to survive, despite the specialized care and support of a fully equipped intensive-care nursery.

At the end of six months, your baby will have completed two-thirds of its stay within its warm, sheltering home in your uterus. The next three months are crucial. Scientists believe poor nutrition in the early months of pregnancy affects the development of the embryo and its ability to survive. Poor nutrition in the latter part of pregnancy affects fetal growth, especially the growth of the brain.

Nutritional Requirements: The Sixth Month

Protein

Your requirement for protein is especially high during the sixth month, so continue eating four servings daily, spread throughout the day for better digestion and absorption. Not only is the fetus growing rapidly this month, but your own bodily needs for this vital nutrient continue increasing until the end of the month. For instance, your uterus is getting bigger, its weight increasing twenty times during the second trimester to make room for the growing size of the baby.

Also, the placenta continues to grow this month, in order to supply the fetus with a greater amount of oxygen, water and proteins. At least until the fetus weighs about seven and one-half-pounds, fetal weight gain is normally accompanied by a comparable increase in the weight of the placenta. So the need for protein continues to be vital in the sixth month and throughout the last three months of pregnancy.

Fortunately, you can choose from a wide variety of protein-rich foods, such as canned tuna or salmon, eggs, cheese, chicken, or steak. All of these foods provide protein and the essential amino acids that are necessary for the birth of a strong, healthy baby.

Calcium

Calcium needs are greatest during the last trimester, and in the sixth month you are building up reserves that will be in demand later. At this time there is still not much calcium deposited in the bones of the fetus. But if your intake is insufficient, the newborn may suffer from fragile bones that are deficient in calcium.

According to *New York Times* science writer Jane Brody, 98 percent of your own body's calcium supply is deposited in the bones, which act as a storage warehouse. Even though most of us think of our bones as solid fixed objects, calcium is constantly moving in and out of them. Within a year, about one-fifth of the calcium in your bones is removed and replaced. If, during pregnancy, your diet doesn't supply enough of this mineral, certain hormones will remove calcium from your bones in order for the life-sustaining role of calcium to continue. As you may remember, calcium must remain in a specific ratio in your blood and in other body fluids. However, nature protects the mother by not allowing all of your body calcium to be depleted for the sake of the fetus. Nevertheless, some scientists feel osteoporosis, a weakening of the bones in older women, may have its origin in calcium depletion from multiple pregnancies.

Therefore, continue with your high intake of this mineral during the sixth month. Drink a quart of milk a day or its equivalent in other milk products. There are, of course, additional foods that will contribute to your calcium intake, other than dairy foods. For example, calcium is found in high amounts in canned sardines with the bones, and in lesser amounts in oysters, canned salmon with the bones, cooked kale, cooked broccoli, and fresh oranges.

Trace Minerals

For many years trace element nutrition was thought to be limited to just two elements, iron and iodine, both of which have been extensively studied. However, one of the more recent advances in nutritional research is the discovery that there are other minerals necessary for human health, growth, and reproduction. These trace minerals, also called trace elements, are only now being investigated as more sophisticated instruments become available to detect and study their presence.

Why are they called trace minerals? Essential minerals are classified by the amounts necessary for the human body. The macrominerals like calcium, phosphorus, magnesium, potassium, and sodium are required in relatively large amounts. The microminerals or trace minerals are needed only in very small amounts, but this doesn't mean they're unimportant for growth and development. In fact, we still have much to learn about their functions in the human body.

In addition to iron and iodine, the trace elements include zinc, copper, chromium, selenium, molybdenum, fluoride and manganese. Furthermore, animal laboratory experiments suggest nickel, vanadium, tin, arsenic, and possibly cadmium may also eventually be added to the list of trace minerals that are necessary in humans. In 1980, for the first time, the Food and Nutrition Board of the National Academy of Sciences established some general guidelines for adequate and safe dietary intake of the elements copper, manganese, fluoride, chromium, selenium, and molybdenum.

Perhaps the study of trace minerals will shed new light on our understanding of nutrition and its role in "making" healthy babies.

Zinc

Zinc has recently been recognized as a highly important trace element in pregnancy. Scientists have evidence this mineral is necessary for cell growth, as it plays a crucial role in the metabolism of various nutrients, especially protein. Therefore, we have made provision for ample zinc intake in your diet from the very first month of pregnancy.

The most devastating effect of a zinc deficiency is failure to grow, and obviously, this would spell disaster at any stage of embryonic or fetal development. In fact, pregnant rats who were fed a diet containing only minimal amounts of zinc gave birth to stunted babies with skeletal defects, misshapen heads, and other serious abnormalities.

In view of the importance of zinc for fetal development, the Food and Nutrition Board advises an increase in zinc intake (from 15 milligrams per day to 20 milligrams per day) during pregnancy. For it's believed only about 15 percent of the dietary zinc is actually absorbed by your body.

Fortunately, eating a high-protein diet with plenty of meat, liver, eggs, poultry, and seafood will give you ample zinc. And the quart of milk you drink daily plus nuts and legumes and the whole-grain bread and cereals that are part of your pregnancy diet are also limited sources of zinc.

Copper

What does copper do for babies? It's believed this mineral facilitates the use of iron for making hemoglobin, but exactly how this happens remains a mystery. Unfortunately, there are still many gaps in our knowledge of trace elements.

However, we do know the concentration of copper in the normal human fetus increases substantially during pregnancy, so that the amount of copper in the liver of your newborn baby will be five to ten times greater than the copper found in your own liver. Nature, in its wisdom, cleverly makes provision to tide the little infant over during the period when it drinks only milk, which is low in copper. Furthermore, copper deficiency has been reported in premature babies who lack the copper stores available to the full-term baby.

Dr. Kamran Moghissi reports that in several animal studies copper deficiency in pregnant rats resulted in skeletal defects in the rat babies. Other researchers have shown copper deficiency in animals leads to a variety of abnormalities, including anemia, degeneration of the nervous system, defects in the color and structure of the hair, and even cardiovascular problems.

The sixth month is an important time to build up fetal copper reserves. Excellent sources of this mineral include organ meats, dry beans, lima beans, bitter chocolate, cocoa, oysters, almonds, walnuts, pecans, mushrooms, and beef liver. Oats, dried peas, rye and whole-wheat flour, and dark-meat turkey are also good sources of copper.

Chromium

This trace element has been shown to be required for maintaining normal glucose metabolism levels in experimental animals. And it has a similar function in humans. A dietary lack of chromium could possibly result in abnormal carbohydrate metabolism.

Good sources of chromium are meat products, whole-grain cereals and breads, peanuts, cheeses, and Brewer's yeast. Until more precise recommendations can be made in the future,

eating a varied, well-balanced diet (as we have provided for you in the menus) remains the best assurance that you are receiving a safe, adequate amount of chromium.

Selenium

The best-known function of selenium is that it protects vital parts of the cell against damage. It is also believed to interact with vitamin E to prevent the breakdown of body chemicals.

Recently, Dr. P. Jack Collipp, director of pediatrics at Nassau County Medical Center, in Long Island, successfully treated a seriously ill two-year-old girl with four weeks of a selenium supplement. The child's problem was initially diagnosed as myocardiopathy, a potentially fatal disease of the heart muscles often caused by a viral infection. When tests showed no apparent virus, Dr. Collipp traced the child's problem to a selenium deficiency in her diet. She was cured, seemingly miraculously.

Apparently, lack of selenium was a serious problem in China, where the deficiency is called Keshan disease. Thousands of Chinese have suffered from the disease because the foods they ate lacked selenium due to selenium-poor soil. Treatment with selenium supplements drastically cut the rate of death from this disease in China, says Dr. Collipp.

Although an imbalanced diet, without selenium, may be harmful to the human fetus, too much of this trace element taken in fortified mineral tablets can also potentially harm your unborn baby. So get your intake of selenium from foods, not pills or tablets. Good sources are seafood and meat (especially liver). Whole-wheat grains and cereals are variable sources of this mineral depending upon the region in which they were grown. Fruits and vegetables contain little selenium.

Molybdenum

Little is known about molybdenum (except that it's very hard to pronounce). But a deficiency of this mineral in animals can cause decreased weight gain and a shortened life span. It's not known, however, whether this holds true for humans.

Molybdenum is found in legumes, cereal grains, liver, and some dark green vegetables. Any good diet would give you sufficient amounts of this trace mineral. The Food and Nutrition Board cautions you, nevertheless, *not* to take additional supplements. For too much molybdenum causes a significant loss of copper from the body.

Fluoride

Fluoride is a trace element most of us are somewhat familiar with, due to the fluoridation of drinking water in certain communities and the addition of fluoride to toothpastes. The main areas affected by fluoride in humans are the bones and the enamel of the teeth.

According to the Food and Nutrition Board, fluoride mainly affects the pre-eruptive phase of the teeth since it becomes incorporated into the structure of the tooth and strengthens it against decay (cavities). And research studies have shown that youngsters whose mothers drank fluoridated water *during pregnancy* and who continued to drink it through their mid-teens have, in general, two-thirds less cavities then children who did not have fluoridated water. Fluoride also combines with the calcium of bones and helps to prevent loss of calcium from the bones in later life.

Fish, most animal foods, fluoridated water, and food grown with or cooked in fluoridated water will provide you and the fetus with a sufficient amount of this trace element. Fluoride too is toxic when consumed in excessive amounts. However, the daily amount required to cause a problem is generally *far* in excess of the average amount you could possibly drink or eat.

Manganese

We know that manganese is an essential element for many animal species, because many baby animals show signs of retarded growth, abnormal bone formation, and other congenital birth defects when their mothers are fed diets deficient in this single mineral.

And it's believed manganese is necessary in humans as well for normal bone structure and proper functioning of the central nervous system. We have, therefore, provided you with foods that contain manganese in the daily menus: nuts and whole grains, vegetables and fruits, and meats and seafood.

Iron

This trace element has long been recognized for its importance during pregnancy, for if you lack sufficient iron when you are expecting a baby, you may not only feel weak and tired, but you will also be less able to tolerate blood loss during birth. Further, anemic women generally have poorer resistance to infection.

You should not only be eating iron-rich foods but continuing to take supplements to meet the greatly increased demands for iron in pregnancy. Most experts believe that without supplementation, more than one-half of pregnant women lack sufficient iron.

It's particularly important that you have enough iron from now on, for the fetus accumulates iron during the last three months of pregnancy. Also, during the sixth month your circulating blood volume must rise to meet the needs of the placenta and other increased tissue growth for you and the baby.

Iron is an essential part of hemoglobin, the substance in the blood that carries oxygen from the lungs to the body cells. Without enough iron you will have a reduced amount of hemoglobin and will have to increase your cardiac output in order to have enough oxygen for the placental and fetal cells. This extra work may make you feel physically exhausted and worn-out.

However, the baby is not usually anemic at birth (unless it's premature). Until very recently doctors believed the removal of iron from the mother was one of the few instances when the fetus still remained a true parasite, assuring its own iron supplies by withdrawing the mother's iron. But Dr. Pedro Rosso comments that earlier studies did not show or test for the fact that full-term babies of anemic mothers had reduced iron stores as well. He believes "a significant reduction of iron stores at term makes the infant more susceptible to become iron-deficient during the first year of life," because in the early months after birth, the baby drinks milk that contains little iron.

Therefore, eating iron-rich foods and taking your daily iron supplement during pregnancy will be beneficial to the baby not only at birth but also long afterward. And you will feel better, stronger, and more energetic. Dr. Sue Rodwell Williams advises that up to two years of a normal diet are needed to replace the iron lost during a pregnancy!

As you may remember from the first month, iron is found in liver, liver sausage, red meats, shellfish, egg yolk, green leafy vegetables, dried fruits such as apricots, prunes, and raisins, dried peas and beans, dark molasses, potatoes, and enriched and whole-grain cereals, and cereal products.

THE SEVENTH MONTH

Fetal malnutrition has emerged as a significant health problem over the past decade.

Dr. Warren Crosby

Getting Ready

In the seventh month the fetus is absorbing a great deal of nutrients from your body through the growing placenta. At birth, the normal placenta is generally eight inches in diameter and weighs about two pounds. Remember, just three months ago the diameter of this organ was only three inches!

The fetus is also continuing to put on weight: about three-quarters of a pound or so a week, so that the baby weighs between two and three pounds at the beginning of the month. In fact, the uterus is beginning to get crowded, and it's more difficult for the fetus to move around.

There are other developments as well. The testes usually descend into the scrotum of most male fetuses. The brain makes tremendous gains in growth during this month. The surface of the brain develops fissures and depressions that every normal person has in precisely the same place.

By the beginning of this month your unborn baby can already suck its tiny thumb, and some doctors have reported delivering babies with calluses on one thumb from so much sucking before birth. In addition, the baby's skin, which had been wrinkled and reddish last month, begins to smooth out.

During the seventh month there are "personality" differences in fetal behavior, mainly as a result of the master blueprint transmitted through heredity. We began to see this minimally at the end of the third month, but it's more marked four months later. Some babies, for example, suck their thumbs in the uterus; others do not.

If you're having a second or third child, you may have noticed other differences in fetal behavior. Certain babies are constantly moving around, kicking and thumping as if they can't wait to get out. If you stay still, you can see the movements of a little foot pushing against your abdomen, especially when you lie down. Other fetuses are somewhat quieter and less restless.

Although the seventh-month fetus is generally strong and lively in the uterus, if it's born prematurely it immediately becomes a frail, delicate infant. Still, it has a fair chance of survival outside of your body when it receives excellent specialized care in a neonatal nursery. Nevertheless, each additional day the fetus can remain in your uterus during the seventh month gives it a better chance to grow and develop normally.

The Premature Baby

Sometimes a baby is born before it's ready to survive on its own. Until recently such an infant was defined as one that weighed less than five and one-half pounds at birth, but doctors are now much more concerned with the baby's maturity and functional development rather than its birth weight alone.

Why are we so anxious to prevent a premature birth? "Unfortunately," says Dr. Leonard Glass, director of Neonatology at Brooklyn's Downstate Medical Center, "most babies born prematurely, before full-term, have problems. In the majority, these problems can be overcome by modern medical care and the infants will survive and grow up normally. Yet a significant number have very serious disorders, such as imperfectly developed lungs, bowel, bladder obstructions, and other crippling defects."

What Causes Premature Labor?

The causes of prematurity are not always known. We still have much to learn about what actually triggers labor and how to stop it when it starts too soon. Poor health, poor nutrition, heavy smoking, a serious accident, and even a severe emotional shock may cause you to go into premature labor. And certain specific diseases such as diabetes, toxemia, thyroid disturbances, and syphilis have all been known to cause prematurity on occasion. Giving birth to more than one baby may also result in an early delivery.

Statistics reveal that poor women who eat poorly and receive inadequate prenatal care are much more likely to deliver prematurely than middle- and upper-class women who eat well and receive good prenatal care.

However, due to the tremendous medical advances that have been made within the past ten years, many of these babies, born at thirty or thirty-one weeks, are surviving. "In the past," says Dr. Nathan Dor, "we just gave up on them. Now they are being born and being maintained." However, the cost of saving a premature baby weighing under 2.2 pounds at birth is staggering: $40,000 for an average case and more than $100,000 for some problem cases requiring specialized hospital care.

Small-for-Gestational-Age Babies

For a long time doctors referred to *all* babies as premature if they weighed less than five or five and one-half pounds at birth. Yet this definition doesn't take into consideration the time the baby has spent in your uterus. Some full-term babies who weigh less than five and one-half pounds at birth are not "premature" babies but underweight full-term babies.

Drs. Kenneth Scott and Robert Usher studied 240 newborns who weighed under five and one-half pounds and found 39 percent of them were stunted nine-month babies. These infants were not only low in birth weight for gestational age, but they showed physical signs of malnutrition and soft tissue "wasting" at birth, such as loose skin, decreased muscle mass, and absence of normal fat deposits. Recently there's been a sizable increase in the number of low birth-weight babies born in the United States; according to the March of Dimes Birth Defects Foundation, this is a serious national problem.

Why has there been such a dramatic upsurge in these low birth-weight babies with retarded fetal growth? And what is the reason they seem to be at even greater risk than babies of the same weight who are born prematurely?

Unfortunately, we don't have all the answers. But we've learned fetal growth is affected by the quality and the quantity of nutrients, and that a nutritional deficiency can strike anywhere and everywhere in the baby's body. The large number of teenage mothers who don't take good care of themselves during pregnancy, as well as the greater numbers of young women who smoke and drink may be partly responsible for the sudden rise. One maternal factor that is significantly associated with a growth-retarded baby is an average weight gain of less than one-half pound per week during the last six months of pregnancy. Other known causes of infant malnutrition while in the uterus are smoking, certain genetic defects, intrauterine infections, uncontrolled hypertension, or a combination of these factors. Each of them deprives the baby, in one way or another, of sufficient nutrition for optimal growth and development

Dr. Richard Naeye and his associates at Babies Hospital in New York City performed autopsies on 1,000 stillborn or low birth-weight babies who died and found certain organ structures in many of these infants were abnormal. They had a smaller thymus, spleen, adrenal glands, and liver than average-weight babies. In addition, the infant suffering from intrauterine impoverishment often has permanent brain damage, which can be expected to impede learning processes throughout life. This may explain why growth-retarded babies often have a poorer prognosis than a "premie" of the same weight.

In mothers where there was no evidence of genetic defects or intrauterine infections, Dr. Herbert Miller and his colleagues at the University of Kansas Medical Center found growth-retarded babies were associated with two or more of these maternal factors: poor maternal weight gain, lack of prenatal care, unmarried, chronic major illness, obesity, and toxemia. However, Dr. Miller also confirmed that a maternal factor positively associated with well-nourished infants is an average weight gain of one pound or more per week during the last two months of pregnancy. Here again, we find proof you do have some control over your baby's good health.

Nutritional Requirements: The Seventh Month

Calories

During the fourth, fifth, and sixth months, your weight gain involved the growth of your breasts and uterus, a large blood volume increase, and the accumulation of fat storage in your body. However, from now on, your weight gain will primarily involve the growth of the fetus, the placenta, and an increase in the volume of amniotic fluid.

During the seventh month, your baby normally gains about three-quarters of a pound a week. So please don't short-change your baby by cutting back on your consumption of calories. Because your baby must have additional amounts of food to continue to grow and develop normally, you should be maintaining a steady weight gain of about three-quarters to one pound a week.

In fact, the greatest need for ample amounts of high-quality foods take place within the last trimester, when cells are increasing in both size and number. At this time, even a mild restriction could cause a problem to the baby. And not all defects show up in early infancy.

Calcium

Most of the accumulation of calcium in your baby's skeleton will take place during the last three months of fetal development. Body calcium will increase in the bones and teeth, with about 1 percent present in the soft tissues and body fluids. Obviously, this is no time to let up on your intake of calcium, as your unborn baby needs this mineral now more than ever.

Sodium

Although there's a good deal of justifiable concern that Americans, in general, eat too much salt, pregnancy is one time your body really needs it. As the placenta increases in size from now on to provide the unborn baby with greater nourishment, it must have more blood flowing through it to work at an optimal level. Salt helps with this necessary expansion of blood volume by allowing you to retain fluid in the bloodstream. Without the resulting increase in blood flow, the placenta is unable to make the growing exchange of nutrients and waste products between yourself and the baby. Furthermore, the formation of new tissues and cells in the body of the fetus during the seventh month requires additional amounts of fluid.

Protein

Your need for protein and amino acids, the "building blocks" of your baby's body, is at an all-time high during the next three months. Nutritional requirements are at their maximum because this is the time when the bulk of the baby's tissues develop. And additional protein storage in your own body is necessary to prepare you for labor, birth, and breast feeding.

Although the Recommended Daily Allowance for protein is 74 grams per day during pregnancy, we're increasing it to 80 to 85 grams per day, as some researchers, such as Dr. Thomas Brewer, recommend. Dr. Kamran Moghissi also suggests there's no harm in increasing the intake of protein for an extra margin of safety. You will, therefore, be getting five servings of protein per day in the monthly menus plus four cups of milk per day. (Each eight-ounce cup of milk contributes 8.8 grams of protein)

Dr. Kamran Moghissi has done a fascinating study on 129 women during the last three months of pregnancy. On two occasions he took blood samples from each of the women, for analysis of the proteins and amino acids in their blood. His findings suggest specific proteins and amino acids contribute to the baby's physical growth, whereas others are related to infant mental or motor development. This is, perhaps, the first time we've had scientific data on the subject, rather than relying upon dietary information from mothers.

What's more, the lack of certain amino acids in the diet of pregnant women (and their absence in the mother's blood) appears to have a damaging effect on their babies. Dr. Moghissi concludes there seems to be a positive correlation between particular amino acids and proteins in the mother's blood and normal fetal development.

But your protein increase doesn't have to "break the bank." Too many of us still see protein mainly in terms of expensive cuts of meat like lamb chops, steaks, and rare roast beef. Yet in many countries in the world where meat is scarce, pregnant women eat ample amounts of quality protein. For instance, Dr. Nathan Dor, a native of Israel, says that Israeli women eat little meat due to its high cost. However, chick-peas, a staple food in their diet, is often combined either with complementary vegetable proteins or small amounts of chicken or fish to provide perfectly balanced protein. And bread in Israel is also highly protein-enriched with soya flour.

How can you make these food combinations work? We've done it for you in some of the daily menus. Some good tasting combinations are Spaghetti with Meat Sauce, Three-Cheese Baked Macaroni, and Salmon and Noodle Bake, or a bowl of split pea soup with frankfurters.

Trace Elements

These microminerals, which are widely distributed in foods, perform a vital function during the last trimester of pregnancy. Some of them function in enzyme systems, acting as biochemical catalysts to speed up cell metabolism. And it's possible there are additional trace elements needed by the fetus for optimal growth, which we have yet to discover.

To make sure you have an adequate daily intake of the trace elements, the daily menus stress variety at mealtime. Although you may occasionally want to substitute different vegetables, fruits, or meats, depending upon their price and availability—learn to stretch your food horizons by varying your diet with a variety of fruits and vegetables. And experiment with recipes and foods you may not have cared for or tasted before.

Folacin

Because the requirement for folacin increases markedly at this time, it is not surprising that the greatest number of folacin deficiencies also occur during the last three months of pregnancy. According to the National Research Council, pregnant women need twice as much folacin as women who are not pregnant. The reasons for this are still not completely understood. However, it's believed folacin plays an important part in the growth processes of pregnancy.

Dr. Myron Winick states a deficiency of this B vitamin is implicated in abnormal brain development in the human baby. With the brain making such tremendous gains in growth during the seventh month, your intake of folacin assumes greater importance, because if it's lacking, cell division does not proceed normally.

Therefore, if your doctor has placed you on folacin supplements, please continue to take them. This vitamin nutrient is also found in a wide variety of foods included in the daily menus. Perhaps you may remember that liver, nuts, dried peas and beans dark green leafy vegetables, wheat germ, whole-grain cereals, oranges and orange juice are all sources of folacin. It is also found in asparagus, broccoli, cauliflower, and endive.

Biotin

Biotin, another of the B vitamins, helps in the synthesis of some of the fatty acids and amino acids in your body. In addition, it aids in releasing energy from carbohydrates. And due to the greatly expanded needs for energy and the increasing nutritional demands of your baby in the latter months of pregnancy, biotin plays an important role in metabolism.

Many scientists believe bacteria in the intestines "manufacture" some of the biotin and that the rest comes from your dietary intake. In this respect, biotin resembles vitamin K, which you'll read about in the next chapter.

The best food sources of biotin are *cooked* eggs, liver, peanuts, green beans, dried peas and beans, chocolate, cauliflower, and mushrooms. All of these are foods that have been used in the daily menu section of this book.

Hemorrhoids

During the latter part of pregnancy, hemorrhoids are a fairly common complaint. These are enlarged rectal veins that dilate and often protrude through the rectum, usually caused by the increased weight of the fetus and the downward pressure it causes.

As a result of hemorrhoids the rectal area may itch, burn, and feel uncomfortable. Often constipation aggravates the hemorrhoids and they bleed a little, so you will want to try to avoid constipation by increasing the amount of liquids and fresh fruits and vegetables in your diet, or by drinking nature's own laxative—prune juice with a slice of lemon.

Warm baths will make you feel better. Afterward, gently pat the sore area with a triple-size cotton ball fluffed in plain corn starch. After a bowel movement, wipe yourself with Tucks pads. Some women find cotton soaked in witch hazel or even a little petroleum jelly helps to get rid of the itching and the irritation.

THE EIGHTH MONTH

The quality of ingested food during gestation may exert important effects on the functional capacity of the brain in later life.

Dr. Kamran S. Moghissi

Getting Set
The Growth of Your Baby's Brain

Nutritional Requirements:
*   The Eighth Month*
Amniotic Fluid

Getting Set

The fetus must continue to absorb increasing amounts of oxygen and nutrients of all kinds in the eighth month. Protein, vitamins, minerals, and calories are vital for your baby's growth and development. Cells are still increasing in number and size in many fetal organs. The brain of the fetus is especially vulnerable to nutritional deprivation at this time, because its development during the last eight weeks is occurring at the most rapid rate yet.

The fetus also gains at least two more pounds this month, so that it weighs about four or five pounds by the end of the month. Most of the weight your baby gains is a protective padding of fat deposited under the skin, making the baby chubbier, less wrinkled, and a lot more appealing-looking. The extra fat, however, is not to enhance appearances, but rather to help control your infant's body temperature.

By now, both you and the baby are beginning to get a bit uncomfortable as the unborn baby occupies more and more of the available space in the enlarging womb and has less room to wiggle around in. The surrounding amniotic fluid diminishes in proportion to baby's growth. With less space and fluid available for the infant to stretch out full length, the little one curls up in what is known as the fetal position. About 97 percent of all babies settle head down into this position late in pregnancy, because it's roomier and they feel more comfortable that way.

No, your baby does not feel dizzy as you or I would continually lying head down, because it's still in a state of weightlessness, despite the loss of some amniotic fluid. However, your baby can no longer do its tumbling and "sitting-up exercises" in such crowded quarters.

A lot of women can't wait for the baby to be born by this time. But an eighth-month baby is still not complete according to Mother Nature's timetable. If you understand what's happening inside your uterus and why, it may help you to be more patient with your increasing size and awkwardness.

If the baby is born prematurely, however, it has a good chance of surviving with special care, although there are problems related to the infant's too early appearance outside of your womb. All systems are *not* ready and set to go. Breathing may be difficult because the infant's lungs haven't matured sufficiently to absorb the necessary quantity of oxygen. The baby can also have trouble with its digestive tract, which is not working perfectly yet. And an eighth-month baby often loses more weight after birth than a full-term baby. In addition, during the eighth month the fetus receives immune substances from you that will protect it from certain diseases early in life, therefore a baby born a month early is more vulnerable to infection.

The Growth of Your Baby's Brain

Although some questions regarding maternal nutrition and fetal growth still remain unresolved, many experts believe the development of your baby's brain can be severely restricted by "comparatively mild undernutrition" *during the period of its fastest growth,* the last two months of pregnancy.

There are, apparently, three stages of brain-cell growth. At first the number of cells in the brain multiply by dividing with enormous rapidity through cell division, although the size of the cells remain unchanged. The eighth month is a period of rapid cell division. During the second stage of development, the number of brain cells continues to increase (but not quite as rapidly as before), and cell size also increases. During the final stage of brain-cell growth, cell division stops, but the weight and protein content of the cells continue to rise as maturational changes take place within each cell.

The Role of Nutrition in Brain Development

If you understand the stages of brain growth, it becomes easier to figure out why your baby's brain is so vulnerable to poor nutrition during the periods of rapid cell division. *For a critical stage in brain development takes place before birth,* and interference with that growth during the phases of active cell division usually results in permanent stunting of the brain (an insufficient number of brain cells).

Sadly, once the precise biological "timer" that regulates the division of brain cells is turned off, it is lost forever. Brain cells don't regenerate themselves like skin or bone cells, which heal and mend by growing additional cells.

Therefore, fetal nutrition expert Dr. Myron Winick believes it's the *timing* of the nutritional deprivation that can be so devastating to the infant's brain development. And as Dr. Kamran Moghissi points out, "The greatest increase in mass of the human fetus and particularly that of its brain, occurs during the last few weeks of gestation and continues during the first few months after birth." (What's more, your baby will be possessed, at birth, of many billions of brain cells!)

Furthermore, Dr. Winick says, researchers have tried in many animal experiments to nourish newborn rat babies *after* they were exposed to prenatal undernutrition, hoping to reverse the cellular effects. Yet animal babies of protein-restricted mothers, for example, remain with a deficit in the total number of brain cells, even if they're nursed by normal "foster rat mothers" and receive adequate nourishment after birth.

However, researchers have discovered that if optimal nutrition is given during the final prenatal stage of brain growth, *this growth impairment can be reversed*. And permanent stunting in animals, which is caused by early malnutrition, can be prevented—if good nutrition is begun while cell division in the brain is still occurring.

The cells of the brain are tremendously active metabolically. Even though they weigh only about 2 percent of the total body weight, they use up approximately 25 percent of the total energy of the body, according to biochemist Dr. Roger Williams. Obviously the needs of the brain cells for quality nutrition are high. Finally, it is hoped that what scientists have learned within the past decade about prenatal brain growth will, once again, put to rest the myth of the fetus as a "perfect parasite."

As you can see from the way brain cells develop, the fetus is unable to withdraw from your body all of the vital nutrients to provide for its needs if they aren't present in sufficient amounts. The high-quality daily diets we've provided for you, with all of the known essential nutrients, will meet that need.

Nutritional Requirements: The Eighth Month

Calories

Check your weight between visits to the doctor. If you're gaining over one pound a week, you can make certain substitutions in your diet, as you don't want to gain excessively. Putting on a lot of additional weight will make it harder for you to take it off after the baby is born.

Skim milk, for example, is just as good for the baby in terms of vitamin and mineral content but has a lower fat and calorie count than whole milk. An eight-ounce glass of skim milk has only ninety calories; a glass of regular milk contains one hundred fifty calories. So you can easily save two hundred forty calories a day by drinking a quart of skim milk instead of whole milk. And once you get used to it, you may never go back to regular milk.

Hard cheeses are also generally higher in calories than soft cheeses like pot cheese, cottage cheese, and farmer cheese, although there are hard skim-milk cheeses you may like. Lorraine Swiss, for instance, is a delicious alternative. Nuts can be deleted from your diet as well, if your weight is zooming up rapidly, for their calorie content is very high.

But *if you are gaining less than three-quarters of a pound a week in the eighth month, you are not gaining enough to provide for your baby's needs!* You may want to include a small amount of foods made with sugar, such as jam, jellies, or ice cream *in addition to your balanced diet* to provide extra calories. The fetus must continue to absorb greater amounts of nutrients of all kinds this month. Your baby's growth is occurring at its most rapid rate from now until the time of birth.

Iron

Anemia is seen more frequently in late than in early pregnancy, as the growing fetus makes greater demands upon you now for iron. As you know, the total red blood cell volume and hemoglobin mass increases by about 25 percent in pregnancy. This increase begins during the sixth month and peaks close to the time of your baby's birth. This is why taking iron supplements and eating iron-rich foods is essential throughout pregnancy.

What's the big fuss about anemia in late pregnancy? According to Dr. John McFee, the pregnant anemic woman is much less able to withstand a significant loss of blood during labor and delivery, and can more quickly go into shock as a result.

Folacin

As we have seen, folacin helps in the formation of hemoglobin. In addition, it's necessary for the synthesis of DNA in the cells—the basic blueprint of life. The huge growth of new cells taking place in the baby's body during the eighth month makes this B vitamin essential.

Thiamin, Niacin, and Riboflavin

The process of producing energy involves several other nutrients in addition to those that yield calories. Thiamin, riboflavin, and niacin are vitally concerned with energy production and therefore are very important in your diet, especially during the eighth month.

Protein

Increasing amounts of protein are required now to form the structural basis of all new cells. You should be eating enough calories so that the protein can be spared for building tissue instead of being used for energy requirements.

Vitamin B_6 (Pyridoxine)

Pyridoxine is necessary for amino acid metabolism and protein synthesis. And *New York Times* science writer Jane Brody reports that some pregnant women need larger amounts of B_6 for the normal development of their babies' central nervous system.

Apparently, researchers at Purdue University found a number of mothers with sick newborns had significantly lower levels of B_6 in their blood than the mothers of normal, healthy babies. Yet these mothers had eaten more than the recommended amounts of vitamin B_6. How can this be explained? It seems that in some women, because of their own biological differences, this level of vitamin B_6 is inadequate.

We are recommending an ample intake of this vitamin daily. But as it's found in many of the foods we have used in our menus, such as liver, green beans, bananas, poultry, fish, meat, nuts, potatoes, leafy green vegetables and whole grain breads and cereals, you won't have difficulty meeting your requirement.

Vitamin K

Vitamin K is known as the "antihemorrhagic vitamin," because it aids in the synthesis of substances necessary in blood clotting. Its presence is essential when your baby is born, as it helps to prevent you from bleeding excessively.

Liver studies have shown that about one-half of the vitamin K in our bodies is manufactured by bacteria in the intestines, and that the other half comes from our diets. Unless you've been treated with antibiotics for a while (which can upset the normal bacterial environment of the intestines) or you have gall bladder disease or some other liver problem, a deficiency is, fortunately, uncommon.

But your baby's intestines will not contain the K-producing bacteria at birth. It takes a few days before the bacteria are available to make vitamin K. Therefore, to prevent possible bleeding because of the cutting of the umbilical cord, some doctors routinely give vitamin K to the newborn baby.

The best dietary sources of vitamin K are green, leafy vegetables. Fruit, cereals, dairy products, and meat provide lesser amounts of it.

Fats

There's a difference between body fat and dietary fat. You don't have to eat much fat in order to gain body fat, for your body can "manufacture" it when you eat extra calories from protein and carbohydrates. Yet dietary fats, in small amounts, serve a nutritional purpose.

In the first place, they're needed to transport fat-soluble vitamins, like vitamin K, in your body. Without some fat in your diet, you're unable to absorb the fat-soluble vitamins. Secondly, polyunsaturated fats, from most vegetable oils, are a good source of linoleic acid, the fatty acid that is essential for growth. Moreover, some fat in the diet makes your food taste better and gives you a "satisfied feeling" after eating.

About 1 to 2 percent of your day's calories should be from vegetable oils, such as corn oil, safflower oil, or soybean oil, which contain linoleic acid.

Zinc

The continuation of the trace element zinc in your diet is vital not only for your baby's further development but also apparently, for labor. According to Dr. Pedro Rosso, a study of 234

women showed a relationship between the mother's blood levels of zinc and the outcome of pregnancy. Women with low zinc levels tend to have more complicated and prolonged labors. Your high-protein diet will, therefore, protect you and your unborn baby from the consequences of a zinc deficiency.

Vitamin E

Vitamin E is an essential nutrient whose deficiency can cause abnormal fragility of the infant's red blood cells. The normal vitamin E concentration in your newborn baby's blood plasma will be about one-third that of adults, and that of the low birth-weight infant is even lower. By one month of age the baby should have normal childhood concentrations of vitamin E. Interestingly enough, vitamin E levels rise more rapidly in breast-fed babies. The best food sources are the polyunsaturated fats in vegetable oils, and margarine.

Amniotic Fluid

The fetus starts to drink small quantities of amniotic fluid as early as twelve to fourteen weeks after conception, "practicing" how to suck and swallow to insure its survival when it has to enter the outside world. Yet drinking amniotic fluid gives your baby more than just practice, as this liquid contains both protein and glucose.

Dr. H. M. Liley, obstetrician and mother of five children herself, points out that individual babies drink different amounts of amniotic fluid. "The very active ones drink as much as six to eight pints of fluid per day, by the eighth or ninth month. This averages about five ounces an hour and is the caloric equivalent of drinking about three and one-half ounces of milk a day."

It's fascinating to realize that no matter how much the baby drinks, the fluid is always present and constantly replaces itself! Most of the fluid is believed to be secreted by the fetal kidneys, but there's still a lot we haven't figured out about this marvelous process.

THE NINTH MONTH

There is no question but that the mother's diet is crucial for her, her fetus, and for her child during its first year.

Dr. Landrum B. Shettles
Dr. Robert Rugh

All Systems Are Ready and Set to Go

Because the baby is continuing to grow and gain weight (about an ounce a day) during the ninth month, you should *not* be on a low-calorie, low-salt diet—even if you think you've gained too much already.

The baby's needs for increased nutrients are still at a very high level. The fetus is now about nineteen to twenty inches long, and should weigh between six and eight pounds by the end of the month. Boy babies are generally a little heavier than girl babies.

The greatest increase in the size of the fetus, including that of its brain, occurs during these last few weeks of gestation. What else is happening this month? The gums in the mouth become ridged, and the tiny breasts are firm and protruding in both sexes. Certain organs in the body, such as the lungs, liver, and kidneys, grow larger. The fetus also receives antibodies from your blood to protect it against certain diseases for the first six months of life. This temporary immunity is nature's way of safe-guarding the infant until it can slowly develop its own immune system to infection.

About two weeks before delivery, the placenta changes its structure. It becomes tough rather than fibrous and its blood vessels degenerate. The placenta's usefulness is finally at an end.

The baby will shortly be mature enough to take care of its own bodily functions, independent of its mother. At last, the onset of labor is near and a new human life is about to begin. One nearly microscopic cell, the egg, has become 200 billion or more cells, weighing 6 billion times more than the fertilized egg. The genetic plan that was signed and sealed at the moment of conception is about to be delivered!

Nutritional Requirements: The Ninth Month

Calories

Although you may feel like an overstuffed teddy bear, continue to gain three-quarters to one pound per week during the ninth month. This is particularly important in view of the rapid brain development that is taking place during the last few weeks of pregnancy. You will also need increased calories for energy requirements in labor and birth as well as for the maintenance of milk in breast feeding.

By now, you should have gained about twenty to twenty-five pounds. Women who were underweight before pregnancy should be at least thirty pounds heavier. Weight control that results in a smaller baby can be harmful to you as well as to your baby. Dr. Tom Brewer points out that there's often prolonged labor in such women and the uterus must be artificially stimulated by drugs into further contractions.

Protein

Our menus are high in protein content throughout your pregnancy, but protein is especially needed at this stage of brain development. Dr. Pedro Rosso of Columbia University's College of Physicians and Surgeons has shown that "fetuses from protein-restricted mothers have an overall reduction in the cell division of the brain." In addition, other organs of the baby's body are growing larger as well, and protein is vital for this additional tissue growth.

Iron

There is a need for continued iron intake during the ninth month, as the baby is building up its own iron stores at this time. In fact, Dr. Roy M. Pitkin advises you to *continue with iron supplements for at least two to three months after the baby is born, even if you're not breast feeding.* The mildly depressed feeling some new mothers experience can be the result of an iron defi-

ciency anemia combined with the fatigue of caring for a new baby.

Copper

Since the trace element copper is believed to stimulate the absorption of iron, it's particularly important now. You are also building up the copper content of the fetal liver; the newborn normally has a much higher amount of copper at birth than it will have later on.

Some excellent sources of copper include almonds, walnuts, pecans, bitter chocolate, cocoa, lima and dry beans, mushrooms, and beef liver. Additional good sources of copper include oats, dried peas, corn, dark meat turkey, rye, and whole-wheat flour.

Vitamin C

This vitamin is essential during pregnancy because it enhances the body's use of iron, folic acid, and vitamin A. It's present in many fruits and vegetables, such as oranges, grapefruit, lemons, and citrus fruit juices, tomatoes, green peppers, and cabbage.

However, *do not take* excessive amounts of vitamin C in tablets, as they may be harmful to your baby. "Megadoses during pregnancy create a dependency on high doses of C in the unborn child," says Jane Brody. "After birth, the baby may suffer from scurvy (vitamin C deficiency disease) when consuming normal amounts of vitamin C."

Zinc

An adequate supply of the trace element zinc is vital for your unborn baby, even during the last month of its development. Researchers now believe a zinc deficiency *at any time* during pregnancy can cause problems in the infant.

Fortunately, by eating animal protein, eggs, or seafood daily, you will meet your baby's requirement for zinc. It's difficult, however, to ingest enough of it without eating some animal protein. Whole grain products like whole wheat or rye bread, oatmeal, and corn contain this mineral as well, but not in a form that is readily available for your body's use.

Iodine

The fetus is now making its own thyroid hormone, but it must receive its iodine requirements and stores from you. And your own needs and those of the fetus are at an all-time high. The continued use of iodized table salt and regular eating of seafood are the best ways to insure that you and the fetus are getting enough iodine.

Magnesium

The mineral magnesium is involved in both the building of your baby's bones and in the manufacture of proteins, so it's essential during the ninth month of pregnancy, when increased bone formation in the baby's skeleton plus a tremendous amount of tissue growth are taking place.

Although scientists still have a lot to learn about the exact role of magnesium in the human body, associations have been made between low levels of magnesium and tremors and convulsions in infants and young children.

Eating lettuce and other leafy, green vegetables, nuts, soybeans, and whole grains will protect you and your baby against a magnesium deficiency.

Vitamin D

This vitamin also plays an important role in your baby's bone development, as it's responsible for regulating the metabolism of calcium and phosphorus and promoting the intestinal absorption of these minerals as well. Without it the baby will suffer from abnormal bone growth, even if you've had an adequate intake of calcium and phosphorus!

Vitamin D is found naturally in fatty fish, eggs, liver, butter, fortified margarine and vitamin D-enriched milk.

Vitamin A

Your increased need for vitamin A continues until the baby's birth. Although vitamin A is efficiently stored in the liver, your allowance during pregnancy is increased by 25 percent to compensate for its storage in the baby's liver. Vitamin A is necessary for healthy skin and mucous membranes, plus normal bone growth. In addition, Dr. Yoko I. Takahashi points out vitamin A is essential for *all* fetal cell development and the growth of enamel-forming cells in tooth formation. But *do not take excessive amounts of vitamin A* in pills or tablets; overdoses of this vitamin are toxic!

Some of the foods richest in vitamin A are organ meats, cantaloupe, cooked broccoli, raw carrots, turnip greens, tomatoes, and cooked green beans.

Thiamin, Niacin, and Riboflavin

These B vitamins are indispensable during the last month of pregnancy due to the great increase in the size of the fetus and particularly that of its brain. Niacin, as you may remember, is a coenzyme in protein metabolism; riboflavin and thiamin are both coenzymes for energy metabolism. A deficiency in *any* of these vitamins can be harmful to your unborn child.

Whole-grain and enriched cereals and breads are good sources of the B triplets.

Vitamins B_6 and B_{12}

Vitamins B_6 and B_{12} are also coenzymes in protein metabolism. What's more, they are necessary for the formation of increasing numbers of red blood cells for you and your baby. The plentiful supply of meat, fish, poultry, milk, and vegetables we have provided in the menus should take care of your needs for these vitamins.

Potassium

Another nutrient that helps your body to release energy from carbohydrates, protein, and fats is the mineral potassium. Insufficient potassium in your diet can make you feel weak and fatigued. And since most mothers by this time are pretty tired normally, you can see why this condition should be avoided for your sake and the baby's.

But if you have been eating our daily menus, which contain oranges, orange juice, dried peas and beans, potatoes, bananas, and dried fruits, you have been provided with a sufficient amount of potassium.

By eating a high-quality diet before and during pregnancy, with ample amounts of calories, proteins, vitamins, minerals, trace elements, and fluids, you have provided your baby with the best possible nutritional environment for its optimal growth and development. And by applying the scientific facts we already know about prenatal growth, you can eliminate some of the tragedy and misery caused by "reproductive failures." So if you've stopped smoking, drinking alcohol, and taking pills and drugs throughout these nine crucial months, you've given your unborn baby a "pollution-free" environment and the opportunity to reach his highest genetic potential. What's more, your precious baby has received from you the greatest gift of all, the chance for a healthy, satisfying life.

Congratulations, mom!

BREAST FEEDING

Breast milk is not a gift; the nutrients contained in milk do not materialize out of thin air. Either directly or indirectly they must come from the mother's diet.

Dr. R. G. Whitehead

To Breast Feed or Not: That Is the Question

Although we know with certainty that breast feeding is, in nutritional terms, the best feeding for the human baby, cultural factors have strongly influenced our decision whether or not to breast feed. Before World War II it was common for babies to be breast fed, unless their mothers were unable to produce sufficient milk.

However, our attitudes changed about thirty or thirty-five years ago with the introduction of "scientific" infant formulas, and even doctors and hospitals discouraged women from breast feeding. In fact, when my daughters were born, I didn't know a single friend or acquaintance who had breast fed a baby! It all seemed "messy," "old-fashioned," "unnecessary," and "embarrassing" to most of the young mothers of my generation.

But due to an increasing awareness of the advantages of mother's milk, thanks to some doctors and such organizations as La Leche League, breast feeding has come back into style for a generation weaned on nature and ecology. According to a recent article in the *New York Times*, about 54 percent of American women were breast feeding their babies in 1980. This is in marked contrast to a survey done by Ross Laboratories, manufacturer of the infant formula, Similac, which showed that only 23 percent of women were breast feeding their babies in 1971.

It's true, however, that many young mothers must return to work soon after giving birth, which makes formula the simplest feeding method. And millions of mothers through the years have raised healthy, contented bottle-fed babies, though it is nutritionally second best.

Why Breast Feeding Is Best Feeding

Biochemical Makeup

Breast feeding benefits both you and the baby for a number of reasons. Breast milk is nutritionally superior to any manufactured formula, because of its biochemical composition, which makes it ideally suited to a baby's needs.

For example, the protein in your milk is completely compatible with your baby and she will not become allergic to it. However, proteins in formulas based on cow's milk can cause a potential problem for certain infants who become sensitized to these "foreign proteins." An allergic baby may, therefore, react with a variety of symptoms, such as a stuffy nose or the symptoms of intestinal infection. And most of us know a baby who had to be switched from one formula to another or even to goat's milk or a soybean formula. Some infants who cannot tolerate any other food have no trouble digesting breast milk.

Dr. Derrick Jelliffe, Professor of Public Health and Pediatrics at the University of California, explains that one of the enzymes in human milk is lipase, which starts the digestion of the milk fat while it is in the baby's mouth, esophagus, and stomach. Human milk is also much richer in lactose, a milk sugar, and cystine, an amino acid produced in the digestion of protein. And Dr. Jelliffe suspects cystine and lactose are related to the rapid continuing development of the newborn baby's brain.

Furthermore, no formula can match the gradual biochemical changes that occur in colostrum and human milk following childbirth. Colostrum is the thin fluid in your breasts that comes out of the nipples, generally late in pregnancy or immediately after childbirth, before the "true milk" comes in. There is simply no manufactured formula that can exactly duplicate the more than one hundred components in human breast milk.

Immune Factors

Breast milk provides the infant with important antibodies against certain diseases and infections. According to Dr. L. A. Hanson, respiratory infections, earaches, and intestinal infections that cause diarrhea are much less common in breast-fed infants. Colostrum is especially high in protective antibodies to fight harmful infections in the newborn. It is so valuable for the baby, some doctors put the newborn to the mother's breast almost immediately after delivery. For the sucking reflex of the little infant is very strong at birth, if the mother hasn't received a lot of anesthesia during childbirth.

"Too-Fat" Babies

Breast feeding guards the infant against early childhood obesity, and the protective effect may be long-lasting. Breast feeding mothers cannot coax or push their babies to take more milk. There aren't any ounces marked on your breasts to tell you how much the baby drank, and you can't force a reluctant baby to finish a half hour later.

What's more, the fat content of breast milk changes throughout a single feeding. At the start the milk has a comparatively low amount of fat, but as the baby continues to nurse, the milk becomes richer, with a higher fat content, until the baby feels full and satisfied without overeating. The infant, with Mother Nature's help, learns to regulate her own appetite. Therefore, many doctors now believe breast feeding can help to prevent childhood obesity, even if there's a tendency in your family to being overweight.

Contraception

Many experts feel successful unsupplemented breast feeding has a definite contraceptive effect that lasts for months after the baby's birth. However, this "natural protection" declines with the introduction of supplementary bottles of formula and with time. So discuss your need for contraception with your doctor. Don't rely upon breast feeding as a fail-safe method of preventing pregnancy. (Though it's been helpful to women in undeveloped countries without access to additional means of birth control.) Neither oral contraceptives nor the chemically treated IUD are advisable when you're breast feeding, as they may both seriously affect the quantity and quality of your milk.

The Cost of Breast Feeding

Although it's true you have to eat more and better to produce sufficient breast milk, the expense is less than buying monthly cases of formula and purchasing sets of baby bottles. And the cost of formula, like everything else, is going up.

Convenience

The breast is readily available to pacify a hungry baby (or you can express your milk in a bottle, which can be fed to your baby by a baby-sitter). There aren't any formulas to mix, no bottles to scrub, boil, and cool. And on a cold winter's night, you don't have to jump out of a warm bed to get a bottle and heat it for the 2 A.M. feeding!

Getting Back Into Shape

When the infant nurses, it stimulates contractions of the muscles of the uterus, which helps to return the expanded uterus to its prepregnant size. Mothers who have breast fed often mention experiencing slight cramps in the lower abdomen, in the beginning. This is nature's way of getting your uterus back to normal.

Psychological Factors

Some experts feel there's a warmth, closeness, and a psychological intimacy between mothers and their breast-fed babies. This doesn't mean a bottle-fed infant, who is held and cuddled during feeding, will eventually wind up on a psychiatrist's couch! It just means breast feeding is special, and a lot of researchers feel there are emotional advantages for you and the baby.

Can I Breast Feed?

Although breast feeding is a "natural" function, it's not instinctive behavior. And most of us have to feel relaxed about it to learn how to do it successfully. Fortunately, *almost all women* who want to breast feed find that they can. Breast feeding usually fails, says Dr. Frederick Goodrich, Jr., because of "a lack of proper understanding of the normal development of the baby, a lack of knowledge of the technique and practice of nursing, and inadequate help and encouragement."

But a lot of mothers become tense and anxious because "true" breast milk doesn't generally come in until the third to the fifth day after delivery. Some women become panicky that their baby isn't gaining enough. However, it's normal for the breast-fed infant to gain more slowly than the bottle-fed infant during this initial period.

An organization that helps breast-feeding mothers in over 1,000 cities and towns throughout the United States is La Leche League International. Made up of groups of young women who are enthusiastic and experienced about breast feeding, La Leche League can help you on a mother-to-mother basis. To contact a branch of La Leche League, look in your local phone directory or call 1-312-455-7730.

The league also publishes an informative, easy-to-read, beautifully illustrated paperback book on breast feeding, called *The Womanly Art of Breastfeeding*, newly revised in 1981. You can purchase the book from La Leche League International, 9616 Minneapolis Avenue, Franklin Park, Illinois, 60131.

Where Does Breast Milk Come From?

The breasts make milk out of substances extracted from the plasma, glucose, amino acids, and minerals in your body. While you breast-feed you need not only the nutrients available for the milk and its energy value, but also nutrients to supply the energy to combine the fat, proteins, and lactose. Although the composition of human milk varies between mothers, it provides, over a period of time, a reliable source of the basic nutrients required by the human infant. We don't yet know why these variations occur, but we do know the composition of breast milk changes depending upon what you eat.

Fortunately, fat laid down during pregnancy can now be used to supply a portion of the extra energy that's required (about four to eight pounds is used in this way), for much of the nutritional preparation for breast feeding has already been accomplished earlier.

However, in a woman who hasn't gained sufficiently, breast feeding will sacrifice the mother's tissues in order to provide for the baby. In fact, the protein and calorie count of milk produced by malnourished mothers isn't that different from the milk of well-nourished mothers. But the volume of the milk production is markedly diminished, so that it's often not enough to provide for the needs of a growing infant.

Dr. Margaret Whichelow of Guy's Hospital in London studied two groups of mothers who wanted to breast feed. All of the twenty-six mothers in the study who were successfully breast feeding were eating considerably more than usual. The unsuccessful mothers, who had an insufficient milk supply, were eating little more than normal. What's more, when three of the successful mothers tried to diet, they developed an immediate reduction in their milk supply.

Nutritional Requirements: Breast Feeding

Calories

After living for weeks on three or four hours of interrupted sleep with my first baby, I clung to the hope that life had to get better. And, of course, it did. But finding the time to eat well will make a big difference in how you cope these first few months.

Breast feeding makes great physical demands upon you. Approximately nine hundred calories of energy are required to produce about one quart of milk. Storage fat will give you about one-third of the energy cost (three hundred calories a day) for the first three months of breast feeding. Therefore, you'll need about six hundred or more additional calories a day during this period. The amount should be increased if you breast feed for longer than three months or if your weight begins to drop below normal for your height. Of course, allowances must be greater if you were lucky enough to have given birth to twins!

But it's very difficult to tell you *exactly* how many calories you'll need. According to Dr. R. G. Whitehead, "Any recommendations can only be a rough guide." There's no magic caloric formula that works for every mother, because there are many variables: How much fat have you laid down during pregnancy? What kind of work do you do? Are you extremely active, running around after two or three other children in addition to the new baby? So there has to be a generous allowance for individual differences.

Many women understandably want to lose weight quickly and regain their prepregnancy figures. Yet Dr. Bonnie Worthington says reducing calories, especially in the early weeks of breast feeding, isn't a good idea. "Lactating [breast feeding] women," she cautions, "should accept a gradual rate of weight loss in the first six months after childbirth." Otherwise you may not produce enough breast milk.

Protein

The Food and Nutrition Board of the National Research Council advises an additional twenty grams of protein a day over the normal dietary allowance for breast-feeding mothers. The amino acids in protein are necessary to produce human milk. However, the March of Dimes Birth Defects Foundation recommends you eat four servings of protein a day, and this is what our menus are based upon during the period you are breast feeding.

Calcium

Twelve hundred milligrams of calcium are required daily to provide the calcium that is released into breast milk. Therefore, some authorities, like Dr. Benjamin Burton, author of *Human Nutrition*, advise new mothers to drink six cups of milk a day, while breast feeding. But please don't add chocolate to the milk, because it reduces your body's ability to absorb calcium.

Luckily you can substitute many foods made with milk to satisfy your requirements. Women who find drinking so much milk each day a bit much can substitute ice cream, ice milk, yogurt, milk puddings, sour cream, soft cheeses such as farmer, pot, and cottage cheese, hard cheeses such as Muenster, Swiss, Edam, Cheddar, and cream soups as part of the calcium requirement. And our menus continue to supply high amounts of this important mineral (five servings a day) during breast feeding.

What happens if you don't include a sufficient intake of this mineral in your diet? The skeleton apparently serves as a calcium reservoir when the demand cannot be met by daily dietary intake. Unfortunately, calcium will be taken away from your own skeletal system, making it more susceptible to bone fracture.

How do we know this? Drs. P. J. Atkinson and R.R. West, using a scanning technique to measure calcium loss in mothers who were breast feeding, observed small bone mineral losses. Moreover, though we don't yet have definite proof, many specialists believe an inadequate calcium intake while breast feeding contributes to the development of osteoporosis in older women. This disease affects about one woman in four after menopause. Its symptoms are weak bones that break easily as a result of the loss of bony tissue.

Vitamins

Researchers believe vitamin deficiencies affect breast milk. According to the Food and Nutrition Board, if you're breast feeding you should increase your intake of vitamins A, D, E, C, and all of the B vitamins over prepregnancy levels. Furthermore, the Recommended Dietary Allowances for vitamins A, C, E, riboflavin, thiamin, and niacin are even somewhat higher than the amounts recommended during pregnancy.

Your physician may want you to take a vitamin-mineral supplement during the months you're nursing your baby. But pills are never a substitute for good food or your own good cooking.

Vitamin A

As you may remember, vitamin A is necessary for proper bone growth and tooth development. The Recommended Dietary Allowance for this vitamin during breast feeding is increased considerably over pregnancy levels to provide for the vitamin A secreted in breast milk. Fortunately many foods contain vitamin A: liver, eggs, cheese, butter, fortified margarine and milk, yellow fruits and vegetables, oranges, carrots, sweet potatoes, cantaloupes and dark-green vegetables are among them.

Vitamin A is efficiently stored in the liver, and well-nourished women have at least several months supply that the body can use. We've listed foods in our menus that contain a good supply of vitamin A from the prepregnancy diet on through pregnancy and breast feeding.

The B Vitamins

The levels of all the water-soluble B vitamins in breast milk are directly related to your own dietary intake. These vitamins, as you may remember, are: riboflavin, niacin, thiamin, pyridoxine, biotin, pantothenic acid, folic acid, and vitamin B_{12}. The Food and Nutrition Board recommends that you slightly increase your daily intake of all these vitamins while breast feeding.

Good sources for almost all of the B vitamins include liver, whole-grain cereals and breads, wheat germ, milk, and nuts. And we have provided you with ample amounts of these foods in the daily menus.

Vitamin C

If your diet is a good one, your breast milk will contain a plentiful supply of vitamin C. Vitamin C-enriched fruit juices, which are recommended for bottle-fed babies in the early months, are unnecessary for the breast-fed baby.

However, unless your diet has ample amounts of vitamin C, your milk will be low in this important nutrient. Dr. Bonnie Worthington believes a certain kind of anemia can conceivably develop in the infant because of combined folic acid and vitamin C deficiencies.

One hundred milligrams of vitamin C a day is considered sufficient for breast feeding mothers. Get your daily vitamin C by eating citrus fruits and juices, melons, tomatoes, green peppers, and raw cabbage. Three servings a day of food rich in this vitamin should be enough. Vitamin C tablets are unnecessary, and excessive amounts may even be harmful.

Vitamin D

The importance of vitamin D in human nutrition lies in its role in regulating calcium and phosphate metabolism. *Without vitamin D, these two minerals cannot be effectively used by the body.* Therefore, you will need to maintain the same increased level of vitamin D while breast feeding as you did during your pregnancy.

In the early 1900s rickets, a disease often caused by a lack of vitamin D, was common in children of women who switched to artificial infant feeding. Until recently, scientists thought breast milk was deficient in vitamin D, even though rickets, which causes an abnormal bowing of the legs was a rare condition in fully breast-fed babies. Apparently, researchers were looking for vitamin D in the wrong place—the fat portion of the milk. In 1976 British scientists discovered vitamin D in the watery portion of breast milk. It had been present after all.

Each eight-ounce glass of milk is generally fortified with vitamin D and will give you 25 percent of the recommended daily allowance for this vitamin. (Check to make sure the milk you're drinking is vitamin D fortified.) Vitamin D also occurs naturally in such animal foods as eggs, liver, butter, and fatty fish.

Vitamin E

During breast feeding, the increased intake of calories normally adds enough vitamin E, which is secreted in breast milk. And breast-fed infants more rapidly develop higher levels of this vitamin in their bodies than babies fed cow's milk formulas. Your best sources of vitamin E are vegetable oils, margarine, and shortening.

Fluids

Nursing mothers usually feel thirstier than normal and should drink additional fluids. Without enough liquids, your milk supply will fall off. Drink plenty of water, fruit and vegetable juices, and soups. Some experts advise breast-feeding mothers to increase their intake of liquids to about three quarts of fluids a day, including a quart of skim or regular milk. So add extra fluids in-between meals to the high quality diets we've provided for you each day.

As in pregnancy, avoid the empty calories of sodas and fruit drinks that contain sugar; they fill you up but have little else that's nutritionally worthwhile. Coffee and tea are okay occasionally, but they shouldn't be your main source of liquids because they're diuretics.

How do you know if you're drinking enough? Urine is one indicator. If your urine is pale yellow in color and you produce large amounts, you're drinking all you need. However, if your urine is darker and concentrated, increase your fluid intake, no matter how busy you are.

Iron

At birth the normal full-term baby should have its own iron stores. In addition, the iron in breast milk is in a highly absorbable form. Therefore, according to Dr. Myron Winick, "iron deficiency in breast-fed infants is very rare." But providing the iron in breast milk may deplete your own iron stores even further, so you must continue to eat iron-rich foods and take supplements. Feeling blue and tired as a result of an iron deficiency anemia is something you want to avoid, as most newborns are exhausting enough to care for, in the beginning.

Iodine

It's important for you to have ample amounts of iodine when you're breast feeding. In fact, the requirement for it now is double the increase you need during pregnancy. Iodine affects the thyroid gland, which regulates the rate at which your body uses energy—and obviously, the continual production of breast milk requires a great deal of energy. Seafood and iodized salt are the two best sources of this mineral in your diet.

Zinc

The requirement for this trace mineral, like iodine, increases during breast feeding. The Food and Nutrition Board advises a daily intake of twenty-five milligrams per day, which is five milligrams higher than your needs during pregnancy. It's believed you will lose about three milligrams per day of zinc in your breast milk.

Although human milk contains less zinc than cow's milk, what is present is much more easily absorbed by your baby. In fact, according to the La Leche League International, scientists discovered in 1978 that breast milk is the best treatment for a rare, genetic metabolic disease called acrodermatitis enteropathica.

Babies with this unfortunate skin problem suffer from a zinc deficiency due to an inherited reduced ability to absorb zinc. Infants prone to this disease, however, develop it on cow's milk, which has *more* zinc. Yet babies who are switched to breast milk, which has an even *lower* zinc content, are cured! This is another of those amazing examples of the interrelationship between nature and nurture.

Zinc is found in meat, eggs, poultry, seafood, milk and whole grains.

Magnesium

Human milk contains about forty milligrams of magnesium per quart. Although we don't know too much about the requirements for this mineral during breast feeding, the Food and Nutrition Board advises an additional intake of one hundred fifty milligrams per day for nursing mothers, the same allowance as in pregnancy.

If you are eating whole-grain breads and cereals, and salads made of leafy green vegetables, you will have little difficulty obtaining sufficient amounts of magnesium.

Fluoride

This trace mineral, as you may remember, contributes to strong teeth and fewer cavities. Some doctors feel that although breast milk does contain fluoride, it's not present in high enough amounts. However, the newly revised handbook of La Leche League International, *The Womanly Art of Breastfeeding*, advises against the use of fluoride drops for breast-fed babies. "A supplement may be potentially dangerous, since the toxic dose of fluoride is only a little more than double the preventive dose. In any case, there are no data to show that totally breast-fed babies benefit from supplemented fluorides."

There are still contradictions, however, in the medical literature as to nutritional needs during breast feeding and even as to the properties of breast milk itself. As Dr. R. G. Whitehead wisely points out, "Human lactation is such a natural process, it has not really been subjected to the vigorous scientific study it deserves." But in recent years, as great numbers of mothers have insisted on the "natural" way to feed their infants, researchers have begun to intensively study the properties of breast milk. While scientists once were preoccupied with the challenge of making "better formulas" for babies, today many of them are discovering the marvels of human breast milk.

No-No's for the Breast-Feeding Mother

Although an occasional glass of wine or other alcoholic drink will not hurt your baby while you are nursing, any more than that and you will simply not produce sufficient milk for the baby.

In recent years a lot has been learned about drugs in human milk, so here too the word is *caution*. Don't take any drugs without checking with your doctor. You want to avoid unnecessary drugs, as they may change both the composition of the milk and even the milk supply itself. Some drugs that may affect your newborn won't cause any problem with an older, more mature baby. But each situation must be considered individually.

A reprint of the comprehensive report, *Breast-feeding and Drugs in Human Milk*, published in 1980, is available from La Leche League International. And if you have questions regarding the safety of a specific drug during breast feeding, you can address them to the League's Professional Advisory Board through a league leader.

Marijuana and cigarette smoking should be avoided while breast feeding. The use of grass has been found to significantly lower levels of a hormone that insures an adequate milk supply. Besides, your little one deserves clean air to breathe and she will be less likely to develop infections of the nose and throat in a smoke-free atmosphere.

Nursing mothers should *not* take birth control pills. They are known to change both the composition of breast milk and the milk supply itself. No one knows, as yet, how they affect the baby.

Working Mothers and Breast Feeding

Some working mothers can and do breast feed their babies. They use a breast pump to express their breast milk and bottle it to be fed to the baby while they're at work. Other mothers supplement breast milk with formula or adjust their working hours to the baby's schedule. Some women have even been able to move closer to where they work and nurse the baby on their lunch hour. Still others postpone going back to work or find a job they can do at home.

Perhaps Betty Wagner, executive director of La Leche League says it best: "It's not easy to work and breast feed but being a mother isn't easy. It's a challenge."

How Long Should I Breast Feed?

Some women begin to worry about when they're going to discontinue breast feeding even before their infant is born! Some women breast feed their babies for only the first few weeks of life; others, like Princess Diana, breast feed for the first few months; and still other mothers allow their children to discontinue feeding at the breast at the baby's own pace. This is an individual matter for you to decide, as no two families are exactly alike.

WHAT'S AHEAD FOR FUTURE MOTHERS?

It is upon health, not upon ill-health, that our sights should be fixed.

Dr. Roger Williams

What Is Amniocentesis?
The Future of Amniocentesis

Gene Therapy
Fetal Surgery
Treating Fetal Malnutrition

For thousands of years the unborn child lay in the darkened room of the uterus. Its growth and development were a deep mystery until it suddenly emerged at the precise moment of birth. Now, thanks to the twin miracles of modern scientific research—amniocentesis and sonography—the light has gone on within that room. And doctors have a "peephole" to observe the incredible drama taking place before birth. These two tests have made it possible to make predictions about certain potentially damaging genetic traits that could endanger your baby's life and well-being.

As a result of these tests, physicians, in rare instances, have begun to treat the fetus before birth. For example, physicians have been able to diagnose and successfully treat a baby with a hereditary enzyme deficiency by giving vitamin B injections to the mother during pregnancy. And we have every reason to hope scientists will soon discover additional cures for genetic biochemical abnormalities, through nutrition.

What Is Amniocentesis?

This procedure (usually performed after the fourteenth week of pregnancy) involves inserting a long thin needle into the mother-to-be's abdomen in order to withdraw a small amount of amniotic fluid. Since the fluid contains fetal cells, it yields valuable information for genetic analysis.

A sonogram of the uterus is generally done at the same time to ensure the needle doesn't puncture the placenta nor harm the fetus. Sonography avoids the harmful aspects of X ray, by using sonar echoes to provide a picture of the soft tissue structures in your body. From this picture doctors can determine the size of the uterus, how long you have been pregnant, or in the case of amniocentesis, the position of the fetus and the placenta.

In experienced hands, amniocentesis carries a low risk for you and the baby, and the discomfort is minimal. However, the procedure does have a slight possibility of both infection and miscarriage. Therefore, it's generally advised only when the mother is thirty-five and over, if there's a family history of genetic defects, or if the parents already have a child with a birth defect.

Fortunately, according to the March of Dimes Birth Defects Foundation, almost one hundred inborn metabolic errors can be detected before birth by analysis of the enzyme levels in fetal cells. And researchers have recently discovered a remarkable method of detecting two devastating problems, spina bifida (open spine) and anencephaly (absence of the brain) by testing the amniotic fluid for the elevation of certain fetal proteins.

The Future of Amniocentesis

Despite the incredible advances in predicting the development of a defective embryo or fetus that have been made within the past few years, amniocentesis has still not yielded all of nature's secrets. "Defects caused by the interplay of environmental and genetic factors—cardiac and intestinal defects, cleft lip and palate, club foot— are missed," says Dr. Richard Morton, associate medical director of the March of Dimes.

And there are also genetic biochemical disorders, such as phenylketonuria (PKU), that cannot be detected prenatally. At present PKU must be detected *after birth* to prevent mental retardation, for if there is too much phenylalanine, one of the essential amino acids in the child's diet, a susceptible youngster will produce poisonous amounts of a chemical that destroys brain cells.

But, in the near future we can look forward to even greater knowledge through the analysis of fetal cells in the amniotic fluid. In fact, doctors at the New York State Institute for Basic Research and Developmental Disabilities have recently detected the presence of the "Fragile X" chromosome in the amniotic fluid of two pregnant women, known to be carriers. (As you may remember, a baby—*especially a male*—with "Fragile X" chromosome will be mentally retarded.) When the tiny fetus is found to be damaged, the parents can choose whether or not to end the pregnancy.

As obstetrician Dr. Richard Schwarz points out, "Much of what we do now is negative, in the sense we determine situations in which we're going to abort a pregnancy because it's got irrevocable problems. Unfortunately, with our present knowledge, we can't do anything about it, except abort the pregnancy." In the future, however, it may be possible to diagnose and change faulty genetic structure before birth.

Gene Therapy

Genetic diseases are among the most tragic of all human ailments. Often just one seemingly unimportant chemical change in a gene will produce physical deformity, hormone problems, heart failure, blood that doesn't clot properly, mental retardation, pain, or early death.

Yet doctors remain powerless to cure almost all genetic defects. This is due to the incredible complexity of nature's control system. For researchers have to determine, among 438 chemical subunits within a single gene, the precise subunit that is malfunctioning. Nevertheless, scientists have already taken the first steps in trying to cure genetic disorders, by transplanting genes in animal experiments. For example, researchers at Yale University have transplanted a human gene into fertilized mouse egg cells. Amazingly, the gene persisted into the next generation of mice!

Some day future generations of scientists may be able to take out the "bad genes" in the fetus by early diagnosis, replacing them with "good genes." But we have a long way to go before human genetic problems can be treated successfully.

Fetal Surgery

Scientists have only recently begun to develop the means and tools to repair the damaged human fetus before birth, after years of research on animal fetuses. Recent pioneering events in fetal surgery include the following:

• An operation was performed by surgeons at the University of Colorado Health Sciences Center to treat a twenty-four-week old fetus with hydrocephalus (fluid on the brain). A tube was inserted to drain the build-up of the fluid, which was causing dangerous pressure to the fetal brain.

• Surgery was done on a twenty-eight-week-old fetus to relieve a life-threatening urinary obstruction. The pediatric surgeon, Dr. Michael Harrison of the University of California-San Francisco, inserted a tube into the fetal bladder to drain liquid into the amniotic sac of this fetus with a urinary tract malformation.

• Even more remarkably, for the first time a fetus has survived out-of-the womb surgery. An operation to correct a urinary-tract obstruction was performed, and the fetus was then safely returned to its mother's uterus by Drs. Michael Harrison, Mitchell Globus, and Roy Filly. Sadly, the baby died after birth because the condition had already caused too much damage to the kidneys and lungs before the surgical procedure.

These are all tremendous milestones in human development, and future mothers can look forward to the refinement of surgical techniques to repair and treat damaged babies *before birth*.

Treating Fetal Malnutrition

Within the past decade scientists have learned a lot about maternal nutrition. We know that prenatal malnutrition may be caused by reduced maternal blood circulation, inadequate nutrients within the mother's circulation, and faulty transport of certain nutrients from the placenta to the fetus.

Our hope, then, is to be able to predict fetal malnutrition with a high degree of accuracy early in pregnancy and then treat the condition to insure normal fetal development *before birth*. Future scientists will be able to identify embryos and fetuses that are growing poorly due to intrauterine malnutrition, through a battery of chemical tests of the mother's urine, blood, and amniotic fluid. Doctors will subsequently treat the unborn baby with specific therapy for specific problems.

Nevertheless, with our present knowledge of fetal growth, your chances of giving birth to a strong, healthy infant are much greater than they were when your mother was pregnant! Many of the myths surrounding pregnancy have crumbled under the light of scientific scrutiny. And scientific research will continue to try and see that *every baby born is a healthy baby*.

Menus

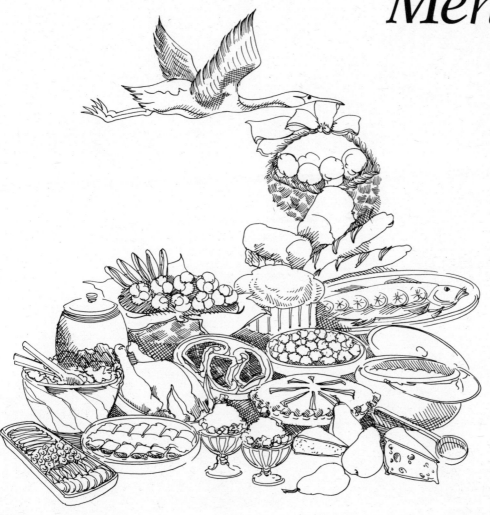

Introduction

The menus that follow are intended to provide you with eleven months of delicious and nutritious eating—not only for the nine months of pregnancy, but also for a "pre-pregnancy" month and a month of breastfeeding. We think that you and your family will enjoy these delicious and easy-to-make recipes, and that you will find yourselves expanding your culinary horizons in healthful and mouth-watering new ways.

The menus have been planned out carefully for you day by day in order to satisfy your nutritional requirements during pregnancy and breastfeeding. However, you should remember they are intended only as suggestions; your own likes and dislikes should be a factor in how you use them. For instance, if a snack of yogurt and fresh fruit doesn't appeal to you on Day 16, you should feel free to substitute another food with the same nutritional value from the Milk Group. Just be sure that you satisfy your daily requirements from the basic food groups (see "Good Nutrition: You Are What You Eat").

So that you can use these menus at any time of the year, we have most often provided you with fruit and vegetable choices that are available year-round. But you may find—particularly in the spring and summer—that seasonal fruits and vegetables (such as peaches, melons, strawberries, plums, cherries, and blueberries, or asparagus, corn, peas, and wax beans) are an appealing and inexpensive alternative to fruits and vegetables listed in the menus. Do take advantage of the many delicious fresh fruits and vegetables available seasonally.

Occasionally, too, you may want to substitute a higher-priced cut of meat for one of our more inexpensive suggestions. If you have an irresistable craving for filet mignon—and your pocketbook can stand it—by all means treat yourself and your family to a steak dinner. The principle remains the same: eat a variety of high-quality, fresh foods from the basic food groups, and you will provide yourself, your family, and your growing baby with a nutritious diet.

The breakfasts, lunches, and snacks have been planned for you, the mother-to-be, only. (The dinner menus, however, are for two or more servings—for you and your family.) Because you will probably be working for at least the first months of your pregnancy, the menus have been designed so that foods for lunch and snacks can be brought to an office from home or purchased from your local coffee shop or delicatessen. If you find that you don't like eating the snacks in the morning and afternoon, you can tack them on to your regular meals or save one of them for an evening snack between dinner and bedtime.

With the nutritional knowledge you have gained in reading the text, you may even find that you enjoy creating your *own* daily menus. Use these menus as an inspiration and guide for your own delicious meals—and enjoy!

Serving Sizes

The recipes provide servings information, but we do not tell you exactly how many nuts you should eat for a snack or how many buttered string beans should be included with your dinner. Again, the menus are not meant to be rigid rules for eating, but instead flexible guidelines. The amount you eat should be determined by appetite, a careful monitoring of your weight, and by making sure you satisfy your daily requirements.

Here's a listing of some common one-serving amounts from the four basic food groups:

Milk and Milk Products
8 oz. milk
1 oz. hard cheese
1 cup yogurt
1 cup creamed
   cottage cheese

Protein Foods
3 oz. meat, poultry,
   fish
½ cup canned tuna
   fish
2 eggs
2 Tbsp. peanut
   butter
1–1⅓ cups nuts,
     sesame seeds,
     sunflower seeds
1½ cups cooked dry
    peas, beans,
    soybeans or
    lentils

Grain Products
1 slice of whole
   wheat bread
½ cup cooked brown
   rice
½ cup cooked pasta
1 pancake
½ cup whole grain
   cereal

Fruits and Vegetables
1 orange, apple,
   pear, peach,
   banana
4 oz. orange juice
½ cup berries
½ cup raisins
¾ cup cooked leafy
   green vegetables
1 cup raw leafy
   green vegetables
½ grapefruit

Salt

The recipes call, in general, for "salt to taste." While it's not good to cut salt out of your diet during pregnancy, it's also not smart to overuse the salt shaker. If you are a *heavy* salt user, you may need to cut down on your use of salt.

Beverages

The menus provide a beverage with every meal and snack, so that you will automatically drink at least five 8-ounce cups of liquid a day. However, as you need seven to eight 8 ounce glasses of liquid each day during pregnancy and breast feeding, you should supplement this beverage intake with additional glasses of water, fruit or vegetable juice, or soup. Mineral water and seltzer can also be refreshing beverage alternatives. (However, seltzer can give you gas and make you feel bloated, so if you get that "too full" feeling, you might want to avoid it.)

Leftovers

It's not a wise idea at any time to let food sit in the refrigerator day after day once you have prepared it, since much of the nutritive value of food is lost through prolonged storage. During pregnancy it's especially important that you eat the freshest foods possible in order to receive their full nutritional benefits. Cooked vegetables in particular quickly lose valuable vitamins and minerals when they are stored. Therefore, we do not advise eating leftover vegetables during pregnancy, nor do we include leftovers of main dishes, desserts, or sandwich spreads in the menus more than a few days after they were first prepared. However it's okay to freeze your own leftovers as long as the food doesn't "sit around" for hours first before freezing. Just be sure that the food is properly defrosted later in your refrigerator.

Variety, Quality, Freshness

These are three key words that you should keep in mind as you use our daily menus or plan your own.

1. Eat a *variety* of foods in order to obtain the maximum nutritional benefit from your diet. For instance, eat a variety of salad greens. Try endive, romaine, escarole, chicory, boston or bibb lettuce as well as the more common iceberg lettuce.

2. Make sure the foods you choose are of the highest possible *quality*. For instance, avoid convenience foods like frozen french fries or cheese spreads, which don't have the same food value as fresh potatoes or real cheese. And be sure to buy only margarine, skim milk or nonfat dry milk that has been fortified with vitamins A and D.

3. Look for *freshness* in the meats, fish, fruits and vegetables you purchase. If you need help, do ask the person at the produce section to show you how to pick ripe sweet fruit. This is especially necessary when choosing plums,

peaches, pears, pineapples, and melons. Cantaloupes, for example, are at their best when they have a slightly sweet aroma and the outside rind responds to the slight pressure of your fingers. A rock-hard unyielding rind indicates the melon isn't ready to be eaten without giving you a possible stomach ache.

Also, be sure to pick the freshest milk or milk products you can find in the dairy case by checking the date on the container.

Here are some more tips on cooking and storing food to help you make sure you are providing the best quality diet for you and your baby:

1. Cook vegetables in a small amount of water in a covered saucepan until just tender. They'll taste better and this method protects their food value.

2. Scrub potatoes before baking and eat the skins. They're delicious, high in vitamins and are served as a delicacy in many expensive restaurants.

3. Don't rinse rice before cooking. You'll wash B vitamins and vitamin C right down the drain.

4. Meats that are broiled, roasted, or fried keep more B vitamins than meat that's stewed or braised. (But if you drink the meat broth in a stew you replace the vitamins lost in the cooking process.)

5. If tomatoes are unripe when you buy them, they'll lose less nutrients if

ripened in your kitchen, *away* from sunlight.

6. Fresh fish must be refrigerated and eaten quickly or frozen.

7. Cooked foods should be chilled immediately. Not only does refrigeration help to maintain the safety of the food, it also helps to protect the nutritive value.

8. The quality of eggs deteriorates rapidly by improper storage at room temperature. Refrigerate them and use up the "older ones" first.

9. If you store fresh fruits and vegetables in the refrigerator for a long time, you'll destroy certain vitamins and minerals. Buy smaller quantities and shop more often.

10. If you can't shop often for fresh fruits and vegetables, buy the frozen ones instead. Freezing is the least damaging method of preserving food. To minimize the vitamin loss of frozen foods, however, your freezer should be kept at 0 degrees F or below. And here too, it's important to use up frozen foods within a month or so.

11. Wash all fruits and vegetables thoroughly but don't let them soak in water, in order to protect their food value.

12. Don't store milk in a clear glass bottle. The B vitamin riboflavin is sensitive to light and may be destroyed.

13. Keeping vegetables warm and reheating them reduces their vitamin C content. This is especially true of frozen foods.

14. Cover food tightly during storage in the refrigerator either in a closed see-through container or sealed well in plastic wrap. Either way the food will stay fresher with less vitamin loss and you can see at a glance what's left.

BON APPETIT!

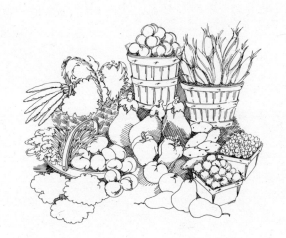

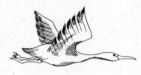 *Pre-pregnancy Month*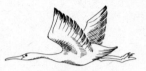

DAY 1

Breakfast
Freshly squeezed orange juice
1 poached egg on buttered whole wheat toast
Milk

Morning Snack
Corn muffin with butter or jelly
Milk

Lunch
3¼ ounces drained canned salmon
Lettuce wedge, tomato wedges, cucumber slices,
and carrot sticks
Apple juice

Afternoon Snack
¼ cup raisins   4 dried apricots
Fruit juice

Dinner
Herbed Veal Chops
Glazed Carrots   Sautéed Mushrooms
Fruit and cheese
Beverage

DAY 2

Breakfast
Freshly squeezed grapefruit juice
¾ cup whole-grain cereal with
sliced banana and milk
Milk

Morning Snack
½ cup plain yogurt with
sliced fresh fruit and wheat germ
Milk

Lunch
Liverwurst sandwich on rye bread
Lettuce and tomato salad with
carrot sticks and celery sticks
Vegetable juice

Afternoon Snack
Cream cheese on 1 slice date-nut bread
Apple juice

Dinner
Broccoli and Bean Soup
Whole wheat bread and butter
Baked Apples   Beverage

DAY 3

Breakfast
1 cup plain yogurt mixed with 1 cup sliced,
unsweetened strawberries
1 slice whole grain bread with butter
Milk

Morning Snack
Peanut butter on whole grain crackers
Apple   Milk

Lunch
Sliced egg, lettuce, and tomato sandwich on
whole grain bread
Cucumber slices   Green pepper strips
Milk

Afternoon Snack
2 slices fresh pineapple or canned pineapple in juice
½ cup cream-style cottage cheese
Fruit juice

Dinner
Cucumber and Tomato Salad
Chicken-Sausage Combo
Cranberry Sauce   Ice cream
Beverage

DAY 4

Breakfast
½ grapefruit   1 scrambled egg
1 slice buttered whole wheat toast   Milk

Morning Snack
Peanut butter on whole grain crackers
Apple slices   Milk

Lunch
Turkey, lettuce, and tomato sandwich on
whole grain bread
Pickle, carrot sticks, and celery stalks
Fruit juice

Afternoon Snack
¼ cup nuts   4 dried apricots   Milk

Dinner
Poached Salmon with mayonnaise
White Bean Salad
Whole wheat rolls and butter
Grapes and pears   Milk

DAY 5

Breakfast
Freshly squeezed grapefruit juice
¾ cup whole grain cereal with sliced banana and milk
Milk

Morning Snack
Cream-style cottage cheese on whole wheat crackers
Grapes   Apple juice

Lunch
2 hard-boiled eggs
Lettuce wedge, tomato wedges, and cucumber slices
Milk

Afternoon Snack
Whole wheat crackers and Cheddar cheese
Apple   Milk

Dinner
Egg Flower Soup
Hunan-style Shredded Lamb   Steamed rice
Fresh pineapple slices
Beverage

DAY 6

Breakfast
½ cantaloupe
½ cup cream-style cottage cheese
1 slice whole grain bread with butter
Milk

Morning Snack
Bran muffin with butter
Milk

Lunch
Sliced chicken, tomato, and lettuce sandwich on
whole wheat bread
Cucumber slices   Green pepper strips
Apple juice

Afternoon Snack
Swiss cheese   Pear   Milk

Dinner
Basil Tomatoes with Oil and Vinegar Dressing
Broccoli Omelet
Whole wheat bread and butter
Apple and Pear Compote
Beverage

DAY 7

Breakfast
Fresh orange segments
1 soft-boiled egg
1 slice whole grain bread with butter
Milk

Morning Snack
Peanut butter and jelly on 1 slice whole grain bread
Milk

Lunch
Tuna Salad, sliced tomato, and lettuce sandwich on
rye bread
Carrot sticks and cucumber slices
Milk

Afternoon Snack
½ cup plain yogurt with raisins
Fruit juice

Dinner
Jambon Normande
Mashed potatoes
Sautéed String Beans   Sliced tomatoes
Apples and cheese   Beverage

DAY 8

Breakfast
½ grapefruit
¾ cup whole grain cereal with milk
Milk

Morning Snack
Cream cheese on 1 slice date-nut bread
Milk

Lunch
Roast beef, tomato, and lettuce sandwich on
rye bread
Carrot sticks and celery stalks
Vegetable juice

Afternoon Snack
Banana
1 slice whole grain bread with butter
Milk

Dinner
Broccoli and Tomato Salad
Salmon Patties
Boiled Potatoes with Sour Cream and Chives
Fresh fruit   Beverage

DAY 9

Breakfast
½ cup cream-style cottage cheese with
Apple and Pear Compote
1 slice whole grain bread with butter
Milk

Morning Snack
1 hard-boiled egg
Tomato wedges
Milk

Lunch
Peanut butter and jelly sandwich on
whole wheat bread
Apple slices
Milk

Afternoon Snack
½ cup plain yogurt sprinkled with wheat germ
Apple juice

Dinner
Tossed salad with Oil and Vinegar Dressing
Skillet Chicken   Crisp rolls and butter
Sautéed Bananas with Honey
Beverage

DAY 10

Breakfast
½ cantaloupe   1 soft-boiled egg
1 slice buttered whole wheat toast
Milk

Morning Snack
Corn muffin with butter or jelly
Milk

Lunch
3¼ ounces drained canned tuna
Lettuce wedge, tomato wedges, cucumber slices, and
carrot sticks
Apple juice

Afternoon Snack
½ cup cream-style cottage cheese with fresh orange
segments and wheat germ
Fruit juice

Dinner
String Beans Vinaigrette   Quiche Lorraine
Whole wheat bread and butter
Fresh fruit   Milk

DAY 11

Breakfast
Freshly squeezed orange juice
¾ cup whole grain cereal with
sliced banana and milk
Milk

Morning Snack
½ cup plain yogurt with ½ cup sliced strawberries
Fruit juice

Lunch
Sliced egg, lettuce, and tomato sandwich on
whole grain bread
Cucumber slices and carrot sticks
Milk

Afternoon Snack
¼ cup raisins   4 dried apricots
Milk

Dinner
Broccoli and Tomato Salad
Roast Beef   Scalloped Potatoes
Stuffed Mushrooms   Ice Cream
Beverage

DAY 12

Breakfast
Orange segments
Tuna Salad sandwich on whole wheat toast
Milk

Morning Snack
Bran muffin with butter
Milk

Lunch
Liverwurst, lettuce, and tomato sandwich on
whole grain bread
Pickle and carrot sticks
Vegetable juice

Afternoon Snack
2 graham crackers with jelly
Fruit juice

Dinner
Cucumber and Tomato Salad
Quiche Lorraine   Steamed Broccoli
Strawberries and cheese
Milk

DAY 13

Breakfast
½ grapefruit
1 scrambled egg on buttered whole wheat toast
Milk

Morning Snack
½ cup plain yogurt with wheat germ
Fruit juice

Lunch
3¼ ounces drained canned salmon
Lettuce wedge, tomato wedges, cucumber slices, and
carrot sticks
Pumpernickel roll with butter
Milk

Afternoon Snack
Whole wheat crackers and Swiss cheese
Grapes
Milk

Dinner
String Beans Vinaigrette
Arroz con Pollo   Crisp rolls and butter
Fresh fruit   Beverage

DAY 14

Breakfast
Vegetable juice
¾ cup whole grain cereal with
sliced banana and milk
Milk

Morning Snack
½ cup cream-style cottage cheese with
fresh orange segments
Milk

Lunch
2 hard-boiled eggs
Coleslaw and carrot sticks
1 slice rye bread and butter   Apple juice

Afternoon Snack
½ cup raw nuts   ¼ cup raisins
Fruit juice

Dinner
Broccoli and Tomato Salad
Shepherd's Pie   Sautéed Mushrooms
Fresh fruit   Beverage

DAY 15

Breakfast
1 cup plain yogurt mixed with
½ cup fresh blueberries
1 slice whole grain bread with butter
Milk

Morning Snack
Cream cheese on 1 slice date-nut bread
Milk

Lunch
Egg Salad with lettuce and tomato in
whole wheat pita
Carrot sticks and cucumber slices
Vegetable juice

Afternoon Snack
¼ cup raisins   4 dried apricots
Milk

Dinner
String Beans Vinaigrette
Pasta with Cauliflower-Veal Sauce
Whole wheat bread and butter
Fresh fruit   Beverage

DAY 16

Breakfast
½ grapefruit
1 poached egg on ½ whole wheat English muffin
Milk

Morning Snack
Homemade Applesauce with raisins
Whole grain crackers   Milk

Lunch
Boiled ham and cream cheese sandwich on
whole wheat bread
Tomato wedges and cucumber slices
Apple juice

Afternoon Snack
Swiss cheese and grapes
Milk

Dinner
Chick-pea Salad
Dorothy Lyons's Savory Mince
Rice Pilaf   Buttered green peas
Fresh fruit   Beverage

DAY 17

Breakfast
Freshly squeezed orange juice
¾ cup whole grain cereal with milk
Milk

Morning Snack
Corn muffin with butter or jelly
Milk

Lunch
Liverwurst, lettuce, and tomato sandwich on
whole grain bread
Apple   Fruit juice

Afternoon Snack
½ cup plain yogurt with
sliced fresh fruit and wheat germ
Pineapple juice

Dinner
Spinach Pie
Cucumber and Tomato Salad
Whole wheat bread and butter
Fresh fruit
Milk

DAY 18

Breakfast
1 cup Apple and Pear Compote with
½ cup cream-style cottage cheese
1 slice buttered whole grain toast
Milk

Morning Snack
Peanut butter on whole grain crackers
Milk

Lunch
Sliced turkey, lettuce, and tomato wedges in
whole wheat pita
Pickle, carrot sticks, and celery stalks
Vegetable juice

Afternoon Snack
Cheddar cheese and pear
Milk

Dinner
Basil Tomatoes with Oil and Vinegar Dressing
Oyster Pilaf   Steamed Broccoli
Fresh fruit   Beverage

DAY 19

Breakfast
Freshly squeezed grapefruit juice
1 fried egg
1 slice buttered whole wheat toast
Milk

Morning Snack
Bran muffin with butter
Milk

Lunch
3¼ ounces drained canned salmon with
lettuce and tomato wedges in whole wheat pita
Carrot sticks and green pepper strips
Vegetable juice

Afternoon Snack
Cream cheese on 1 slice date-nut bread
Milk

Dinner
Marinated Artichokes
Sausages, Peppers, and Potatoes
Whole wheat bread and butter
Fruit and cheese   Beverage

DAY 20

Breakfast
Grilled ham and Swiss cheese sandwich on
rye bread
1 banana   Milk

Morning Snack
½ cup raisins   4 dried apricots
Milk

Lunch
Sliced egg, lettuce, and tomato sandwich on
whole wheat bread
Cucumber slices and carrot sticks
Apple juice

Afternoon Snack
Peanut butter and jelly on whole wheat crackers
Milk

Dinner
Beef Bouillon with Mushrooms and Chives
Spinach Pie   Sliced tomatoes
Whole grain bread and butter
Apple and Pear Compote   Beverage

DAY 21

Breakfast
½ grapefruit
¾ cup whole grain cereal with sliced banana
and milk
Milk

Morning Snack
½ cup cream-style cottage cheese with
½ cup fresh blueberries
Fruit juice

Lunch
Broiled hamburger on enriched-flour roll
Lettuce and tomato salad
Milk

Afternoon Snack
Peanut butter on whole wheat crackers
Grapes
Milk

Dinner
String Beans Vinaigrette
Moorish Chicken   Fresh fruit
Beverage

DAY 22

Breakfast
Orange segments   1 soft-boiled egg
1 slice buttered whole grain bread
Milk

Morning Snack
Swiss cheese and apple slices
Whole grain crackers
Milk

Lunch
Roast beef, tomato, and lettuce sandwich on
whole wheat roll
Milk

Afternoon Snack
½ cup plain yogurt   Grapes
Apple juice

Dinner
Basil Tomatoes with Oil and Vinegar Dressing
Veal Cutlets Florentine
Mashed potatoes   Melon wedge
Beverage

DAY 23

Breakfast
Grilled Swiss cheese sandwich on rye bread
Apple slices   Milk

Morning Snack
½ cup plain yogurt with banana slices and
wheat germ
Fruit juice

Lunch
Tuna Salad with lettuce and tomato wedges in
whole wheat pita
Green pepper strips and carrot sticks
Milk

Afternoon Snack
Cream cheese on 1 slice date-nut bread
Milk

Dinner
Mushroom Salad
Fusilli with Meat Sauce   Bread sticks and butter
Vanilla ice cream with toasted slivered almonds
Beverage

DAY 24

Breakfast
Freshly squeezed orange juice
½ cantaloupe with ½ cup cream-style cottage cheese
1 slice buttered whole grain toast

Morning Snack
1 hard-boiled egg   Tomato wedges
Milk

Lunch
Boiled ham and cream cheese sandwich on
pumpernickel bread
Green pepper strips and carrot sticks
Apple juice

Afternoon Snack
½ cup plain yogurt with sliced fresh fruit and
wheat germ
Milk

Dinner
Hot Salade Niçoise
Whole wheat bread and butter
Fresh pears   Beverage

DAY 25

Breakfast
½ grapefruit
Tuna Salad sandwich on whole wheat toast
Milk

Morning Snack
Bran muffin with butter
Milk

Lunch
Roast beef, lettuce, and tomato sandwich on
rye bread
Pickle, carrot sticks, and cucumber slices
Vegetable juice

Afternoon Snack
Cheddar cheese and apple
Milk

Dinner
Eggplant Salad   Skillet Chicken
Rice Pilaf   Fresh fruit
Beverage

DAY 26

Breakfast
Freshly squeezed orange juice
¾ cup whole grain cereal with milk
Milk

Morning Snack
Corn muffin with butter or jelly
Milk

Lunch
Sliced turkey, lettuce, and tomato sandwich on
whole wheat bread
Cucumber slices and carrot sticks
Apple juice

Afternoon Snack
Peanut butter on whole wheat crackers
Milk

Dinner
Cucumber and Tomato Salad
Sautéed Shrimp
Lima Beans with Blue Cheese
Apple and Pear Compote
Beverage

DAY 27

Breakfast
1 cup plain yogurt and 1 cup sliced, unsweetened
strawberries
1 slice whole grain bread with butter
Milk

Morning Snack
Peanut butter and jelly on whole wheat crackers
Milk

Lunch
3¼ ounces drained canned tuna
¼ cup cream-style cottage cheese
Tomato wedges and cucumber slices
Milk

Afternoon Snack
¼ cup raisins   ¼ cup nuts
Vegetable juice

Dinner
Basil Tomatoes with Oil and Vinegar Dressing
Sautéed Chicken Livers
Rice Pilaf   Sautéed String Beans
Fresh fruit   Beverage

DAY 28

Breakfast
Freshly squeezed orange juice
1 poached egg on buttered whole wheat toast
Milk

Morning Snack
½ cup plain yogurt with raisins
Apple juice

Lunch
Salmon Salad with lettuce and tomato wedges in
whole wheat pita
Cucumber slices and carrot sticks
Milk

Afternoon Snack
Cream cheese on 1 slice date-nut bread
Milk

Dinner
White Bean Salad
Steamed Mussels
Whole wheat rolls and butter
Apple and Pear Compote
Beverage

DAY 29

Breakfast
½ grapefruit
¾ cup whole grain cereal with sliced banana
and milk
Milk

Morning Snack
Bran muffin with butter
Milk

Lunch
1 cup homemade applesauce with
½ cup cream-style cottage cheese
1 slice whole grain bread and butter
Fruit juice

Afternoon Snack
Peanut butter and jelly on 1 slice whole wheat bread
Milk

Dinner
Cream of Mushroom-Barley Soup
Parmesan Hamburger Patty
Tossed salad   Pear and Cheddar cheese
Beverage

DAY 30

Breakfast
Cinnamon-Cheese Toast   Orange segments
Milk

Morning Snack
1 hard-boiled egg
Tomato wedges and cucumber slices
Milk

Lunch
Cream-style cottage cheese, tomato, and lettuce
sandwich on whole wheat bread
Carrot sticks and green pepper strips
Vegetable juice

Afternoon Snack
¼ cantaloupe, cubed, mixed with
½ cup sliced, unsweetened strawberries
Milk

Dinner
Cucumber and Tomato Salad
Baked Tile Fish
Curried Rice   Fresh fruit
Beverage

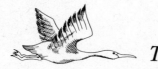 *The First Month*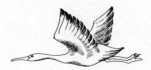

DAY 1

Breakfast
½ grapefruit   1 scrambled egg
1 slice buttered whole wheat bread
Milk

Morning Snack
Cream cheese on 1 slice date-nut bread
Milk

Lunch
Grilled cheeseburger on enriched-flour bun
Lettuce and tomato salad
Apple juice

Afternoon Snack
½ cup plain yogurt with sliced strawberries
Milk

Dinner
Beef Bouillon with Mushrooms and Chives
Chicken Livers Florentine
Rice Pilaf   Sliced tomato
Melon wedges   Beverage

DAY 2

Breakfast
Grilled Swiss cheese sandwich on rye bread
Apple slices
Milk

Morning Snack
Bran muffin with butter
Milk

Lunch
3 slices fresh pineapple or canned pineapple in juice
1 cup cream-style cottage cheese
1 slice whole grain bread with butter
Apple juice

Afternoon Snack
¼ cup raw nuts   ¼ cup raisins
Milk

Dinner
Mushroom Salad
Sautéed Chicken Breasts
Mashed potatoes   Victorian Spinach
Fresh fruit   Beverage

DAY 3

Breakfast
Freshly squeezed orange juice
¾ cup whole grain cereal with
sliced banana and milk
Milk

Morning Snack
Corn muffin with butter or jelly
Milk

Lunch
Liverwurst, lettuce, and tomato sandwich on
whole grain bread
Coleslaw   Apple juice

Afternoon Snack
Cheddar cheese and apple slices
Whole wheat crackers   Milk

Dinner
Basil Tomatoes with Oil and Vinegar Dressing
Asparagus Omelet
Whole wheat bread and butter
Apple and Pear Compote   Beverage

DAY 4

Breakfast
½ cantaloupe
½ cup cream-style cottage cheese
1 slice whole grain bread with butter
Milk

Morning Snack
Peanut butter on whole grain crackers
Pear   Milk

Lunch
Sliced egg, lettuce, and tomato sandwich on
whole grain bread
Cucumber slices and green pepper strips
Vegetable juice

Afternoon Snack
Swiss cheese and apple slices
Milk

Dinner
Lettuce wedges with oil and vinegar dressing
Pork Chops with Chick-peas
Steamed rice   Fresh fruit
Beverage

DAY 5

Breakfast
½ grapefruit   1 poached egg
½ buttered whole wheat English muffin
Milk

Morning Snack
Cream cheese on 1 slice date-nut bread
Milk

Lunch
Sliced turkey, lettuce, and tomato sandwich on
rye bread
Pickle and coleslaw
Fruit juice

Afternoon Snack
Swiss cheese and grapes
Milk

Dinner
White Bean Salad
Sautéed Flounder Fillets
Steamed Broccoli   Ice cream
Beverage

DAY 6

Breakfast
Freshly squeezed orange juice
2 corn muffins with butter and jelly
Milk

Morning Snack
Cream-style cottage cheese on whole wheat crackers
Tangerine
Milk

Lunch
Salmon Salad with lettuce wedge, tomato wedges,
cucumber slices, and carrot sticks
1 slice buttered rye bread
Vegetable juice

Afternoon Snack
Peanut butter on 1 slice pumpernickel bread
Milk

Dinner
Egg Flower Soup
Chicken with Broccoli
Steamed rice   Fresh pineapple slices
Beverage

DAY 7

Breakfast
½ grapefruit   1 soft-boiled egg
1 slice buttered whole wheat toast
Milk

Morning Snack
¼ cup raisins   4 dried apricots
Milk

Lunch
Tuna Salad with lettuce and tomato wedges in
whole wheat pita
Cucumber slices and carrot sticks
Apple juice

Afternoon Snack
Peanut butter and jelly on whole grain crackers
Milk

Dinner
Broccoli and Tomato Salad
Pork Chops with Chick-peas
Steamed rice
Apples and Cheddar cheese
Beverage

DAY 8

Breakfast
¼ cantaloupe
¾ cup whole grain cereal with milk
Milk

Morning Snack
½ cup plain yogurt with ½ cup sliced, unsweetened
strawberries
Fruit juice

Lunch
2 hard-boiled eggs
Tomato wedges, cucumber slices, and celery stalks
1 slice rye bread with butter
Milk

Afternoon Snack
1 corn muffin with butter or jelly
Milk

Dinner
Cucumber and Tomato Salad
Meatloaf   Mashed potatoes
Sautéed Mushrooms   Melon wedges
Beverage

DAY 9

Breakfast
1 cup Apple and Pear Compote mixed with
½ cup cream-style cottage cheese
1 slice buttered whole grain toast
Milk

Morning Snack
1 hard-boiled egg
Tomato wedges and cucumber slices
Milk

Lunch
Meatloaf sandwich on enriched-flour bun
Cucumber slices, carrot sticks, and
green pepper strips
Milk

Afternoon Snack
Swiss cheese and pear
Fruit juice

Dinner
Near-East Chicken Soup
Toasted whole wheat pita and butter
Fresh fruit   Beverage

DAY 10

Breakfast
1 fried egg   1 slice grilled ham
1 slice buttered rye toast
Apple wedges
Milk

Morning Snack
½ cup plain yogurt sprinkled with wheat germ
Apple juice

Lunch
3¼ ounces drained canned salmon
Lettuce wedge, tomato wedges, cucumber slices, and
carrot sticks
Milk

Afternoon Snack
Peanut butter and jelly on whole wheat crackers
Milk

Dinner
White Bean Salad
Sautéed Chicken Livers
Stewed Zucchini   Fruit and cheese
Beverage

DAY 11

Breakfast
½ grapefruit
¾ cup whole grain cereal with
sliced banana and milk
Milk

Morning Snack
½ cup cream-style cottage cheese with
½ cup unsweetened blueberries
Apple juice

Lunch
Sliced turkey and coleslaw sandwich on
whole wheat toast
Sliced cucumbers and tomato wedges
Milk

Afternoon snack
Cream cheese on 1 slice date-nut bread
Milk

Dinner
String Beans Vinaigrette
Roast Beef   Scalloped Potatoes
Glazed Carrots   Melon wedges
Beverage

DAY 12

Breakfast
Freshly squeezed orange juice
1 poached egg
½ toasted whole wheat English muffin with butter
Milk

Morning Snack
¼ cup raisins   4 dried apricots
Milk

Lunch
Roast Beef sandwich on whole wheat bread
Lettuce and tomato salad   Vegetable juice

Afternoon Snack
2 slices fresh pineapple or canned pineapple in juice
½ cup cream-style cottage cheese
Milk

Dinner
Eggplant Salad   Sautéed Veal Chops
Tomato-Rice Pilaf
Sautéed Mushrooms   Fresh fruit
Beverage

DAY 13

Breakfast
Grilled Swiss cheese on rye bread
½ cup sliced peaches
Milk

Morning Snack
1 hard-boiled egg
Tomato wedges
Milk

Lunch
Sliced ham, tomato, and lettuce sandwich on
hard roll
Coleslaw, celery stalks, and green pepper strips
Vegetable juice

Afternoon Snack
Corn muffin with butter or jelly
Milk

Dinner
Cucumber and Tomato Salad
Roast Chicken with Curry Stuffing
Sautéed String Beans
Ice cream   Beverage

DAY 14

Breakfast
Orange segments
Tuna Salad sandwich on whole wheat toast
Milk

Morning Snack
Peanut butter and jelly on whole wheat crackers
Milk

Lunch
Roast beef, lettuce, and tomato sandwich on
whole wheat bread
Carrot sticks
Milk

Afternoon Snack
½ cup cream-style cottage cheese with
½ cup cubed cantaloupe
Fruit juice

Dinner
Broccoli and Tomato Salad
Spaghetti with White Clam Sauce
Whole wheat rolls and butter
Fruit and cheese   Beverage

DAY 15

Breakfast
Freshly squeezed orange juice
1 cup plain yogurt mixed with 1 cup sliced,
unsweetened strawberries
1 slice whole grain bread with butter

Morning Snack
¼ cup raisins   4 dried apricots
Milk

Lunch
Sliced turkey and coleslaw sandwich on rye bread
Carrot sticks and tomato wedges
Milk

Afternoon Snack
Cream cheese on 1 slice date-nut bread
Milk

Dinner
Lamb Kebabs   Rice Pilaf
Apple and Pear Compote
Beverage

DAY 16

Breakfast
½ grapefruit
¾ cup whole grain cereal with milk
Milk

Morning Snack
Bran muffin with butter
Milk

Lunch
Boiled ham and cream cheese sandwich on
whole wheat toast
Lettuce and tomato salad
Milk

Afternoon Snack
½ cup plain yogurt mixed with ½ cup fresh,
unsweetened fruit
Fruit juice

Dinner
Marinated Artichokes
Poached Eggs with Stewed Zucchini
Whole wheat rolls and butter
Fresh fruit   Beverage

DAY 17

Breakfast
Orange segments   1 scrambled egg
1 slice buttered whole grain toast
Milk

Morning Snack
Peanut butter and jelly on 1 slice whole wheat bread
Milk

Lunch
Salmon Salad with lettuce and tomato wedges in
whole wheat pita
Cucumber slices and carrot sticks
Milk

Afternoon Snack
½ cup homemade Applesauce with
½ cup cream-style cottage cheese
Fruit juice

Dinner
Spiced Lamb Chops   Mashed potatoes
Steamed Broccoli   Fruit and cheese
Beverage

DAY 18

Breakfast
Apple juice
French toast
Milk

Morning Snack
1 hard-boiled egg
Tomato wedges and cucumber slices
Fruit juice

Lunch
Broiled cheeseburger in whole wheat pita
Lettuce and tomato salad
Milk

Afternoon Snack
Peanut butter and jelly on whole wheat crackers
Milk

Dinner
Roast Chicken with Curry Sauce
Rice Pilaf   Steamed Cabbage
Fresh fruit   Beverage

DAY 19

Breakfast
Grilled ham and Swiss cheese sandwich on
rye bread
Banana   Milk

Morning Snack
Corn muffin with butter or jelly
Milk

Lunch
Liverwurst, lettuce, and tomato sandwich on
pumpernickel bread
Coleslaw and carrot sticks
Milk

Afternoon Snack
½ cup cream-style cream cheese with
orange segments
Fruit juice

Dinner
Mushroom Salad
Baked Fish with Eggplant
Whole wheat bread and butter
Fruit and cheese   Apple juice

DAY 20

Breakfast
½ grapefruit
¾ cup whole grain cereal with milk
Milk

Morning Snack
Cheddar cheese   Apple   Milk

Lunch
3¼ ounces drained canned tuna
Lettuce wedge, tomato wedges, cucumber slices and
carrot sticks
Hard roll
Vegetable juice

Afternoon Snack
¼ cup raisins   4 dried apricots
Milk

Dinner
Egg Flower Soup
Shredded Pork with Scallions
Steamed rice   Orange sherbet
Beverage

DAY 21

Breakfast
½ cantaloupe
½ cup cream-style cottage cheese
1 slice whole grain bread with butter
Milk

Morning Snack
Bran muffin with butter
Milk

Lunch
Egg Salad with lettuce and tomato wedges in
whole wheat pita
Carrot sticks, celery stalks, and green pepper strips
Milk

Afternoon Snack
Swiss cheese and tangerine
Apple juice

Dinner
White Bean Salad   Stuffed Eggplant
Whole wheat bread and butter
Apple and Pear Compote
Beverage

DAY 22

Breakfast
1 fried egg
2 slices whole wheat toast
Apple   Milk

Morning Snack
¼ cup raisins   4 dried apricots
Milk

Lunch
Cream-style cottage cheese and tomato sandwich on
whole grain toast
Lettuce wedge, carrot sticks, and green pepper
strips
Milk

Afternoon Snack
Orange and grapes
Pineapple juice

Dinner
Marinated Steak
Sautéed Peppers and Potatoes
Pears and cheese   Apple juice

DAY 23

Breakfast
¼ cantaloupe   1 soft-boiled egg
½ toasted whole wheat English muffin with butter
Milk

Morning Snack
½ cup plain yogurt with raisins and nuts
Fruit juice

Lunch
Sliced chicken, lettuce, and tomato sandwich on
pumpernickel bread
Carrot sticks, cucumber slices, and green pepper
strips
Milk

Afternoon Snack
Banana
1 slice whole grain bread with butter
Milk

Dinner
Chick-pea Salad   Spedini
Rice Milanese   Fresh fruit
Beverage

DAY 24

Breakfast
½ grapefruit
Grilled Swiss cheese sandwich on
whole wheat bread
Milk

Morning Snack
1 hard-boiled egg
Tomato wedges and cucumber slices
Milk

Lunch
1 cup homemade Applesauce with
½ cup cream-style cottage cheese
2 slices whole grain bread and butter
Fruit juice

Afternoon Snack
¼ cup raisins   ¼ cup nuts   Milk

Dinner
Tossed salad   Spaghetti with Meat Sauce
Bread sticks and butter
Fruit and cheese   Beverage

DAY 25

Breakfast
Freshly squeezed orange juice
¾ cup whole grain cereal with
sliced banana and milk
Milk

Morning Snack
Peanut butter and jelly on whole wheat crackers
Milk

Lunch
Liverwurst, lettuce, and tomato sandwich on
pumpernickel bread
Apple juice

Afternoon Snack
Swiss cheese and whole grain crackers
Milk

Dinner
Beef Bouillon with Mushrooms and Chives
Roladen   Buttered noodles
Fresh fruit   Beverage

DAY 26

Breakfast
½ grapefruit
Salmon Salad sandwich on whole wheat toast
Milk

Morning Snack
½ cup plain yogurt with raisins
Fruit juice

Lunch
Roast beef and coleslaw sandwich on
pumpernickel bread
Tomato wedges, cucumber slices, and carrot sticks
Milk

Afternoon Snack
Peanut butter and jelly on whole wheat crackers
Milk

Dinner
String Beans Vinaigrette
Pasta with Stewed Zucchini
Sautéed Veal Chops
Whole wheat bread sticks and butter
Fruit and cheese   Beverage

DAY 27

Breakfast
Freshly squeezed orange juice
2 corn muffins with butter and jelly
Milk

Morning Snack
1 hard-boiled egg
Tomato wedges and cucumber slices
Milk

Lunch
3 slices fresh pineapple or canned pineapple in juice
1 cup cream-style cottage cheese
1 slice whole grain bread with butter
Apple juice

Afternoon Snack
¼ cup raisins   ¼ cup nuts
Milk

Dinner
Lemon-basted Roast Chicken
Rice Pilaf   Sautéed Mushrooms
Fruit and cheese   Beverage

DAY 28

Breakfast
¼ cantaloupe
¾ cup whole grain cereal with milk
Milk

Morning Snack
Cream cheese on 1 slice date-nut bread
Milk

Lunch
Sliced turkey and coleslaw sandwich on rye bread
Tomato wedges, cucumber slices, and carrot sticks
Vegetable juice

Afternoon Snack
Cheddar cheese and apple slices
Whole grain crackers
Milk

Dinner
White Bean Salad   Sautéed Bluefish
Mashed potatoes
Asparagus with Butter and Cheese
Apple and Pear Compote
Beverage

DAY 29

Breakfast
½ cup homemade Applesauce with
½ cup cream-style cottage cheese
Bran muffin with butter   Milk

Morning Snack
Peanut butter on whole wheat crackers
Milk

Lunch
3¼ ounces drained canned salmon
Lettuce wedge, tomato wedges, cucumber slices, and
carrot sticks
Whole wheat roll   Milk

Afternoon Snack
½ cup plain yogurt with sliced fresh fruit and
wheat germ
Fruit juice

Dinner
Broccoli and Tomato Salad
Spinach Omelet
Whole wheat bread and butter
Grapes and Cheddar cheese
Apple juice

DAY 30

Breakfast
Orange segments   1 scrambled egg
1 slice toasted whole grain bread with butter
Milk

Morning Snack
Corn muffin with butter or jelly   Milk

Lunch
Cream-style cottage cheese and tomato sandwich on
whole grain toast
Lettuce wedge, carrot sticks, and
green pepper strips
Fruit juice

Afternoon Snack
Banana
Whole wheat crackers   Milk

Dinner
Lemon-basted Roast Chicken
Steamed Broccoli   Sautéed Mushrooms
French bread and butter   Ice cream
Apple juice

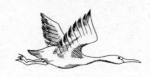 *The Second Month*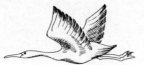

DAY 1

Breakfast
½ grapefruit
¾ cup whole grain cereal with milk
Milk

Morning Snack
½ cup plain yogurt with raisins and nuts
Fruit juice

Lunch
Roast beef, lettuce, and tomato sandwich on rye
bread
Coleslaw
Milk

Afternoon Snack
Cheddar cheese and grapes
Milk

Dinner
Sautéed Scallops   Tomato-Rice Pilaf
Steamed Broccoli with lemon wedges
Apple and Pear Compote
Beverage

DAY 2

Breakfast
½ cantaloupe
½ cup cream-style cottage cheese
1 slice whole wheat bread with butter
Milk

Morning Snack
1 hard-boiled egg
Tomato wedges and cucumber slices
Milk

Lunch
3¼ ounces drained canned salmon
Lettuce wedge, tomato wedges, cucumber slices, and
carrot sticks
Fruit juice

Afternoon Snack
Peanut butter on whole wheat crackers
Apple   Milk

Dinner
Pickled Salad   Chicken Parmigiana
Sautéed String Beans
Whole wheat bread and butter
Ice cream   Beverage

DAY 3

Breakfast
Freshly squeezed grapefruit juice
¾ cup whole grain cereal with milk
Milk

Morning Snack
½ cup plain yogurt and sliced fresh fruit sprinkled
with wheat germ
Fruit juice

Lunch
Boiled ham, Swiss cheese, and lettuce sandwich on
rye bread
Tomato wedges, cucumber slices, and carrot sticks
Apple juice

Afternoon Snack
¼ cup nuts   4 dried apricots
Milk

Dinner
Sliced tomato with lemon juice
Sautéed Veal Cutlets
Mashed potatoes   Sautéed Mushrooms
Fruit and cheese
Beverage

DAY 4

Breakfast
Freshly squeezed orange juice
Salmon Salad sandwich on whole wheat toast
Milk

Morning Snack
Cream-style cottage cheese on whole grain crackers
Banana   Cranberry juice

Lunch
Sliced turkey and coleslaw sandwich on rye bread
Tomato wedges, green pepper strips, and carrot
sticks
Milk

Afternoon Snack
Corn muffin with butter or jelly
Milk

Dinner
Tossed salad with Oil and Vinegar Dressing
Beef Liver and Onions
Whole wheat roll and butter
Fruit and cheese   Beverage

DAY 5

Breakfast
Orange wedges
1 poached egg on ½ buttered, toasted whole wheat
English muffin
Milk

Morning Snack
Bran muffin with butter
Milk

Lunch
Tuna Salad with lettuce and tomato wedges in
whole wheat pita
Cucumber slices and carrot sticks
Milk

Afternoon Snack
½ cup plain yogurt with banana slices
Fruit juice

Dinner
Beef Bouillon with Mushrooms and Chives
Home-style Beef   Steamed rice
Mandarin orange segments
Beverage

DAY 6

Breakfast
Freshly squeezed grapefruit juice
Cream cheese on 1 slice whole grain bread
Milk

Morning Snack
1 hard-boiled egg
Tomato wedges and cucumber slices
Milk

Lunch
Boiled ham, Swiss cheese, lettuce, and tomato
sandwich on whole wheat bread
Apple   Fruit juice

Afternoon Snack
¼ cup raisins   ¼ cup nuts
Milk

Dinner
Marinated Artichokes
Linguini with Red Clam Sauce
Bread sticks and butter
Pears and cheese
Beverage

DAY 7

Breakfast
½ grapefruit
¾ cup whole grain cereal with milk
Milk

Morning Snack
Cream cheese on 1 slice date-nut bread
Milk

Lunch
Salmon Salad, lettuce, and tomato sandwich on
pumpernickel bread
Carrot sticks and pickle
Milk

Afternoon Snack
½ cup plain yogurt with tangerine sections
Fruit juice

Dinner
Tossed salad
Lamb with Stewed Zucchini
Toasted pound cake with ice cream
Beverage

DAY 8

Breakfast
Grilled cheese sandwich on whole wheat bread
Apple slices
Milk

Morning Snack
1 hard-boiled egg
Tomato wedges and cucumber slices
Milk

Lunch
Roast beef, lettuce, and tomato sandwich on rye
bread
Coleslaw and pickle
Fruit juice

Afternoon Snack
Peanut butter on whole wheat crackers
Apple
Milk

Dinner
Chick-pea Salad
Sautéed Flounder Fillets
Steamed Broccoli   Melon wedges
Beverage

DAY 9

Breakfast
1 cup plain yogurt mixed with 1 cup sliced,
unsweetened fruit
1 slice whole grain bread with butter
Milk

Morning Snack
Bran muffin with butter
Milk

Lunch
3¼ ounces drained canned tuna
Coleslaw, tomato wedges, and cucumber slices
Fruit juice

Afternoon Snack
Cheddar cheese and apple slices
Whole wheat crackers   Milk

Dinner
Roast Turkey Breast with Pan Gravy
Scalloped Potatoes   Stuffed Mushrooms
Cranberry Sauce
Ice cream with sliced strawberries
Beverage

DAY 10

Breakfast
½ grapefruit
2 corn muffins with butter and jelly
Milk

Morning Snack
¼ cup raisins   4 dried apricots
Milk

Lunch
Sliced turkey, lettuce, and tomato sandwich on
rye bread
Coleslaw   Milk

Afternoon Snack
½ cup cream-style cottage cheese with
½ cup homemade Applesauce
Fruit juice

Dinner
String Beans Vinaigrette
Spinach Omelet
Whole wheat bread and butter
Tangerines and Cheddar cheese
Beverage

DAY 11

Breakfast
Freshly squeezed orange juice
1 scrambled egg
1 slice whole grain toast with butter
Milk

Morning Snack
Cream cheese on 1 slice date-nut bread
Milk

Lunch
Roast beef sandwich on whole wheat bread
Lettuce and tomato salad
Carrot sticks   Apple juice

Afternoon Snack
Whole wheat crackers with butter and jelly
Milk

Dinner
Tomato slices
Marinated Haddock   Steamed Broccoli
Whole wheat bread and butter
Ice cream   Beverage

DAY 12

Breakfast
¾ cup whole grain cereal with
sliced fresh fruit and milk
Milk

Morning Snack
Peanut butter and jelly on 1 slice whole grain bread
Milk

Lunch
3¼ ounces drained canned tuna
Lettuce wedge, coleslaw, tomato wedges, and
carrot sticks
Bran roll and butter   Milk

Afternoon Snack
½ cup cream-style cottage cheese with
fresh orange segments
Fruit juice

Dinner
Lettuce wedges with oil and vinegar dressing
Cornish Hens Derby
Cranberry Sauce
Baked Apples   Beverage

DAY 13

Breakfast
Cream-style cottage cheese sandwich on
whole wheat bread
Banana   Milk

Morning Snack
1 hard-boiled egg
Tomato wedges and cucumber slices
Milk

Lunch
Liverwurst, lettuce, and tomato sandwich on
pumpernickel bread
Carrot sticks and green pepper strips
Apple juice

Afternoon Snack
¼ cup nuts   4 dried apricots
Milk

Dinner
Tossed salad
Linguini with Red Clam Sauce
Bread sticks and butter
Fruit and cheese   Beverage

DAY 14

Breakfast
Freshly squeezed orange juice
Egg Salad sandwich on whole wheat toast
Milk

Morning Snack
Bran muffin with butter
Milk

Lunch
3 slices fresh pineapple or canned pineapple in juice
1 cup cream-style cottage cheese
1 slice whole grain bread with butter
Apple juice

Afternoon Snack
Cheddar cheese and apple slices
Milk

Dinner
Jambon Normande
Baked sweet potato
Sautéed String Beans
Pound cake   Beverage

DAY 15

Breakfast
½ grapefruit
1 soft-boiled egg
1 slice toasted whole wheat bread with butter
Milk

Morning Snack
¼ cup raisins   ¼ cup nuts
Milk

Lunch
Roast beef and coleslaw sandwich on
whole grain bread
Tomato wedges and cucumber slices
Milk

Afternoon Snack
½ cup cream-style cottage cheese sprinkled with
wheat germ
Banana   Fruit juice

Dinner
Pickled Salad
Eggplant Parmigiana with Marinara Sauce
Bread sticks and butter
Fresh fruit   Beverage

DAY 16

Breakfast
Freshly squeezed grapefruit juice
¾ cup whole grain cereal with milk
Milk

Morning Snack
Cheddar cheese on whole wheat crackers
Tangerine   Milk

Lunch
Egg Salad with lettuce and tomato wedges in
whole wheat pita
Carrot sticks and green pepper strips
Apple juice

Afternoon Snack
Cream cheese on 1 slice date-nut bread
Milk

Dinner
Sliced tomatoes with lemon wedges
Sautéed Chicken Livers
Sautéed Peppers and Potatoes
Melon wedges   Beverage

DAY 17

Breakfast
Grilled Swiss cheese sandwich on rye bread
Apple slices
Milk

Morning Snack
1 hard-boiled egg
Tomato wedges and cucumber slices
Milk

Lunch
Hamburger, lettuce, and tomato on enriched-flour
bun
Coleslaw and pickle
Apple juice

Afternoon Snack
½ cup plain yogurt with raisins
Milk

Dinner
Egg Flower Soup
Honey-basted Chicken Breasts
Sautéed String Beans
Apple and Pear Compote
Beverage

DAY 18

Breakfast
Freshly squeezed grapefruit juice
2 corn muffins with butter and jelly
Milk

Morning Snack
½ cup cream-style cottage cheese with
½ cup Apple and Pear Compote
Milk

Lunch
Sardines, lettuce, and tomato sandwich on rye bread
Carrot sticks and pickle
Fruit juice

Afternoon Snack
Peanut butter on whole wheat crackers
Banana
Milk

Dinner
Lettuce wedges with oil and vinegar dressing
Turkey Fricassee with Biscuit Topping
Pears and Cheese   Beverage

DAY 19

Breakfast
Orange wedges
1 fried egg   1 slice buttered rye toast
Milk

Morning Snack
½ cup plain yogurt with raisins and nuts
Milk

Lunch
Roast beef, lettuce, and tomato sandwich on
whole wheat bread
Carrot sticks, cucumber slices, and green pepper
strips
Apple juice

Afternoon Snack
Cheddar cheese and banana
Milk

Dinner
String Beans Vinaigrette
Eggplant Parmigiana with Marinara Sauce
Whole wheat rolls and butter
Melon wedges   Beverage

DAY 20

Breakfast
½ grapefruit   1 poached egg
1 slice toasted whole wheat bread with butter
Milk

Morning Snack
Peanut butter and jelly on whole grain crackers
Milk

Lunch
Cream-style cottage cheese and tomato sandwich on
whole wheat toast
Lettuce wedge, carrot sticks, and green pepper
strips
Milk

Afternoon Snack
¼ cup raisins   ¼ cup nuts
Apple juice

Dinner
Basil Tomatoes with Oil and Vinegar Dressing
Sautéed Oysters
Victorian Spinach   Glazed Carrots
Ice cream   Beverage

DAY 21

Breakfast
Freshly squeezed orange juice
¾ cup whole grain cereal with milk
Milk

Morning Snack
Banana
1 slice whole grain bread with butter
Milk

Lunch
3¼ ounces drained canned tuna
Coleslaw and carrot sticks
Whole wheat bread and butter
Apple juice

Afternoon Snack
Corn muffin with butter and jelly
Milk

Dinner
Lettuce Wedges with Oil and Vinegar Dressing
Lamb Chops with Brown Rice
Grapes   Beverage

DAY 22

Breakfast
½ cantaloupe
½ cup cream-style cottage cheese
1 slice whole grain bread with butter
Milk

Morning Snack
1 hard-boiled egg
Tomato wedges and cucumber slices
Milk

Lunch
Liverwurst, lettuce, and tomato sandwich on
whole wheat bread
Apple   Milk

Afternoon Snack
½ cup plain yogurt with raisins
Mineral water

Dinner
Egyptian Pea Soup
Sautéed Chicken Breasts
Stewed Cabbage
Whole wheat rolls and butter
Melon wedges   Beverage

DAY 23

Breakfast
Freshly squeezed grapefruit juice
1 scrambled egg
1 slice buttered whole wheat toast
Milk

Morning Snack
½ cup plain yogurt with grapes
Fruit juice

Lunch
Sliced turkey and coleslaw sandwich on
pumpernickel bread
Tomato wedges, cucumber slices, and pickle
Milk

Afternoon Snack
¼ cup raisins   4 dried apricots
Milk

Dinner
Linguini with Marinara Sauce
Sautéed Veal Cutlets   Marinated Artichokes
Whole wheat rolls and butter
Fruit and cheese   Beverage

DAY 24

Breakfast
1 cup plain yogurt mixed with 1 cup sliced,
unsweetened strawberries
1 slice whole grain bread with butter
Milk

Morning Snack
Peanut butter on whole wheat crackers
Milk

Lunch
Roast beef, lettuce, and tomato sandwich on
rye bread
Coleslaw and pickle   Fruit juice

Afternoon Snack
Cheddar cheese and apple slices
Milk

Dinner
Mushroom Salad
Haddock with Capers
Boiled Potatoes with Oil and Parsley
Steamed Spinach
Melon wedges   Beverage

DAY 25

Breakfast
¾ cup whole grain cereal with
sliced banana and milk
Milk

Morning Snack
Bran muffin with butter
Milk

Lunch
Egg Salad with lettuce and tomato wedges in
whole wheat pita
Carrot sticks and green pepper strips
Mineral water

Afternoon Snack
Swiss cheese and pear
Milk

Dinner
Broccoli and Tomato Salad
Beef Stew
Whole grain bread and butter
Fresh pineapple slices   Beverage

DAY 26

Breakfast
Freshly squeezed orange juice
1 scrambled egg
1 slice toasted whole grain bread with butter
Milk

Morning Snack
Cream-style cottage cheese on whole wheat crackers
Apple
Fruit juice

Lunch
Cheeseburger with lettuce and tomato wedges in
whole wheat pita
Coleslaw and pickle
Milk

Afternoon Snack
¼ cup raisins   4 dried apricots
Milk

Dinner
Spicy Chicken and Eggplant
Steamed rice
Fresh orange segments
Beverage

DAY 27

Breakfast
½ cup Apple and Pear Compote mixed with
½ cup cream-style cottage cheese
1 slice whole grain bread with butter
Milk

Morning Snack
Corn muffin with butter or jelly   Milk

Lunch
Tuna Salad, tomato, and lettuce sandwich on
whole wheat bread
Carrot sticks, cucumber slices, and green pepper
strips
Fruit juice

Afternoon Snack
Orange
Whole wheat crackers with butter
Mineral water

Dinner
String Beans Vinaigrette
Lamb Chops with Brown Rice
Bran rolls and butter
Fruit and cheese   Beverage

DAY 28

Breakfast
1 cup plain yogurt mixed with 1 cup sliced,
unsweetened strawberries
1 slice whole grain bread with butter
Milk

Morning Snack
1 hard-boiled egg
Tomato wedges and cucumber slices
Milk

Lunch
Sliced chicken, lettuce, and tomato sandwich on
rye bread
Coleslaw and pickle   Apple juice

Afternoon Snack
¼ cup raisins
Banana   Milk

Dinner
Broccoli and Tomato Salad   Salmon Patties
Boiled Potatoes with Sour Cream and Chives
Fresh fruit   Beverage

DAY 29

Breakfast
Freshly squeezed grapefruit juice
¾ cup whole grain cereal with milk
Milk

Morning Snack
1 bagel with cream cheese
Milk

Lunch
Liverwurst, lettuce, and tomato sandwich on
whole wheat bread
Carrot sticks and pickle
Vegetable juice

Afternoon Snack
Cheddar cheese and apple slices
Whole wheat crackers
Milk

Dinner
Basil Tomatoes with Oil and Vinegar Dressing
Turkey with Mornay Sauce
Buttered noodles
Fresh pineapple slices
Beverage

DAY 30

Breakfast
Freshly squeezed orange juice
1 poached egg on ½ toasted whole wheat English
muffin
Milk

Morning Snack
Bran muffin with butter
Milk

Lunch
Salmon Patty on whole wheat roll
Lettuce and tomato salad
Vegetable juice

Afternoon Snack
Peanut butter and jelly on whole wheat crackers
Milk

Dinner
Lettuce Wedges with Oil and Vinegar Dressing
Beef Stew
Whole wheat bread and butter
Melon wedges   Milk

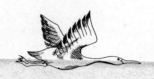 *The Third Month*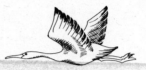

DAY 1

Breakfast
½ cantaloupe
½ cup cream-style cottage cheese
1 slice whole grain toast with butter
Milk

Morning Snack
1 hard-boiled egg
Tomato wedges and cucumber slices
Milk

Lunch
Roast beef, lettuce, and tomato sandwich on
rye bread
Carrot sticks and green pepper strips
Fruit juice

Afternoon Snack
½ cup plain yogurt with ½ cup sliced fresh fruit
sprinkled with wheat germ
Fruit juice

Dinner
Sautéed Shrimp   Victorian Spinach
Sliced tomatoes
Bran rolls and butter   Fresh fruit
Beverage

DAY 2

Breakfast
¾ cup whole grain cereal with sliced banana
and milk
Milk

Morning Snack
Bran muffin with butter or jelly
Milk

Lunch
Egg Salad, lettuce, and tomato sandwich on
whole wheat bread
Apple   Fruit juice

Afternoon Snack
Peanut butter and jelly on whole grain crackers
Milk

Dinner
Beef Liver and Onions
Mashed potatoes   Glazed Carrots
Whole grain bread and butter
Pears and cheese
Beverage

DAY 3

Breakfast
Freshly squeezed grapefruit juice
Egg Salad sandwich on whole wheat toast
Milk

Morning Snack
Corn muffin with butter or jelly
Milk

Lunch
3¼ ounces drained canned tuna
Egyptian Potato Salad
Lettuce wedge and tomato slices
Mineral water

Afternoon Snack
Apple and Cheddar cheese
Milk

Dinner
Pickled Salad
Fusilli with Sauce Bolognese
Whole grain bread with butter
Ice cream   Beverage

DAY 4

Breakfast
1 cup plain yogurt mixed with ½ cup sliced,
unsweetened strawberries, sprinkled
with wheat germ
1 slice whole grain bread with butter
Milk

Morning Snack
½ cup nuts
¼ cup dried fruit
Fruit juice

Lunch
Sliced turkey, lettuce, and tomato sandwich on
pumpernickel bread
Carrot sticks and cucumber slices
Milk

Afternoon Snack
Corn muffin with butter or jelly
Milk

Dinner
Beef Bouillon with Mushrooms and Chives
Baked Veal Chops   Bran rolls and butter
Fresh fruit and cheese   Beverage

DAY 5

Breakfast
Freshly squeezed orange juice
¾ cup whole grain cereal with milk
Milk

Morning Snack
Peanut butter on whole wheat crackers
Grapes   Fruit juice

Lunch
Cream-style cottage cheese and tomato sandwich on
whole wheat toast
Carrot sticks and cucumber slices
Milk

Afternoon Snack
Bran muffin with butter
Milk

Dinner
Eggplant-Gumbo Soup
Broccoli Omelet   Sliced tomatoes
Whole grain bread and butter
Apple-Fig Cream   Beverage

DAY 6

Breakfast
½ grapefruit
1 scrambled egg
1 slice toasted whole grain bread with butter
and jam
Milk

Morning Snack
Cream cheese on 1 slice date-nut bread
Milk

Lunch
Grilled hamburger in whole wheat pita
Lettuce and tomato salad
Carrot sticks   Fruit juice

Afternoon Snack
Orange wedges
Whole wheat crackers   Mineral water

Dinner
Sautéed Chicken Breasts
Egyptian Potato Salad
Sliced tomato   Bran rolls and butter
Apples and Cheddar cheese   Beverage

DAY 7

Breakfast
Freshly squeezed grapefruit juice
Grilled Swiss cheese sandwich on
enriched-flour bread
Milk

Morning Snack
Corn muffin with butter or jelly
Milk

Lunch
3¼ ounces drained canned tuna
¼ cup cream-style cottage cheese
Lettuce wedge, tomato wedges, and cucumber slices
1 piece rye bread and butter   Milk

Afternoon Snack
½ cup plain yogurt with raisins
Fruit juice

Dinner
Lettuce Wedges with Oil and Vinegar Dressing
Spaghetti with Sauce Bolognese
Whole wheat rolls and butter
Sherbet   Beverage

DAY 8

Breakfast
¼ cantaloupe   1 fried egg
1 slice enriched-flour bread with butter and jam
Milk

Morning Snack
½ cup Apple and Pear Compote
Whole wheat crackers with butter
Milk

Lunch
Boiled ham and cream cheese sandwich on
pumpernickel bread
Coleslaw and tomato wedges   Milk

Afternoon Snack
Banana and Cheddar cheese
Fruit juice

Dinner
Basil Tomatoes with Oil and Vinegar Dressing
Shrimp-stuffed Fillets   Steamed Spinach
Baked Cauliflower Beignets
Fresh fruit   Beverage

DAY 9

Breakfast
Freshly squeezed orange juice
¾ cup whole grain cereal with milk
Milk

Morning Snack
Bran muffin with butter or jelly
Milk

Lunch
Roast beef and lettuce sandwich on
whole wheat bread
Tomato wedges and pickle
Orange   Milk

Afternoon Snack
½ cup plain yogurt sprinkled with raw nuts
Fruit juice

Dinner
Cold Cucumber Soup
Pork Chops with Cabbage and Potatoes
Pumpernickel rolls and butter
Apple and Pear Compote   Beverage

DAY 10

Breakfast
½ grapefruit
1 poached egg on buttered whole grain bread
Milk

Morning Snack
Cream cheese on 1 slice date-nut bread
Milk

Lunch
Sliced chicken, tomato, and lettuce on hard roll
Coleslaw and pickle
Milk

Afternoon Snack
½ cup Apple and Pear Compote with
¼ cup cream-style cottage cheese
Fruit juice

Dinner
Beef Bouillon with Mushrooms and Chives
Artichoke Omelet   Stewed Cauliflower
Bran rolls and butter
Fresh fruit and cheese
Beverage

DAY 11

Breakfast
Orange wedges
¾ cup whole grain cereal with milk
Milk

Morning Snack
Peanut butter and jelly on whole grain crackers
Milk

Lunch
Sliced egg, lettuce, and tomato sandwich
on rye bread
Carrot sticks and cucumber slices
Apple   Milk

Afternoon Snack
½ cup plain yogurt with raisins
Fruit juice

Dinner
Cold Cucumber Soup
Chicken Kebabs   Rice Pilaf
Fresh pineapple slices
Beverage

DAY 12

Breakfast
Cranberry juice
Cinnamon-Cheese Toast
Milk

Morning Snack
1 hard-boiled egg
Tomato wedges and cucumber slices
Fruit juice

Lunch
Cream-style cottage cheese, lettuce, and
tomato sandwich on pumpernickel bread
Banana   Milk

Afternoon Snack
Corn muffin with butter or jelly
Milk

Dinner
String Beans Vinaigrette
Lamb Chops with Sautéed Mushrooms
Stewed Cauliflower
Whole grain bread and butter
Fresh fruit and cheese   Beverage

DAY 13

Breakfast
1 cup plain yogurt mixed with ½ cup plain,
unsweetened fruit
1 slice buttered whole wheat toast
Milk

Morning Snack
Bran muffin with butter or jelly
Milk

Lunch
Grilled cheeseburger on enriched-flour roll
Coleslaw, pickle, and tomato wedges
Fruit juice

Afternoon Snack
¼ cup raisins   ¼ cup nuts
Milk

Dinner
Marinated Artichokes
Baked Tile Fish
Asparagus with Butter and Cheese
Whole wheat rolls and butter
Rice Pudding   Beverage

DAY 14

Breakfast
½ grapefruit
1 scrambled egg on buttered whole wheat toast
Milk

Morning Snack
½ cup plain yogurt sprinkled with wheat germ
Milk

Lunch
Sliced turkey, lettuce, and tomato sandwich
on hard roll
Coleslaw and pickle
Orange   Fruit juice

Afternoon Snack
Cream cheese on 1 slice date-nut bread
Milk

Dinner
Eggplant Salad
Linguini with Chicken Liver Spaghetti Sauce
Whole wheat rolls and butter
Fresh fruit and cheese   Beverage

DAY 15

Breakfast
½ cantaloupe
½ cup cream-style cottage cheese
1 slice buttered whole wheat toast
Milk

Morning Snack
Bran muffin with butter or jelly
Milk

Lunch
Roast beef and coleslaw sandwich on hard roll
Tomato wedges and pickle
Orange   Fruit juice

Afternoon Snack
½ cup plain yogurt with ½ cup sliced unsweetened
strawberries sprinkled with wheat germ
Fruit juice

Dinner
Cream of Mushroom-Barley Soup
Avocado Dinner Salad
Pumpernickel rolls and butter
Rice Pudding   Beverage

DAY 16

Breakfast
Freshly squeezed grapefruit juice
¾ cup whole grain cereal with
sliced banana and milk
Milk

Morning Snack
1 hard-boiled egg
Tomato wedges and cucumber slices
Milk

Lunch
Peanut butter and jelly sandwich on whole wheat
bread
Apple   Milk

Afternoon Snack
Cream-style cottage cheese on whole grain crackers
Fruit juice

Dinner
Broccoli and Tomato Salad
Chicken Gumbo   Steamed rice
Whole wheat bread and butter
Fresh fruit   Beverage

DAY 17

Breakfast
½ cup sliced fresh peach or canned peaches in juice
French toast
Milk

Morning Snack
Corn muffin with butter or jelly
Milk

Lunch
Sliced chicken, lettuce, and tomato sandwich on
hard roll
Coleslaw and pickle
Mineral water

Afternoon Snack
Cream cheese on 1 slice date-nut bread
Milk

Dinner
Zucchini Soup à la Eve
Cauliflower Omelet
Sautéed peppers and potatoes
Whole wheat rolls and butter
Melon wedges   Beverage

DAY 18

Breakfast
Freshly squeezed orange juice
1 fried egg
1 slice buttered pumpernickel bread
Milk

Morning Snack
Peanut butter and jelly on whole wheat crackers
Milk

Lunch
Tuna Salad, lettuce, and tomato wedges in
whole wheat pita
Carrot sticks and green pepper strips
Fruit juice

Afternoon Snack
Apple and Swiss cheese
Milk

Dinner
Chick-pea Salad
Sautéed Flounder Fillets   Steamed Broccoli
Melon wedges   Beverage

DAY 19

Breakfast
Freshly squeezed grapefruit juice
¾ cup whole grain cereal with
sliced banana and milk
Milk

Morning Snack
Bran muffin with butter or jelly
Milk

Lunch
Grilled hamburger on enriched-flour bun
Lettuce and tomato salad
Carrot sticks
Milk

Afternoon Snack
½ cup plain yogurt and raisins
Fruit juice

Dinner
Lettuce Wedges with Oil and Vinegar Dressing
Chicken Gumbo   Brown Rice
Whole grain bread and butter
Fresh fruit   Beverage

DAY 20

Breakfast
¼ cantaloupe   1 soft-boiled egg
Bran roll and butter   Milk

Morning Snack
Corn muffin with butter or jelly
Milk

Lunch
Sliced turkey and coleslaw sandwich on
pumpernickel bread
Carrot sticks, tomato wedges, and pickle
Mineral water

Afternoon Snack
Apple and Cheddar cheese
Milk

Dinner
Salmon salad on lettuce leaves
Sliced tomatoes   Sliced cucumbers
Corn Salad
Bran rolls and butter
Chocolate-Raisin Bread Pudding
Beverage

DAY 21

Breakfast
Freshly squeezed orange juice
Grilled ham and Swiss cheese sandwich on
enriched-flour bread
Milk

Morning Snack
1 hard-boiled egg   Tomato wedges
Whole grain crackers with butter
Milk

Lunch
Tuna Salad, lettuce, and tomato wedges in
whole wheat pita
Coleslaw and pickle
Pear   Milk

Afternoon Snack
½ cup plain yogurt sprinkled with wheat germ
Fruit juice

Dinner
Cold Ratatouille on lettuce leaves
Three-Cheese Baked Macaroni
Steamed Broccoli with butter
Whole wheat bread and butter
Baked Apples   Beverage

DAY 22

Breakfast
½ grapefruit
1 poached egg on buttered whole grain toast
Milk

Morning Snack
¼ cup raisins   ¼ cup nuts   Fruit juice

Lunch
Three-Cheese Baked Macaroni
Lettuce and tomato salad
Hard roll and butter
Baked Apple   Milk

Afternoon Snack
Peanut butter and jelly on whole grain crackers
Milk

Dinner
Spanish-style Cod   Rice Pilaf
Sautéed String Beans
Whole wheat bread and butter
Frozen Yogurt Cream   Beverage

DAY 23

Breakfast
Freshly squeezed orange juice
¾ cup whole grain cereal with milk
Milk

Morning Snack
1 hard-boiled egg
Tomato wedges and cucumber slices
Milk

Lunch
Roast beef, lettuce, and tomato sandwich on
rye bread
Carrot sticks, green pepper strips, and pickle
Vegetable juice

Afternoon Snack
Pear and Cheddar cheese
Whole grain crackers
Milk

Dinner
Chicken Livers with Lemon, Oil, and Oregano
Asparagus with Butter and Cheese
Boiled potatoes
Chocolate-Raisin Bread Pudding
Beverage

DAY 24

Breakfast
½ cup plain yogurt with ½ cup unsweetened fruit
Bran roll and butter   Milk

Morning Snack
Cream cheese on 1 slice date-nut bread
Milk

Lunch
Three-Cheese Baked Macaroni
Lettuce wedge, tomato wedges, and carrot sticks
Hard roll and butter   Vegetable juice

Afternoon Snack
Orange
Whole grain crackers with butter
Milk

Dinner
Basil Tomatoes with Oil and Vinegar Dressing
Braised Lamb Shanks with Lentils Provençale
Bran rolls and butter
Fresh fruit and cheese   Beverage

DAY 25

Breakfast
½ cantaloupe
½ cup cream-style cottage cheese
Bran roll and butter
Milk

Morning Snack
Corn muffin with butter or jelly
Milk

Lunch
Sliced egg, tomato, and lettuce sandwich on
whole wheat bread
Coleslaw and pickle   Vegetable juice

Afternoon Snack
Cream cheese and jelly on whole-grain crackers
Milk

Dinner
Egg Flower Soup
Shredded Pork with Scallions
Steamed rice
Gold-topped Ice Cream
Beverage

DAY 26

Breakfast
½ grapefruit
¾ cup whole grain cereal with
sliced banana and milk
Milk

Morning Snack
Bran muffin with butter or jelly   Milk

Lunch
3 slices fresh pineapple or canned pineapple in juice
1 cup cream-style cottage cheese
Whole grain crackers with butter
Apple juice

Afternoon Snack
¼ cup raisins   ¼ cup nuts
Milk

Dinner
Lentil Soup
Grilled hamburger patties
Scalloped Potatoes   Steamed Broccoli
Whole wheat bread and butter
Apples   Beverage

DAY 27

Breakfast
Freshly squeezed grapefruit juice
Grilled Swiss cheese sandwich on whole grain bread
Apple slices
Milk

Morning Snack
Corn muffin with butter or jelly
Milk

Lunch
Sliced turkey, lettuce, and tomato on hard roll
Coleslaw and pickle
Vegetable juice

Afternoon Snack
Tangerine and Cheddar cheese
Milk

Dinner
White Bean Salad
Spinach Omelet   Ratatouille
Whole grain roll and butter
Baked Custard   Beverage

DAY 28

Breakfast
Freshly squeezed orange juice
1 soft-boiled egg
1 slice buttered whole grain bread
Milk

Morning Snack
½ cup plain yogurt with raisins
Fruit juice

Lunch
Liverwurst, lettuce, and tomato sandwich on
whole grain bread
Apple   Milk

Afternoon Snack
Orange
Whole wheat crackers with butter
Fruit juice

Dinner
Sliced Tomato with lemon wedge
Chicken Rollups
Whole wheat bread and butter
Fresh fruit and cheese
Beverage

DAY 29

Breakfast
Freshly squeezed grapefruit juice
¾ cup whole grain cereal with milk
Milk

Morning Snack
¼ cup raisins   ¼ cup dried fruit
Milk

Lunch
Grilled cheeseburger in whole wheat pita
Lettuce and tomato salad
Vegetable juice

Afternoon Snack
Peanut butter on whole grain crackers
Milk

Dinner
Lentil Soup
Stuffed Tomato Salad Plate
Bran roll and butter
Baked Custard   Beverage

DAY 30

Breakfast
Orange wedges
Cinnamon-Cheese Toast
Milk

Morning Snack
1 hard-boiled egg
Tomato wedges and cucumber slices
Milk

Lunch
Sliced chicken and coleslaw sandwich on
pumpernickel bread
Carrots and pickle
Vegetable juice

Afternoon Snack
Corn muffin with butter or jelly
Milk

Dinner
Egg Flower Soup
Shrimp with Garlic Sauce
Steamed rice
Sautéed Asparagus
Chilled mandarin orange segments
Beverage

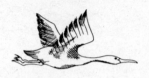 *The Fourth Month*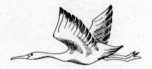

DAY 1

Breakfast
Freshly squeezed grapefruit juice
Cream cheese and boiled ham on 1 toasted
English muffin
Milk

Morning Snack
1 hard-boiled egg
Tomato wedges and cucumber slices
Milk

Lunch
Peanut butter and jelly sandwich on
enriched-flour bread
Milk

Afternoon Snack
½ cup plain yogurt sprinkled with raisins
Fruit juice

Dinner
Egyptian Pea Soup
Sautéed Chicken Breasts
Stewed Zucchini   French bread and butter
Fresh fruit   Beverage

DAY 2

Breakfast
Freshly squeezed orange juice
¾ cup whole grain cereal with sliced banana
and milk
Milk

Morning Snack
Corn muffin with butter or jelly
Milk

Lunch
Roast beef, lettuce, and tomato sandwich
on hard roll
Coleslaw and pickle
Milk

Afternoon Snack
Orange
Whole wheat crackers with butter
Fruit juice

Dinner
Mushroom Salad   Snappy Red Snapper
Rice Pilaf   Steamed Broccoli
Whole grain bread and butter
Apples and cheese   Beverage

DAY 3

Breakfast
½ grapefruit   1 scrambled egg
1 slice buttered enriched-flour toast with jelly
Milk

Morning Snack
Cream cheese on 1 slice date-nut bread
Milk

Lunch
Tuna Salad, lettuce, and tomato sandwich on
pumpernickel bread
Carrot sticks and green pepper strips
Fruit juice

Afternoon Snack
Apple and Muenster cheese
Milk

Dinner
Cucumber and Tomato Salad
Pork Chops with Sauerkraut
Boiled potatoes   Bran rolls and butter
Frozen Yogurt Cream   Beverage

DAY 4

Breakfast
Orange wedges
Tuna Salad sandwich on whole wheat toast
Milk

Morning Snack
¼ cup raisins   ¼ cup nuts
Milk

Lunch
Grilled cheeseburger on enriched-flour bun
Coleslaw, tomato wedges, and cucumber slices
Fruit juice

Afternoon Snack
Bran muffin with butter or jelly
Milk

Dinner
Lentil Soup
Egg Salad on lettuce leaves
Sliced tomatoes   Cucumber slices
Pumpernickel bread and butter
Melon wedges   Beverage

DAY 5

Breakfast
¾ cup whole grain cereal with ½ cup sliced peaches
and milk
Milk

Morning Snack
Peanut butter and jelly on whole wheat crackers
Milk

Lunch
Liverwurst, lettuce, and tomato sandwich on
whole grain bread
Grapes   Milk

Afternoon Snack
Apple and Cheddar cheese
Fruit juice

Dinner
String Beans Vinaigrette
Broccoli and Bean Soup
Bran rolls and butter
Fresh fruit   Beverage

DAY 6

Breakfast
½ grapefruit
Grilled Swiss cheese on English muffin
Milk

Morning Snack
Corn muffin with butter or jelly
Milk

Lunch
Sliced turkey and coleslaw sandwich on hard roll
Tomato wedges and carrot sticks
Vegetable juice

Afternoon Snack
Cream cheese on 1 slice date-nut bread
Milk

Dinner
Lettuce Wedges with Oil and Vinegar Dressing
Herbed Lamb Chops
Mashed potatoes   Buttered green peas
Ice cream   Beverage

DAY 7

Breakfast
Freshly squeezed orange juice
½ cantaloupe
½ cup cream-style cottage cheese
1 slice toasted enriched-flour bread with
butter and jelly

Morning Snack
¼ cup raisins   ¼ cup dried fruit
Milk

Lunch
Roast beef sandwich on rye bread
Lettuce and tomato salad
Apple   Milk

Afternoon Snack
Grapes and Swiss cheese   Milk

Dinner
Cold Cucumber Soup
Avocado Dinner Salad
Whole wheat roll and butter
Apple and Pear Compote   Beverage

DAY 8

Breakfast
Freshly squeezed orange juice
1 soft-boiled egg
1 slice toasted whole wheat bread with
butter and jelly
Milk

Morning Snack
Bran muffin with butter
Milk

Lunch
1 cup Apple and Pear Compote mixed with ½ cup
cream-style cottage cheese
Whole grain crackers
Milk

Afternoon Snack
½ cup plain yogurt sprinkled with wheat germ
Milk

Dinner
Marinated Artichokes
Pot Roast   Brown Rice
Bran roll and butter
Melon wedges   Beverage

DAY 9

Breakfast
Freshly squeezed grapefruit juice
¾ cup whole grain cereal with ½ cup sliced peaches
and milk
Milk

Morning Snack
Apple
Peanut butter on whole grain crackers
Milk

Lunch
Sliced chicken, lettuce, and tomato sandwich
on rye bread
Carrot sticks and cucumber slices
Vegetable juice

Afternoon Snack
¼ cup raisins   ¼ cup nuts
Mineral water

Dinner
Beef Bouillon with Mushrooms and Chives
Asparagus Omelet   Stewed Cabbage
Whole wheat bread and butter
Fruit and cheese   Beverage

DAY 10

Breakfast
Orange wedges
Cream cheese and boiled ham on 2 halves of a
toasted English muffin
Milk

Morning Snack
Bran muffin with butter or jelly
Milk

Lunch
Sliced egg, lettuce, and tomato sandwich on
enriched-flour bread
Coleslaw and pickle   Vegetable juice

Afternoon Snack
Apple and Cheddar cheese   Milk

Dinner
White Bean Salad
Coconut Chicken
Glazed Carrots   Sautéed Mushrooms
Hard rolls and butter
Sherbet   Beverage

DAY 11

Breakfast
½ grapefruit
2 corn muffins with butter or jelly
Milk

Morning Snack
½ toasted bagel with cream cheese
Milk

Lunch
3 slices fresh pineapple or canned pineapple in juice
½ cup cream-style cottage cheese
Whole grain crackers with butter
Milk

Afternoon Snack
Peanut butter and jelly on whole wheat bread
Vegetable juice

Dinner
String Beans Vinaigrette
Beef Liver Sauté
Brown Rice   Bran rolls and butter
Fresh fruit   Beverage

DAY 12

Breakfast
Freshly squeezed orange juice
1 poached egg on ½ toasted English muffin
Milk

Morning Snack
Cream cheese on 1 slice date-nut bread
Milk

Lunch
Coconut Chicken   Lettuce and tomato salad
Hard roll and butter
Apple   Mineral water

Afternoon Snack
Melon wedge
Whole grain crackers with butter
Milk

Dinner
Lettuce Wedges with Oil and Vinegar Dressing
Baked Rolled Flounder
Linguini with Marinara Sauce
Steamed Broccoli with butter
French bread and butter
Ice cream with banana slices   Beverage

DAY 13

Breakfast
Pineapple juice
¾ cup whole grain cereal with sliced banana
and milk
Milk

Morning Snack
¼ cup raisins   ¼ cup dried fruit
Milk

Lunch
Sliced turkey, lettuce, and tomato sandwich on a
hard roll
Orange   Milk

Afternoon Snack
Grapes
½ cup cream-style cottage cheese
Fruit juice

Dinner
Basil Tomatoes with Oil and Vinegar Dressing
Jambon Normande   Mashed potatoes
Sautéed String Beans
Apples and cheese   Beverage

DAY 14

Breakfast
½ cantaloupe
½ cup cream-style cottage cheese
1 slice buttered whole grain toast
Milk

Morning Snack
1 hard-boiled egg
Tomato wedges and cucumber slices
Milk

Lunch
Sliced chicken, lettuce and tomato sandwich on
whole wheat bread
Cucumber slices and carrot sticks
Vegetable juice

Afternoon Snack
Pear and Swiss cheese   Milk

Dinner
Pickled Salad
Rotelle with Eggplant Sauce
Bran rolls and butter
Sherbet   Beverage

DAY 15

Breakfast
½ grapefruit
Cream cheese on ½ toasted bagel
Milk

Morning Snack
Bran muffin with butter or jelly
Milk

Lunch
Roast beef sandwich on hard roll
Coleslaw, tomato wedges, and pickle
Vegetable juice

Afternoon Snack
Apple
Peanut butter on whole grain crackers
Milk

Dinner
Cottage Cheese Salad with sliced tomato
Near-East Chicken Soup
Whole grain bread and butter
Fresh fruit   Beverage

DAY 16

Breakfast
Freshly squeezed orange juice
¾ cup whole grain cereal with raisins and milk
Milk

Morning Snack
Corn muffin with butter or jelly
Milk

Lunch
Cream-style cottage cheese and tomato sandwich on
pumpernickel bread
Grapes   Vegetable juice

Afternoon Snack
1 slice of pizza
Milk

Dinner
Marinated Artichokes   Stuffed Eggplant
Bran rolls and butter
Fresh pineapple slices
Beverage

DAY 17

Breakfast
½ grapefruit   1 scrambled egg
Bran roll with butter or jelly
Milk

Morning Snack
½ cup cream-style cottage cheese with
diced fresh pineapple
Milk

Lunch
Cream cheese and boiled ham sandwich on
pumpernickel bread
Apple   Fruit juice

Afternoon Snack
¼ cup raisins   ¼ cup nuts
Milk

Dinner
Pickled Salad with tomato wedges
Sautéed Chicken Livers
Mashed potatoes   Steamed Spinach
Melon wedges   Beverage

DAY 18

Breakfast
½ cantaloupe
½ cup cream-style cottage cheese
1 slice buttered whole wheat toast
Milk

Morning Snack
Peanut butter on whole grain crackers
Milk

Lunch
Sliced egg, lettuce, and tomato sandwich
on rye bread
Carrot sticks and cucumber slices
Vegetable juice

Afternoon Snack
Corn muffin with butter or jelly
Milk

Dinner
Lentil Salad
Spaghetti with Meat Sauce
Whole wheat bread and butter
Fruit and cheese   Beverage

DAY 19

Breakfast
½ grapefruit
2 bran muffins with butter or jelly
Milk

Morning Snack
Cream cheese on 1 slice date-nut bread
Milk

Lunch
Grilled hamburger, lettuce, and tomato wedges in
whole wheat pita
Coleslaw and pickle   Vegetable juice

Afternoon Snack
Apple and Cheddar cheese
Milk

Dinner
Broccoli and Tomato Salad
Artichoke Omelet
Bran rolls and butter
Fresh pineapple slices   Beverage

DAY 20

Breakfast
Freshly squeezed orange juice
¾ cup whole grain cereal with sliced strawberries
and milk
Milk

Morning Snack
1 hard-boiled egg
Tomato wedges
Whole wheat crackers with butter
Milk

Lunch
Tuna Salad, cucumber slices, carrot sticks, and
green pepper strips on lettuce leaves
Hard roll and butter
Vegetable juice

Afternoon Snack
Peanut butter and jelly on whole grain crackers
Milk

Dinner
Cottage Cheese Salad
Lamb and String Bean Stew
Whole wheat bread and butter
Apple-Fig Cream   Beverage

DAY 21

Breakfast
Apple juice
Tuna Salad sandwich on rye toast
Milk

Morning Snack
Corn muffin with butter or jelly
Milk

Lunch
½ cantaloupe
½ cup cream-style cottage cheese
Pumpernickel roll and butter
Vegetable juice

Afternoon Snack
Apple
Peanut butter on whole grain crackers
Milk

Dinner
Chicken-Potato Salad on lettuce leaves
Marinated Artichokes
Sliced tomatoes
Bran rolls and butter
Fresh fruit   Beverage

DAY 22

Breakfast
Freshly squeezed grapefruit juice
1 poached egg on toasted whole grain bread
Milk

Morning Snack
Cream cheese on 1 slice date-nut bread
Milk

Lunch
Sliced turkey and coleslaw on hard roll
Lettuce and tomato salad
Milk

Afternoon Snack
½ cup plain yogurt with sliced fresh fruit
Vegetable juice

Dinner
Egg Flower Soup
Salmon Patties   Tomato-Rice Pilaf
Sautéed String Beans
Whole grain bread and butter
Apple-Fig Cream   Beverage

DAY 23

Breakfast
¾ cup whole grain cereal with sliced
banana and milk
Milk

Morning Snack
Bran muffin with butter or jelly
Milk

Lunch
Salmon Patty on pumpernickel roll
Lettuce and tomato salad
Grapes   Vegetable juice

Afternoon Snack
¼ cup raisins   ¼ cup nuts
Milk

Dinner
Cucumber and Tomato Salad
Cauliflower Omelet
Sautéed Peppers and Potatoes
Hard rolls and butter
Ice cream   Beverage

DAY 24

Breakfast
Orange wedges
Grilled Swiss cheese sandwich on rye bread
Milk

Morning Snack
½ cup cream-style cottage cheese with
applesauce and cinnamon
Fruit juice

Lunch
Egg Salad, lettuce, and tomato on hard roll
Carrot sticks and green pepper strips
Pear   Milk

Afternoon Snack
Peanut butter and jelly on whole grain crackers
Milk

Dinner
Chicken Parmigiana
Linguini   Steamed Broccoli
French bread and butter
Fruit and cheese   Beverage

DAY 25

Breakfast
Apple juice
Cream cheese and boiled ham on
toasted English muffin
Milk

Morning Snack
Corn muffin with butter or jelly
Milk

Lunch
Liverwurst, lettuce, and tomato sandwich on
whole wheat bread
Coleslaw and pickle
Apple   Vegetable juice

Afternoon Snack
Grapes and Swiss cheese
Milk

Dinner
Lettuce Wedges with Oil and Vinegar Dressing
Beef Stew   Sautéed String Beans
Bran rolls and butter
Fresh fruit   Beverage

DAY 26

Breakfast
½ grapefruit
1 scrambled egg
1 slice buttered whole grain toast with jelly
Milk

Morning Snack
¼ cup raisins   ¼ cup dried fruit
Milk

Lunch
Roast beef, lettuce, and tomato sandwich
on hard roll
Pear   Vegetable juice

Afternoon Snack
Cream cheese and jelly on whole grain crackers
Milk

Dinner
Sautéed Veal Cutlets
Rice Salad and sliced tomatoes on lettuce leaves
Buttered green peas
Whole wheat roll and butter
Melon wedges   Beverage

DAY 27

Breakfast
Freshly squeezed orange juice
¾ cup whole grain cereal with raisins and milk
Milk

Morning Snack
1 hard-boiled egg
Tomato wedges and cucumber slices
Milk

Lunch
Cream-style cottage cheese, lettuce, and tomato
on hard roll
Carrot sticks and cucumber slices
Apple   Fruit juice

Afternoon Snack
Pear
Cheddar cheese and whole grain crackers
Milk

Dinner
Lentil Soup   Hot Salad Niçoise
Whole grain bread and butter
Chocolate-Raisin Bread Pudding   Beverage

DAY 28

Breakfast
Freshly squeezed grapefruit juice
2 corn muffins with butter and jelly
Milk

Morning Snack
Banana and Cheddar cheese   Fruit juice

Lunch
3¼ ounces drained canned tuna
½ cup cream-style cottage cheese
Tomato wedges and cucumber slices
Whole grain crackers with butter
Milk

Afternoon Snack
Orange
Peanut butter on whole grain crackers
Milk

Dinner
Cucumber and Tomato Salad   Meatloaf
Stuffed Mushrooms   Sautéed Zucchini
Hard rolls and butter
Fresh fruit   Beverage

DAY 29

Breakfast
Freshly squeezed orange juice
Grilled Cheddar cheese sandwich on rye bread
Milk

Morning Snack
Cream-style cottage cheese on raisin bagel
Tomato wedges
Whole wheat crackers with butter
Milk

Lunch
Meatloaf, lettuce, and tomato sandwich on hard roll
Coleslaw and carrot sticks
Vegetable juice

Afternoon Snack
Cream cheese on 1 slice date-nut bread
Milk

Dinner
Cornish Hen with Scallions
Steamed rice   Sautéed Asparagus
Cucumber Relish
Ice cream   Beverage

DAY 30

Breakfast
¾ cup whole grain cereal with sliced
berries and milk
Milk

Morning Snack
Corn muffin with butter or jelly
Milk

Lunch
3¼ ounces drained canned tuna, lettuce, and
tomato wedges in whole wheat pita
Carrot sticks and pickle
Vegetable juice

Afternoon Snack
Grapes and Swiss cheese
Milk

Dinner
White Bean Salad
Linguini with Marinara Sauce
Steamed Broccoli
French bread and butter
Sherbet   Beverage

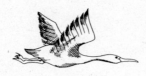 *The Fifth Month*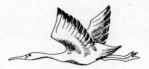

DAY 1

Breakfast
Freshly squeezed grapefruit juice
1 soft-boiled egg
1 slice buttered whole wheat toast
Milk

Morning Snack
Bran muffin with butter or jelly
Milk

Lunch
Grilled cheese and tomato sandwich on
whole wheat bread
Coleslaw, tomato wedges, and pickle
Vegetable juice

Afternoon Snack
Peanut butter and jelly on whole grain crackers
Milk

Dinner
Zucchini Soup à la Eve   Sautéed Shrimp
Boiled Potatoes with Oil and Parsley
Steamed Broccoli   Fresh fruit
Beverage

DAY 2

Breakfast
Apple juice
¾ cup whole grain cereal with raisins and milk
Milk

Morning Snack
½ cup plain yogurt with nuts
Milk

Lunch
Sliced turkey and coleslaw sandwich on
pumpernickel bread
Tomato wedges and pickle
Vegetable juice

Afternoon Snack
Pear
Peanut butter on whole grain crackers
Milk

Dinner
Eggplant-Gumbo Soup   Spinach Omelet
Sliced tomatoes   Bran rolls and butter
Gold-topped Ice Cream
Beverage

DAY 3

Breakfast
½ grapefruit
2 corn muffins with butter and jelly
Milk

Morning Snack
Cream-style cottage cheese on 1 slice
whole wheat toast
Milk

Lunch
Sliced egg, lettuce, and tomato sandwich
on rye bread
Coleslaw and pickle   Vegetable juice

Afternoon Snack
¼ cup raisins   ¼ cup nuts
Milk

Dinner
Lentil Soup
Grilled hamburger patties
Scalloped Potatoes   Steamed Broccoli
Baked Apples   Beverage

DAY 4

Breakfast
Freshly squeezed orange juice
Cream cheese and jelly on toasted English muffin
Milk

Morning Snack
Cheddar cheese on whole wheat crackers
Tomato juice

Lunch
Tuna Salad, lettuce, and tomato sandwich
on hard roll
Cucumber slices, carrot sticks, and green
pepper strips
Grapes   Milk

Afternoon Snack
Baked Apple
Milk

Dinner
Marinated Artichokes
Chicken in Mustard Sauce
Rice Pilaf   Steamed Spinach
Whole wheat bread and butter
Fresh fruit   Beverage

DAY 5

Breakfast
Freshly squeezed grapefruit juice
Tuna Salad sandwich on whole wheat toast
Milk

Morning Snack
Peanut butter and jelly on whole grain crackers
Milk

Lunch
Grilled cheeseburger in whole wheat pita
Lettuce and tomato salad
Vegetable juice

Afternoon Snack
Melon wedge
Milk

Dinner
Eggplant-Gumbo Soup
Herbed Veal Chops
Glazed Carrots   Sautéed Mushrooms
Bran rolls and butter
Fresh fruit   Beverage

DAY 6

Breakfast
Apple juice
1 poached egg on whole wheat toast
Milk

Morning Snack
Cream cheese on 1 slice date-nut bread
Milk

Lunch
Tuna Salad, cream-style cottage cheese, tomato
wedges, and cucumber slices on lettuce leaves
Pumpernickel roll and butter
Vegetable juice

Afternoon Snack
¼ cup raisins   ¼ cup nuts
Milk

Dinner
Lettuce Wedges with Oil and Vinegar Dressing
Beef Liver Sauté
Cauliflower with Pasta
Broiled tomato halves
French bread and butter
Stewed Fruit   Beverage

DAY 7

Breakfast
Stewed Fruit   French toast
Milk

Morning Snack
1 hard-boiled egg
Tomato wedges and cucumber slices
Vegetable juice

Lunch
Sliced chicken, lettuce, and tomato sandwich on
whole grain bread
Coleslaw and pickle   Milk

Afternoon Snack
Peanut butter on whole grain crackers
Milk

Dinner
String Beans Vinaigrette
Pork Chops with Chick-peas
Rice Pilaf
Hard rolls and butter
Ice cream   Beverage

DAY 8

Breakfast
Freshly squeezed orange juice
¾ cup whole grain cereal with raisins and milk
Milk

Morning Snack
Bran muffin with butter or jelly
Milk

Lunch
Roast beef, lettuce, and tomato sandwich
on rye bread
Cucumber slices and carrot sticks
Vegetable juice

Afternoon Snack
Apple
Peanut butter on whole wheat crackers
Milk

Dinner
Eggplant Salad
Sautéed Flounder Fillets
Bengal Beans   Cucumber Relish
Sautéed Bananas with Honey
Milk

DAY 9

Breakfast
Apple juice
1 scrambled egg
1 slice toasted whole grain bread with butter

Morning Snack
Corn muffin with butter or jelly
Milk

Lunch
½ cantaloupe
1 cup cream-style cottage cheese
1 slice whole wheat bread with butter
Milk

Afternoon Snack
Fresh Fruit   Milk

Dinner
Pickled Salad
Lemon-basted Roast Chicken
Steamed Cabbage and Potatoes
Whole wheat bread and butter
Fruit and cheese   Beverage

DAY 10

Breakfast
½ grapefruit
Cream cheese and boiled ham on
1 toasted English muffin
Milk

Morning Snack
Peanut butter on whole wheat crackers
Milk

Lunch
3¼ ounces drained canned salmon
Coleslaw, tomato wedges, cucumber slices, and
carrot sticks
Hard roll and butter   Vegetable juice

Afternoon Snack
Apple and Swiss cheese
Milk

Dinner
Egg Flower Soup
Noodle Salad   Sliced tomatoes
Onion Relish   Bran rolls and butter
Mandarin orange sections
Beverage

DAY 11

Breakfast
Freshly squeezed orange juice
3¼ ounces drained canned salmon in
whole wheat pita
Milk

Morning Snack
1 hard-boiled egg
Whole grain crackers with butter
Milk

Lunch
Lemon-basted Roast Chicken
Lettuce and tomato salad
Hard roll and butter
Apple   Vegetable juice

Afternoon Snack
Cream cheese and jelly on whole wheat crackers
Milk

Dinner
Sliced tomatoes with lemon wedge
Beef Liver and Onions
Mashed potatoes   Steamed Spinach
Fresh pineapple slices
Beverage

DAY 12

Breakfast
¾ cup whole grain cereal with sliced
banana and milk
Milk

Morning Snack
Cream cheese on 1 slice date-nut bread
Milk

Lunch
Noodle Salad   Tomato wedges
Bran roll and butter
Apple juice

Afternoon Snack
1 slice of pizza   Milk

Dinner
Lentil Soup
Quiche Lorraine   Pickled Salad
Bran roll and butter
Stewed Fruit   Beverage

DAY 13

Breakfast
Apple juice
1 buttered whole wheat English muffin with jelly
Milk

Morning Snack
½ cup cream-style cottage cheese with blueberries
Milk

Lunch
Quiche Lorraine
Tomato wedges and carrot sticks
Whole grain bread and butter
Fruit juice

Afternoon Snack
¼ cup raisins   ¼ cup dried fruit
Milk

Dinner
Broccoli and Tomato Salad
Beef Stew
Whole wheat bread and butter
Fruit and cheese   Beverage

DAY 14

Breakfast
½ grapefruit
1 scrambled egg
1 slice buttered whole wheat toast and jelly
Milk

Morning Snack
½ cup plain yogurt with sliced fresh fruit
and wheat germ
Milk

Lunch
Roast beef, lettuce and tomato sandwich
on hard roll
Green pepper strips and carrot sticks
Vegetable juice

Afternoon Snack
Cream cheese on 1 slice date-nut bread

Dinner
Shredded Pork with Scallions
Steamed rice   Sautéed Asparagus
Fresh pineapple slices
Beverage

DAY 15

Breakfast
Apple juice
¾ cup whole grain cereal with raisins and milk
Milk

Morning Snack
Toasted corn muffin with butter or jelly
Milk

Lunch
Grilled cheese sandwich on rye bread
Lettuce and tomato salad
Pumpernickel roll and butter
Freshly squeezed orange juice

Afternoon Snack
Apple
Peanut butter on whole wheat crackers
Milk

Dinner
Tossed salad   Sautéed Oysters
Caribbean Red Beans
Onion Relish
Rice Pudding   Beverage

DAY 16

Breakfast
Freshly squeezed orange juice
Cream cheese and boiled ham sandwich on
pumpernickel bread
Milk

Morning Snack
1 hard-boiled egg
Tomato wedges and cucumber slices
Milk

Lunch
Chicken salad sandwich on whole wheat bread
Coleslaw, carrot sticks, and green pepper strips
Vegetable juice

Afternoon Snack
Rice Pudding   Apple juice

Dinner
Mushroom Salad
Spaghetti with Olives and Tomatoes
Steamed Broccoli
Whole wheat bread and butter
Fruit and cheese   Beverage

DAY 17

Breakfast
½ cantaloupe
½ cup cream-style cottage cheese
1 slice buttered whole wheat toast
Milk

Morning Snack
Banana
Milk

Lunch
Sliced egg, lettuce, and tomato sandwich on
pumpernickel bread
Carrot sticks, green pepper strips, and cucumber
slices
Fruit juice

Afternoon Snack
Orange
Peanut butter on whole grain crackers
Milk

Dinner
Broccoli and Tomato Salad
Beef Stew   Bran rolls and butter
Frozen Yogurt Cream
Beverage

DAY 18

Breakfast
Freshly squeezed grapefruit juice
1 poached egg on ½ toasted English muffin
Milk

Morning Snack
Cream cheese and jelly on 1 slice whole wheat bread
Milk

Lunch
Roast beef and lettuce on hard roll
Coleslaw and pickle
Vegetable juice

Afternoon Snack
Rice Pudding   Apple juice

Dinner
Cucumber and Tomato Salad
Chicken with Artichokes
Rice Pilaf
French bread and butter
Fresh fruit   Beverage

DAY 19

Breakfast
Freshly squeezed orange juice
¾ cup whole grain cereal with raisins and milk
Milk

Morning Snack
Corn muffin with butter or jelly
Milk

Lunch
Liverwurst, lettuce, and tomato sandwich on
whole wheat bread
Coleslaw and pickle
Vegetable juice

Afternoon Snack
Grapes and Cheddar cheese
Milk

Dinner
Lentil Soup
Egg Salad on lettuce leaves
Sliced tomatoes   Cucumber slices
Bran rolls and butter
Pound cake with ice cream
Beverage

DAY 20

Breakfast
Grilled Swiss cheese sandwich on rye bread
Tangerine
Milk

Morning Snack
½ cup plain yogurt sprinkled with
wheat germ and raisins
Cranberry juice

Lunch
½ cantaloupe
1 cup cream-style cottage cheese
1 slice whole wheat bread with butter
Milk

Afternoon Snack
Peanut butter and jelly on whole wheat crackers
Milk

Dinner
Lentil Salad   Lamb Kebab
Curried Rice   Onion Relish
Applesauce   Beverage

DAY 21

Breakfast
1 cup cream-style cottage cheese with
1 cup unsweetened fresh fruit
1 slice toasted enriched-flour bread with butter
Milk

Morning Snack
¼ cup raisins   ¼ cup nuts
Milk

Lunch
Grilled hamburger on enriched-flour bun
Lettuce and tomato salad
Vegetable juice

Afternoon Snack
Grapes
Whole grain crackers with butter
Milk

Dinner
String Beans Vinaigrette
Poached Eggs with Stewed Zucchini
Whole wheat bread and butter
Fruit and cheese   Beverage

DAY 22

Breakfast
½ grapefruit
¾ cup whole grain cereal with sliced banana
and milk
Milk

Morning Snack
½ toasted bagel with cream cheese
Milk

Lunch
Sliced egg, lettuce, and tomato sandwich
on hard roll
Coleslaw and pickle
Vegetable juice

Afternoon Snack
1 slice of pizza
Milk

Dinner
Egg Flower Soup
Shrimp with Garlic Sauce
Steamed rice   Steamed Spinach
Fresh fruit   Beverage

DAY 23

Breakfast
Apple juice
Cream cheese and boiled ham on 1 toasted
English muffin   Milk

Morning Snack
1 hard-boiled egg
Tomato wedges and cucumber slices
Milk

Lunch
Roast beef and Coleslaw sandwich on rye bread
Pickle   Vegetable juice

Afternoon Snack
Cheddar cheese on whole grain crackers
Milk

Dinner
Cottage Cheese Salad
Sautéed Chicken Breasts   Stewed Zucchini
Pumpernickel rolls and butter
Sherbet   Beverage

DAY 24

Breakfast
½ grapefruit
1 soft-boiled egg
Toasted English muffin with butter or jelly
Milk

Morning Snack
Cream cheese on 1 slice date-nut bread
Milk

Lunch
Sliced turkey, lettuce, and tomato sandwich on
pumpernickel roll
Carrot sticks, cucumber slices, and green
pepper strips
Milk

Afternoon Snack
Orange
Whole grain crackers with butter
Fruit juice

Dinner
Split Pea Soup   Anytime Dinner Salad
Whole wheat roll and butter
Chocolate-Raisin Bread Pudding
Beverage

DAY 25

Breakfast
Freshly squeezed orange juice
¾ cup whole grain cereal with milk
Milk

Morning Snack
Peanut butter and jelly on whole grain crackers
Milk

Lunch
Sliced chicken sandwich on hard roll
Lettuce and tomato salad
Banana   Vegetable juice

Afternoon Snack
Apple and Cheddar cheese
Milk

Dinner
Beef Bouillon with Mushrooms and Chives
Pork Hocks and Collard Greens
Brown Rice   Bran rolls and butter
Fresh fruit   Beverage

DAY 26

Breakfast
Freshly squeezed grapefruit juice
Grilled Cheddar cheese sandwich on
whole wheat bread
Milk

Morning Snack
¼ cup raisins   ¼ cup dried fruit
Milk

Lunch
Sliced egg, ½ cup cream-style cottage cheese,
cucumber slices, and carrot sticks on lettuce leaves
Hard roll and butter
Apple   Milk

Afternoon Snack
Grapes
Whole grain crackers with butter
Fruit juice

Dinner
Sliced tomato with lemon wedges
Haddock with Capers
Stuffed Mushrooms   Steamed Spinach
Baked Custard   Beverage

DAY 27

Breakfast
1 cup plain yogurt with ½ cup unsweetened
fresh fruit
Bran roll and butter
Milk

Morning Snack
Corn muffin with butter or jelly
Milk

Lunch
Peanut butter and jelly sandwich on
whole wheat bread
Orange   Milk

Afternoon Snack
Apple and Swiss cheese
Fruit juice

Dinner
Veal Rolls with Mustard
Mashed potatoes   Glazed Carrots
French bread and butter
Fresh Fruit   Beverage

DAY 28

Breakfast
Freshly squeezed orange juice
¾ cup whole grain cereal with sliced banana
and milk
Milk

Morning Snack
Bran muffin with butter or jelly
Milk

Lunch
Grilled cheeseburger in whole wheat pita
Lettuce and cucumber salad
Vegetable juice

Afternoon Snack
1 slice of pizza
Milk

Dinner
Split Pea Soup   Cauliflower Omelet
Stewed Zucchini
Whole wheat bread and butter
Jam Parfait   Beverage

DAY 29

Breakfast
Freshly squeezed grapefruit juice
1 scrambled egg
1 slice whole wheat toast with butter and jelly
Milk

Morning Snack
Cream cheese on 1 slice date-nut bread
Milk

Lunch
Roast beef, lettuce, and tomato sandwich
on hard roll
Carrot sticks and cucumber slices
Apple   Vegetable juice

Afternoon Snack
Orange
Peanut butter on whole grain crackers
Milk

Dinner
Marinated Artichokes
Baked Stewed Cauliflower with Shells
Sautéed Chicken Livers   French bread and butter
Fruit and cheese   Beverage

DAY 30

Breakfast
Orange wedges
Grilled Swiss cheese sandwich on whole grain bread
Milk

Morning Snack
1 hard-boiled egg
1 slice whole wheat bread with butter
Milk

Lunch
½ cantaloupe   1 cup cream-style cottage cheese
Whole grain crackers with butter   Fruit juice

Afternoon Snack
¼ cup raisins and dried fruit
¼ cup nuts   Milk

Dinner
Split Pea Soup
Tuna Salad on lettuce leaves
Sliced tomatoes   Corn Salad
Bran rolls and butter
Baked Custard   Beverage

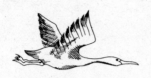 *The Sixth Month*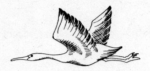

DAY 1	**DAY 2**
Breakfast ½ grapefruit ¾ cup whole grain cereal with raisins and milk Milk	*Breakfast* Freshly squeezed orange juice Cream cheese and boiled ham on toasted English muffin Milk
Morning Snack Corn muffin with butter or jelly Milk	*Morning Snack* Peanut butter and jelly on whole wheat crackers Milk
Lunch Sliced egg, lettuce, and tomato sandwich on enriched-flour bread Coleslaw and pickle Apple juice	*Lunch* Sliced turkey and lettuce sandwich on hard roll Carrot sticks, cucumber slices, and pickle Milk
Afternoon Snack ½ cup plain yogurt with nuts Milk	*Afternoon Snack* Apple and Cheddar cheese Milk
Dinner String Beans Vinaigrette Chicken Breasts Florentine Mashed potatoes Whole wheat rolls and butter Fruit and cheese Beverage	*Dinner* Basil Tomatoes with Oil and Vinegar Dressing Salmon and Noodle Bake Sautéed Asparagus Bran rolls and butter Fresh pineapple slices Beverage

DAY 3

Breakfast
1 cup Applesauce with 1 cup cream-style
cottage cheese
1 slice whole grain bread and butter
Milk

Morning Snack
Blueberry muffin with butter or jelly
Milk

Lunch
Grilled hamburger on enriched-flour bun
Lettuce wedges and celery sticks
Vegetable juice

Afternoon Snack
¼ cup raisins and dried fruit
¼ cup raw nuts   Milk

Dinner
Lentil Soup   Broccoli Omelet
Sliced tomato
Whole wheat bread and butter
Baked Apples   Beverage

DAY 4

Breakfast
½ grapefruit   1 scrambled egg
1 slice whole wheat toast and butter
Milk

Morning Snack
Cream cheese on 1 slice date-nut bread
Milk

Lunch
3 slices fresh pineapple or canned pineapple in juice
1 cup cream-style cottage cheese
Pumpernickel roll and butter
Fruit juice

Afternoon Snack
Orange
Peanut butter on whole grain crackers
Milk

Dinner
Marinated Artichokes
Veal Stew   Wide noodles
Sautéed Zucchini
French bread and butter
Fresh fruit   Beverage

DAY 5

Breakfast
Freshly squeezed orange juice
¾ cup whole grain cereal with
sliced banana and milk
Milk

Morning Snack
Toasted English muffin with butter or jelly
Milk

Lunch
Roast beef and coleslaw sandwich on rye bread
Tomato wedges, celery sticks, and
green pepper strips
Vegetable juice

Afternoon Snack
1 slice pizza
Milk

Dinner
Salmon and Noodle Bake
Sautéed String Beans   Glazed Carrots
Whole grain bread and butter
Baked Apples   Beverage

DAY 6

Breakfast
Orange segments
Cream cheese on a pumpernickel bagel
Milk

Morning Snack
Grapes
Peanut butter on whole grain crackers
Milk

Lunch
Tuna Salad, lettuce, and tomato wedges in
whole wheat pita
Carrot sticks and pickle   Apple juice

Afternoon Snack
½ cup cream-style cottage cheese with
½ cup unsweetened fresh fruit
Milk

Dinner
Home-style Beef Liver
Sliced tomatoes   Steamed rice
Steamed Cabbage
Ice cream   Beverage

DAY 7

Breakfast
Orange wedges
Tuna Salad on 1 toasted English muffin
Milk

Morning Snack
½ cup plain yogurt with sliced fresh fruit and
wheat germ
Fruit juice

Lunch
Sliced turkey, lettuce, and tomato sandwich
on hard roll
Carrot sticks and cucumber slices
Milk

Afternoon Snack
Apple and Swiss cheese
Whole grain crackers with butter
Milk

Dinner
Eggplant Salad
Broccoli and Bean Soup
Bran rolls and butter
Melon wedges   Beverage

DAY 8

Breakfast
½ grapefruit
¾ cup whole grain cereal with milk
Milk

Morning Snack
Bran muffin with butter or jelly
Milk

Lunch
Tuna Salad on lettuce leaves
Tomato wedges, carrot sticks, and pickle strips
Hard roll and butter   Vegetable juice

Afternoon Snack
½ cup Applesauce mixed with ½ cup cream-style
cottage cheese
Milk

Dinner
Veal Stew   Rice Milanese
Sautéed String Beans
French bread and butter
Jam Parfait   Beverage

DAY 9

Breakfast
Grapefruit juice
1 poached egg on buttered whole wheat toast
Milk

Morning Snack
½ cup plain yogurt with raisins
Milk

Lunch
Swiss cheese and tomato sandwich on
pumpernickel bread
Grapes   Milk

Afternoon Snack
Peanut butter and jelly on 1 slice whole wheat bread
Milk

Dinner
Beef Bouillon with Mushrooms and Chives
Spareribs with Cabbage and Potatoes
Whole wheat rolls and butter
Apple and Pear Compote
Beverage

DAY 10

Breakfast
1 cup Apple and Pear Compote with
1 cup cream-style cottage cheese
1 slice buttered whole grain toast
Milk

Morning Snack
Corn muffin with butter or jelly
Milk

Lunch
Grilled cheeseburger in whole wheat pita
Lettuce and tomato salad
Vegetable juice

Afternoon Snack
¼ cup raisins   ¼ cup nuts
Milk

Dinner
Pan-fried Cornish Hen
Cinnamon-Almond Pilaf
Steamed Broccoli
Whole grain bread and butter
Sherbet   Beverage

DAY 11

Breakfast
¼ melon
¾ cup whole grain cereal with milk
Milk

Morning Snack
Cream cheese on 1 slice date-nut bread
Milk

Lunch
Egg Salad, lettuce, and tomato sandwich on
whole wheat bread
Banana
Milk

Afternoon Snack
Peanut butter and jelly on whole grain crackers
Fruit juice

Dinner
Chick-pea Salad   Sautéed Shrimp
Stewed Cabbage   Hard rolls and butter
Apple and Pear Compote   Beverage

DAY 12

Breakfast
Freshly squeezed orange juice
Cream cheese and boiled ham on
1 toasted English muffin
Milk

Morning Snack
½ bagel with cottage cheese and chives
Fruit juice

Lunch
Egg Salad on lettuce leaves
Tomato wedges, cucumber slices, carrot sticks,
and pickle
Pumpernickel roll and butter
Milk

Afternoon Snack
1 slice of pizza
Milk

Dinner
Broccoli and Tomato Salad
Gandules with Rice   Glazed Carrots
Hard rolls and butter   Stewed Fruit
Beverage

DAY 13

Breakfast
½ grapefruit   1 soft-boiled egg
Bran roll with butter
Milk

Morning Snack
Fresh Fruit   Milk

Lunch
Roast beef and coleslaw sandwich on
pumpernickel bread
Lettuce and tomato salad
Fruit juice

Afternoon Snack
Blueberry muffin with butter or jelly
Milk

Dinner
Eggplant-Gumbo Soup   Spinach Pie
Sliced tomatoes with lemon wedges
Hard rolls and butter
Melon wedges   Beverage

DAY 14

Breakfast
Freshly squeezed orange juice
¾ cup whole grain cereal with sliced banana
and milk
Milk

Morning Snack
Cream cheese on 1 slice date-nut bread
Milk

Lunch
Spinach Pie
Whole grain crackers with butter
Apple   Fruit juice

Afternoon Snack
Peanut butter on 1 slice whole wheat bread
Milk

Dinner
Pickled Salad
Spaghetti with Veal Sauce
Whole wheat rolls and butter
Fruit and cheese   Beverage

DAY 15

Breakfast
½ grapefruit
Cream cheese on 1 pumpernickel bagel
Milk

Morning Snack
1 hard-boiled egg
Carrot sticks and cucumber slices
Milk

Lunch
Liverwurst, lettuce, and tomato sandwich on
whole wheat bread
Celery sticks   Apple   Milk

Afternoon Snack
Grapes and Cheddar cheese
Whole grain crackers with butter
Fruit juice

Dinner
Basil Tomatoes with Oil and Vinegar Dressing
Gandules with Rice   Steamed Broccoli
Bran rolls and butter
Chilled mandarin orange segments   Beverage

DAY 16

Breakfast
Orange segments
Grilled Cheddar cheese sandwich on
whole grain bread
Milk

Morning Snack
½ cup plain yogurt with raisins
Fruit juice

Lunch
Sliced turkey and coleslaw sandwich on
pumpernickel bread
Lettuce and tomato salad   Milk

Afternoon Snack
Peanut butter and jelly on whole grain crackers
Milk

Dinner
Eggplant-Gumbo Soup
Salmon Salad on lettuce leaves
Pickled Salad   Sliced tomatoes
Whole wheat bread and butter
Ice milk   Beverage

DAY 17

Breakfast
½ grapefruit
¾ cup whole grain cereal with raisins and milk
Milk

Morning Snack
1 hard-boiled egg   Tomato wedges
Whole grain crackers with butter
Milk

Lunch
Roast beef, lettuce, and tomato sandwich on
rye bread
Coleslaw and pickle   Vegetable juice

Afternoon Snack
Apple and Swiss cheese   Milk

Dinner
Lettuce Wedges with Oil and Vinegar Dressing
Cranberry Chicken Breasts
Rice Pilaf   Sautéed Mushrooms
Hard rolls and butter   Fresh fruit
Beverage

DAY 18

Breakfast
Freshly squeezed orange juice
1 scrambled egg
1 slice buttered whole wheat toast
Milk

Morning Snack
Bran muffin with butter or jelly   Milk

Lunch
3½ ounces drained canned tuna
Lettuce wedge, tomato wedges, cucumber slices, and
carrot sticks
2 slices whole wheat bread and butter
Milk

Afternoon Snack
½ cup plain yogurt sprinkled with sliced fresh fruit
and wheat germ
Apple juice

Dinner
Cold Cucumber Soup
Bean Sprout Fritters   Ratatouille
Whole wheat bread and butter
Jam Parfait   Beverage

DAY 19

Breakfast
Apple juice
2 corn muffins with butter and jelly
Milk

Morning Snack
Peanut butter on whole wheat crackers
Orange   Milk

Lunch
3¼ ounces drained canned tuna
½ cup cream-style cottage cheese
Lettuce wedge, carrot sticks, and green
pepper strips
Pumpernickel roll and butter
Vegetable juice

Afternoon Snack
Cream cheese on 1 slice date-nut bread
Milk

Dinner
Cucumber and Tomato Salad
Spaghetti with Veal Sauce   Steamed Broccoli
Whole wheat bread and butter
Fruit and cheese   Beverage

DAY 20

Breakfast
Freshly squeezed grapefruit juice
¾ cup whole grain cereal with sliced banana
and milk
Milk

Morning Snack
Bran muffin with butter or jelly   Milk

Lunch
½ cantaloupe   1 cup cream-style cottage cheese
1 slice whole grain bread and butter
Milk

Afternoon Snack
Banana
Peanut butter on whole grain crackers
Milk

Dinner
Tossed Salad with Oil and Vinegar Dressing
Sautéed Chicken Livers   Mashed potatoes
Steamed Spinach   Bran rolls and butter
Apple-Fig Cream   Beverage

DAY 21

Breakfast
Freshly squeezed orange juice
Cream cheese and boiled ham sandwich on
pumpernickel bread
Milk

Morning Snack
½ cup plain yogurt with raisins
Fruit juice

Lunch
Sliced turkey and lettuce sandwich on rye bread
Coleslaw, tomato wedges, and pickle
Mineral water

Afternoon Snack
Cheddar cheese on whole wheat crackers
Apple   Milk

Dinner
Egg Flower Soup
Sautéed Flounder Fillets
Lima Beans with Blue Cheese
Whole wheat bread and butter
Fresh fruit   Beverage

DAY 22

Breakfast
½ grapefruit
1 poached egg on buttered whole grain toast
Milk

Morning Snack
Corn muffin with butter or jelly
Milk

Lunch
Grilled hamburger on enriched-flour bun
Lettuce and tomato salad
Pear   Vegetable juice

Afternoon Snack
¼ cup raisins   ¼ cup nuts
Milk

Dinner
Lettuce Wedges with Oil and Vinegar Dressing
Lamb and String Bean Stew
Bran rolls and butter
Apple-Fig Cream   Beverage

DAY 23

Breakfast
Vegetable juice
¾ cup whole grain cereal with sliced peaches
and milk
Milk

Morning Snack
Cream cheese on 1 slice date-nut bread
Milk

Lunch
Peanut butter and jelly sandwich on
whole wheat bread
Apple   Milk

Afternoon Snack
Grapes and Cheddar cheese
Whole grain crackers with butter
Fruit juice

Dinner
Egyptian Pea Soup
Egg Salad on lettuce leaves
Corn Salad   Sliced tomatoes
Pickles   Bran rolls and butter
Melon wedges   Beverage

DAY 24

Breakfast
Freshly squeezed orange juice
2 bran muffins with butter and jelly
Milk

Morning Snack
1 hard-boiled egg   Tomato wedges
Whole grain crackers with butter
Milk

Lunch
1 cup plain yogurt with 1 cup sliced, unsweetened
fresh fruit
Hard roll and butter   Milk

Afternoon Snack
½ cup ice milk   Fruit juice

Dinner
Tossed salad with Oil and Vinegar Dressing
Chicken Valenciana   Rice Pilaf
French bread and butter
Fresh fruit   Beverage

DAY 25

Breakfast
½ grapefruit
Grilled Swiss cheese and boiled ham sandwich on
rye bread
Milk

Morning Snack
½ cup cream-style cottage cheese sprinkled with
sliced berries and wheat germ
Fruit juice

Lunch
Roast beef, lettuce, and tomato sandwich on
hard roll
Carrot sticks and cucumber slices
Milk

Afternoon Snack
Peanut butter and jelly on whole grain crackers
Milk

Dinner
Mushroom Salad   Eggplant Parmigiana
Linguini   French bread and butter
Tangerines   Beverage

DAY 26

Breakfast
Freshly squeezed orange juice
¾ cup whole grain cereal with sliced peaches
and milk
Milk

Morning Snack
1 corn muffin with butter or jelly
Milk

Lunch
Boiled ham and Swiss cheese sandwich on
whole wheat bread
Lettuce and tomato salad
Vegetable juice

Afternoon Snack
1 slice of pizza
Milk

Dinner
Egg Flower Soup
Sea Scallops with Cucumber   Steamed rice
Sautéed Asparagus   Fresh pineapple slices
Beverage

DAY 27

Breakfast
Apple juice   1 soft-boiled egg
1 slice buttered whole wheat toast
Milk

Morning Snack
½ cup cream-style cottage cheese with blueberries
Milk

Lunch
Tuna Salad, lettuce, and tomato sandwich on
hard roll
Coleslaw and pickle   Vegetable juice

Afternoon Snack
¼ cup dried apricots   ¼ cup nuts   Milk

Dinner
Tossed salad with Oil and Vinegar Dressing
Parmesan Hamburger Patties
Sautéed Peppers and Potatoes
Hard rolls and butter
Chocolate-Raisin Bread Pudding
Beverage

DAY 28

Breakfast
Freshly squeezed grapefruit juice
Tuna Salad on 1 toasted English muffin
Milk

Morning Snack
1 hard-boiled egg   Tomato wedges
Whole grain crackers with butter
Milk

Lunch
Sliced turkey and coleslaw sandwich on
pumpernickel roll
Carrot sticks and green pepper strips
Apple juice

Afternoon Snack
Peanut butter and jelly on 1 slice whole wheat bread
Milk

Dinner
Beef Bouillon with Mushrooms and Chives
Sautéed Veal Chops   Brown Rice
Buttered green peas
Bran rolls and butter
Fresh fruit and cheese   Beverage

DAY 29

Breakfast
Freshly squeezed orange juice
2 bran muffins with butter or jelly
Milk

Morning Snack
½ raisin bagel with cream cheese   Milk

Lunch
Liverwurst, lettuce, and tomato sandwich
on rye bread
Coleslaw and pickle
Vegetable juice

Afternoon Snack
Banana and Cheddar cheese
Whole grain crackers with butter
Milk

Dinner
Broccoli and Tomato Salad
Eggplant Parmigiana   Linguini
Hard rolls and butter
Fruit and cheese   Beverage

DAY 30

Breakfast
½ grapefruit
¾ cup whole grain cereal with raisins and milk
Milk

Morning Snack
Cream cheese on 1 slice date-nut bread
milk

Lunch
1 cup plain yogurt mixed with 1 cup sliced,
unsweetened fresh fruit
Bran roll and butter   Fruit juice

Afternoon Snack
Peanut butter on whole grain crackers
Milk

Dinner
Egyptian Pea Soup
Poached Salmon with mayonnaise and
lemon wedges
String Beans Vinaigrette
Whole wheat bread and butter
Chocolate-Raisin Bread Pudding
Beverage

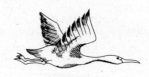 *The Seventh Month*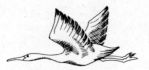

DAY 1

Breakfast
Freshly squeezed orange juice
1 scrambled egg
1 slice whole wheat toast with
farmer cheese and jelly
Milk

Morning Snack
Corn muffin with butter or jelly
Milk

Lunch
Salmon Salad, lettuce, and tomato sandwich on
pumpernickel bread
Coleslaw and pickle   Apple juice

Afternoon Snack
Pear
Peanut butter on whole grain crackers
Milk

Dinner
Egg Flower Soup
Sliced Chicken with Scallions
Steamed rice   Steamed Spinach
Chilled mandarin orange segments
Beverage

DAY 2

Breakfast
Apple juice
Salmon Salad sandwich on whole wheat toast
Milk

Morning Snack
½ cup plain yogurt with raisins
Fruit juice

Lunch
Grilled cheeseburger on enriched-flour bun
Lettuce and tomato salad
Orange   Milk

Afternoon Snack
Cream cheese on 1 slice date-nut bread
Milk

Dinner
Egyptian Pea Soup   Cauliflower Omelet
Stewed Zucchini   Bran rolls and butter
Fruit and cheese   Beverage

DAY 3

Breakfast
Orange segments
¾ cup whole grain cereal with milk
Milk

Morning Snack
1 hard-boiled egg
Tomato wedges and cucumber slices
Milk

Lunch
Liverwurst, lettuce, and tomato sandwich on
whole wheat bread
Coleslaw and pickle   Milk

Afternoon Snack
Peanut butter and jelly on whole grain crackers
Milk

Dinner
Pickled Salad   Zucchini Lasagna
Steamed Broccoli with butter
Whole wheat bread and butter
Fresh fruit   Beverage

DAY 4

Breakfast
½ grapefruit
Grilled ham and Swiss cheese sandwich
on rye bread
Milk

Morning Snack
Bran muffin with butter or jelly
Milk

Lunch
Sliced egg, lettuce, and tomato on hard roll
Coleslaw and pickle
Fruit juice

Afternoon Snack
½ cup cream-style cottage cheese with sliced,
unsweetened fresh fruit
Milk

Dinner
Lettuce Wedges with Oil and Vinegar Dressing
Roast Beef   Baked Cauliflower Beignets
Sautéed Mushrooms   Hard rolls and butter
Apple-Fig Cream   Beverage

DAY 5

Breakfast
Freshly squeezed orange juice
Cinnamon-Cheese Toast
Milk

Morning Snack
½ cup plain yogurt sprinkled with sliced fresh fruit
and wheat germ
Fruit juice

Lunch
Roast beef and coleslaw sandwich on hard roll
Tomato wedges, cucumber slices, and carrot sticks
Milk

Afternoon Snack
¼ cup raisins   ¼ cup nuts
Milk

Dinner
Mushroom Salad   Zucchini Lasagna
Steamed Spinach
French bread and butter
Fruit and cheese   Beverage

DAY 6

Breakfast
Freshly squeezed grapefruit juice
¾ cup whole grain cereal with sliced banana
and milk
Milk

Morning Snack
Cream cheese on 1 slice date-nut bread
Milk

Lunch
Sliced turkey, lettuce, and tomato sandwich on
whole wheat bread
Potato salad   Fruit juice

Afternoon Snack
Apple and Swiss cheese
Whole grain crackers with butter
Milk

Dinner
Pickled Salad   Roast Beef
Tomato-Rice Pilaf
Lima Beans with Blue Cheese
Bran rolls and butter
Apple-Fig Cream   Beverage

DAY 7

Breakfast
Freshly squeezed orange juice
1 poached egg on whole grain toast
Milk

Morning Snack
Corn muffin with butter or jelly
Milk

Lunch
Chicken salad, lettuce, and tomato wedges in whole
wheat pita
Coleslaw and pickle
Vegetable juice

Afternoon Snack
Peanut butter on whole grain crackers
Milk

Dinner
White Bean Salad   Salmon Patties
Stewed Zucchini
Whole wheat bread and butter
Melon wedges with ice milk
Beverage

DAY 8

Breakfast
½ grapefruit
Egg Salad sandwich on enriched-flour toast
Milk

Morning Snack
Peanut butter and jelly on whole wheat crackers
Milk

Lunch
Salmon Patty on hard roll
Lettuce and tomato salad
Banana   Fruit juice

Afternoon Snack
Grapes   Wedge of Cheddar cheese
Milk

Dinner
Marinated Artichokes
Potted Lamb Shanks   Brown Rice
Bran rolls and butter
Fresh fruit   Beverage

DAY 9

Breakfast
½ cantaloupe with ½ cup cream-style cottage cheese
1 slice whole wheat bread with butter and jelly
Milk

Morning Snack
Bran muffin with butter or jelly
Milk

Lunch
Grilled cheeseburger on enriched-flour bun
Lettuce and tomato salad
Coleslaw and pickle
Fruit juice

Afternoon Snack
½ cup ice milk with sliced fresh fruit
Fruit juice

Dinner
Lentil Soup   Chicken-Potato Salad
Sliced tomatoes   Cucumber slices
Whole wheat rolls and butter
Sherbet   Beverage

DAY 10

Breakfast
½ grapefruit
¾ cup whole grain cereal with raisins and milk
Milk

Morning Snack
Cream cheese on 1 slice date-nut bread
Milk

Lunch
Salmon Patty on enriched-flour bun
Coleslaw, tomato wedges, and cucumber slices
Fruit juice

Afternoon Snack
Orange
Whole grain crackers with butter and jelly
Milk

Dinner
Tossed Salad with Oil and Vinegar Dressing and
feta cheese chunks
Jambon Normande   Mashed potatoes
Stuffed Mushrooms
Whole grain bread and butter
Fresh fruit   Beverage

DAY 11

Breakfast
Freshly squeezed orange juice
2 corn muffins with butter or jelly
Milk

Morning Snack
1 hard-boiled egg   Tomato wedges
Whole grain crackers with butter   Milk

Lunch
3¼ ounces drained canned tuna
½ cup cream-style cottage cheese
Lettuce wedge, tomato wedges, cucumber slices, and
carrot sticks
Pumpernickel roll with butter
Fruit juice

Afternoon Snack
¼ cup raisins   ¼ cup nuts   Milk

Dinner
Tossed salad with Oil and Vinegar Dressing
Eggplant Patties   Brown Rice
Bengal Beans   Bran rolls and butter
Frozen Yogurt Cream   Beverage

DAY 12

Breakfast
½ grapefruit   1 soft-boiled egg
Toasted English muffin with butter and jelly
Milk

Morning Snack
½ cup plain yogurt with sliced fresh fruit and
wheat germ
Fruit juice

Lunch
Liverwurst, lettuce, and tomato sandwich on
pumpernickel bread
Carrot sticks, green pepper strips, and pickle
Milk

Afternoon Snack
Peanut butter and jelly on whole wheat bread
Milk

Dinner
Lentil Soup   Chicken Rollups
Hard rolls and butter
Baked Apples   Beverage

DAY 13

Breakfast
Freshly squeezed orange juice
Cream cheese and boiled ham sandwich on
pumpernickel bread
Milk

Morning Snack
Bran muffin with butter or jelly
Milk

Lunch
3¼ ounces drained canned tuna, lettuce, and
tomato wedges in whole wheat pita
Cucumber slices, carrot sticks, and celery sticks
Fruit juice

Afternoon Snack
Baked Apple   Milk

Dinner
Eggplant-Gumbo Soup
Avocado Dinner Salad
Sliced tomatoes   Coleslaw
Bran rolls and butter
Fresh fruit with cheese   Beverage

DAY 14

Breakfast
Freshly squeezed grapefruit juice
¾ cup whole grain cereal with sliced banana
and milk
Milk

Morning Snack
Peanut butter and jelly on 1 slice whole-wheat bread
Milk

Lunch
Sliced turkey and coleslaw on hard roll
Lettuce and tomato salad
Fruit juice

Afternoon Snack
Pear and Cheddar cheese
Milk

Dinner
Lettuce Wedges with Oil and Vinegar Dressing
Fish Primavera   Hard rolls and butter
Fruit and cheese   Beverage

DAY 15

Breakfast
½ cantaloupe with ½ cup cream-style cottage cheese
Toasted English muffin with butter and jelly
Milk

Morning Snack
½ cup plain yogurt with raisins
Fruit juice

Lunch
Boiled ham and Swiss cheese sandwich on rye bread
Lettuce and tomato salad
Fruit juice

Afternoon Snack
1 slice of pizza
Milk

Dinner
Eggplant-Gumbo Soup   Asparagus Omelet
Victorian Spinach
Bran rolls and butter
Jam Parfait   Beverage

DAY 16

Breakfast
½ grapefruit   1 scrambled egg
1 slice whole grain toast with butter and jelly
Milk

Morning Snack
Corn muffin with butter or jelly
Milk

Lunch
Grilled hamburger on enriched-flour bun
Lettuce and tomato salad
Coleslaw and pickle
Fruit juice

Afternoon Snack
Grapes
Whole grain crackers with cream cheese
Milk

Dinner
Lentil Salad   Sicilian Cutlets
Rice Milanese   Sautéed String Beans
Hard rolls and butter
Fruit and cheese
Beverage

DAY 17

Breakfast
Freshly squeezed orange juice
Cinnamon-Cheese Toast
Milk

Morning Snack
1 hard-boiled egg
Tomato wedges and cucumber slices
Milk

Lunch
Salmon Salad and lettuce sandwich on hard roll
Coleslaw, pickle, and carrot sticks
Vegetable juice

Afternoon Snack
Apple and Cheddar cheese
Milk

Dinner
Broccoli and Tomato Salad
Sautéed Chicken Livers
Mashed potatoes   Sautéed Zucchini
Whole wheat bread and butter
Stewed Fruit   Beverage

DAY 18

Breakfast
Stewed Fruit
Salmon Salad on 1 toasted English muffin
Milk

Morning Snack
Cream cheese on 1 slice date-nut bread
Milk

Lunch
Peanut butter and jelly sandwich on
whole wheat bread
Apple
Milk

Afternoon Snack
½ cup plain yogurt sprinkled with wheat germ
Vegetable juice

Dinner
Tossed salad with Oil and Vinegar Dressing
Chili Beans and Tofu
Bran rolls and butter
Sautéed Bananas with Honey
Beverage

DAY 19

Breakfast
½ grapefruit
¾ cup whole grain cereal with raisins and milk
Milk

Morning Snack
Cheddar cheese and apple   Milk

Lunch
Chicken salad, lettuce, and tomato sandwich on
whole wheat bread
Coleslaw, pickle, and carrot sticks
Vegetable juice

Afternoon Snack
Peanut butter and jelly on whole grain crackers
Milk

Dinner
Egg Flower Soup
Shrimp in Lobster Sauce
Steamed rice   Sautéed Asparagus
Chilled mandarin orange segments
Beverage

DAY 20

Breakfast
Freshly squeezed orange juice
Cream cheese and jelly sandwich on
pumpernickel bread
Milk

Morning Snack
1 hard-boiled egg
Tomato wedges and cucumber slices
Milk

Lunch
Tuna Salad and lettuce sandwich on hard roll
Coleslaw and carrot sticks
Banana   Vegetable juice

Afternoon Snack
Swiss cheese on whole wheat crackers
Milk

Dinner
Marinated Artichokes
Near-East Chicken Soup
Bran rolls and butter
Chocolate-Raisin Bread Pudding
Beverage

DAY 21

Breakfast
½ grapefruit
Egg Salad on 1 toasted English muffin
Milk

Morning Snack
½ cup plain yogurt with raisins
Fruit juice

Lunch
Boiled ham, Swiss cheese, lettuce, and tomato
sandwich on whole wheat bread
Carrot sticks and pickle
Milk

Afternoon Snack
Apple with Cheddar cheese   Milk

Dinner
Basil Tomatoes with Oil and Vinegar Dressing
Beef Liver and Onions
Steamed Cabbage and Potatoes
Whole grain bread and butter
Fresh fruit   Beverage

DAY 22

Breakfast
Freshly squeezed grapefruit juice
¾ cup whole grain cereal with sliced
banana and milk
Milk

Morning Snack
Cream cheese and jelly on 1 slice whole wheat bread
Milk

Lunch
Egg Salad, lettuce, and tomato wedges in
whole wheat pita
Coleslaw and carrot sticks   Vegetable juice

Afternoon Snack
½ cup cream-style cottage cheese with
raisins and nuts
Milk

Dinner
Corn Salad   Chili Beans and Tofu
Steamed Spinach
Whole wheat bread and butter
Chocolate-Raisin Bread Pudding
Beverage

DAY 23

Breakfast
Freshly squeezed orange juice
1 poached egg on toasted whole grain bread
Milk

Morning Snack
½ cup plain yogurt with raisins and nuts
Fruit juice

Lunch
Sliced turkey and coleslaw sandwich on
pumpernickel bread
Tomato wedges, cucumber slices, and pickle
Milk

Afternoon Snack
Bran muffin with cream cheese and jelly
Milk

Dinner
Spiced Lamb Chops   Rice Pilaf
Bengal Beans   Cucumber Relish
Applesauce   Beverage

DAY 24

Breakfast
1 cup cream-style cottage cheese with
1 cup Applesauce
1 slice toasted whole grain bread with butter
Milk

Morning Snack
Sliced peaches with milk

Lunch
Roast beef, lettuce, and tomato sandwich on
rye bread
Potato salad and pickle
Milk

Afternoon Snack
Tangerine and Cheddar cheese
Milk

Dinner
String Beans Vinaigrette
Linguini with Marinara Sauce
French bread and butter
Fruit and cheese   Beverage

DAY 25

Breakfast
½ grapefruit
Grilled Cheddar cheese sandwich on rye bread
Milk

Morning Snack
½ cup plain yogurt with raisins
Fruit juice

Lunch
½ cantaloupe with 1 cup cream-style cottage cheese
Bran roll with butter
Milk

Afternoon Snack
Blueberry muffin with butter or jelly
Milk

Dinner
Cucumber and Tomato Salad with
feta cheese chunks
Meat Balls with Eggplant
Rice Pilaf
Whole wheat bread and butter
Applesauce   Beverage

DAY 26

Breakfast
Apple juice
¾ cup whole grain cereal with raisins and milk
Milk

Morning Snack
Cream cheese on 1 slice raisin bread
Milk

Lunch
Grilled cheeseburger on enriched-flour bun
Lettuce and tomato salad
Coleslaw and pickle   Vegetable juice

Afternoon Snack
Orange
Peanut butter on whole grain crackers
Milk

Dinner
Zucchini Soup à la Eve
Sautéed Chicken Breasts
Mashed potatoes   Steamed Spinach
Hard rolls and butter   Fresh fruit
Beverage

DAY 27

Breakfast
Freshly squeezed orange juice
1 scrambled egg
1 slice whole grain bread with butter and jelly
Milk

Morning Snack
½ cup plain yogurt with raisins and nuts
Fruit juice

Lunch
Boiled ham, Swiss cheese, and lettuce sandwich on
hard roll
Potato salad and cucumber slices
Milk

Afternoon Snack
Orange
½ cup cream-style cottage cheese
Mineral water

Dinner
Pasta and Salmon Salad   Sliced tomatoes
Cucumber Relish   Bran rolls and butter
Melon wedges   Beverage

DAY 28

Breakfast
½ grapefruit
2 bran muffins with cream cheese and jelly
Milk

Morning Snack
1 hard-boiled egg
Tomato wedges and cucumber slices
Milk

Lunch
Pasta and Salmon Salad
Carrot sticks and green pepper strips
Pumpernickel roll with butter
Vegetable juice

Afternoon Snack
Peanut butter and jelly on 1 slice whole wheat bread
Milk

Dinner
Twice-cooked Tofu and Vegetables
Sautéed Asparagus
Sherbet   Beverage

DAY 29

Breakfast
Freshly squeezed orange juice
Grilled ham and Swiss cheese sandwich on
rye bread
Milk

Morning Snack
Corn muffin with butter or jelly   Milk

Lunch
Sliced egg, lettuce, and tomato sandwich on
pumpernickel bread
Coleslaw and pickle   Milk

Afternoon Snack
½ cup plain yogurt with raisins
Apple juice

Dinner
Marinated Artichokes
Meat Balls with Eggplant   Thin egg noodles
Bran rolls and butter
Fruit and cheese   Beverage

DAY 30

Breakfast
Apple juice
¾ cup whole grain cereal with
sliced peaches and milk
Milk

Morning Snack
1 hard-boiled egg
1 slice whole grain bread with butter
Milk

Lunch
Roast beef, lettuce, and tomato sandwich on
rye bread
Potato salad   Vegetable juice

Afternoon Snack
Grapes with Swiss cheese
Whole grain crackers with butter   Milk

Dinner
Chicken Livers with Lemon, Oil, and Oregano
Mashed potatoes
Asparagus with Butter and Cheese
Whole wheat bread and butter
Brown Sugar-Banana Custard
Beverage

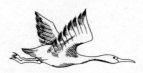 *The Eighth Month*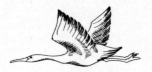

DAY 1

Breakfast
½ grapefruit
Cinnamon-Cheese Toast
Milk

Morning Snack
½ cup yogurt with sliced peaches and wheat germ
Fruit juice

Lunch
Cream-style cottage cheese and tomato sandwich on
whole wheat toast
Lettuce wedge, celery sticks, and carrot sticks
Milk

Afternoon Snack
Peanut butter on whole wheat crackers
Apple   Milk

Dinner
Cucumber and Tomato Salad
Pork Chops with Sauerkraut
Scalloped Potatoes
Pumpernickel bread and butter
Applesauce   Beverage

DAY 2

Breakfast
Freshly squeezed orange juice
1 soft-boiled egg
Toasted English muffin with butter and jelly

Morning Snack
Corn muffin with butter or jelly
Milk

Lunch
Liverwurst and lettuce sandwich on
pumpernickel bread
Coleslaw and pickle
Mineral water

Afternoon Snack
Apple and Swiss cheese
Milk

Dinner
Lettuce Wedges with Oil and Vinegar Dressing
Roast Beef   Brown Rice
Bran rolls and butter
Brown Sugar-Banana Custard
Beverage

DAY 3

Breakfast
Apple juice
¾ cup whole grain cereal with raisins and milk
Milk

Morning Snack
Toasted English muffin with cottage
cheese and chives
Milk

Lunch
Grilled hamburger on enriched-flour bun
Lettuce and tomato salad
Cucumber slices and carrot sticks
Fruit juice

Afternoon Snack
Apple
Peanut butter on whole grain crackers
Milk

Dinner
Split Pea Soup   Artichoke Omelet
Ratatouille   Whole wheat rolls and butter
Fruit and cheese   Beverage

DAY 4

Breakfast
Freshly squeezed orange juice
½ cup cream-style cottage cheese with 2 slices fresh
pineapple or canned pineapple in juice
1 slice buttered whole wheat toast   Milk

Morning Snack
1 hard-boiled egg
Tomato wedges and cucumber slices
Milk

Lunch
Roast beef, coleslaw, and lettuce sandwich on
pumpernickel bread
Carrot sticks, green pepper strips, and pickle
Vegetable juice

Afternoon Snack
¼ cup raisins   ¼ cup nuts   Milk

Dinner
String Beans Vinaigrette
Sautéed Chicken Breasts   Brown Rice
Hard rolls and butter
Frozen Yogurt Cream   Beverage

DAY 5

Breakfast
Freshly squeezed orange juice
Grilled ham and Swiss cheese sandwich on
rye bread
Milk

Morning Snack
Cream cheese on 1 slice date-nut bread   Milk

Lunch
2 hard-boiled eggs
Lettuce and tomato salad
Coleslaw, cucumber slices, and carrot sticks
Pumpernickel roll and butter
Vegetable juice

Afternoon Snack
Corn muffin with butter or jelly
Pear   Milk

Dinner
Split Pea Soup   Sautéed Bluefish
Boiled Potatoes with Oil and Parsley
Sautéed Zucchini
Bran rolls and butter   Baked Apples
Beverage

DAY 6

Breakfast
½ grapefruit
¾ cup whole grain cereal with sliced
banana and milk
Milk

Morning Snack
Cream cheese and jelly on 1 slice whole wheat bread
Milk

Lunch
Salmon Salad, lettuce, and tomato sandwich on
hard roll
Coleslaw and pickle   Vegetable juice

Afternoon Snack
Grapes and Swiss cheese   Milk

Dinner
Tossed salad with Oil and Vinegar Dressing
Pot Roast   Mashed potatoes
Whole wheat bread and butter
Baked Apples with softened vanilla ice cream
Beverage

DAY 7

Breakfast
Freshly squeezed orange juice
Salmon Salad on 1 toasted English muffin
Milk

Morning Snack
½ cup plain yogurt sprinkled with wheat germ
Cranberry juice

Lunch
Boiled ham, lettuce, and tomato sandwich on
whole wheat toast
Coleslaw and pickle   Milk

Afternoon Snack
Peanut butter and jelly on whole grain crackers
Milk

Dinner
Pickled Salad   Baked Ziti
French bread and butter
Fruit and cheese   Beverage

DAY 8

Breakfast
½ grapefruit
1 poached egg on buttered whole wheat toast
Milk

Morning Snack
½ cup cream-style cottage cheese with applesauce
Fruit juice

Lunch
Pot Roast, lettuce, and tomato sandwich on
whole wheat bread
Carrot sticks, green pepper strips, and pickle
Milk

Afternoon Snack
¼ cup raisins and dried fruit
¼ cup nuts   Milk

Dinner
Eggplant and Rice Salad on lettuce leaves
Grilled Hamburger   Sliced tomato
Bran rolls and butter
Baked Custard   Beverage

DAY 9

Breakfast
Apple juice
Cream cheese and boiled ham sandwich on
pumpernickel bread
Milk

Morning Snack
Graham crackers with jelly
Milk

Lunch
Sliced turkey, Swiss cheese, and coleslaw on
hard roll
Vegetable juice

Afternoon Snack
1 slice of pizza
Milk

Dinner
Broccoli and Tomato Salad
Sautéed Flounder Fillet
Glazed Carrots   Steamed Spinach
Whole wheat bread and butter
Fresh pineapple slices   Beverage

DAY 10

Breakfast
Freshly squeezed orange juice
¾ cup whole grain cereal with raisins and milk
Milk

Morning Snack
Bran muffin with butter or jelly
Wedge of cheese   Milk

Lunch
Sliced egg, lettuce, and tomato sandwich on
hard roll
Coleslaw and pickle   ¼ cup raw nuts
Apple   Vegetable juice

Afternoon Snack
½ bagel with cream cheese
Milk

Dinner
Marinated Artichokes
Baked Ziti with Meat Sauce
Hard rolls and butter
Fresh fruit   Beverage

DAY 11

Breakfast
½ cantaloupe with 1 cup cream-style cottage cheese
1 slice buttered whole wheat toast   Milk

Morning Snack
Banana
Peanut butter and jelly on whole wheat crackers
Milk

Lunch
Roast beef, lettuce, and tomato sandwich on
hard roll
Coleslaw and pickle   Fruit juice

Afternoon Snack
Apple and wedge of cheese   Milk

Dinner
Lentil Soup
Egg Salad on lettuce leaves
Marinated Potato Salad
Sliced tomato   Cucumber slices
Bran rolls and butter
Fresh pineapple slices   Beverage

DAY 12

Breakfast
Freshly squeezed grapefruit juice
1 scrambled egg
1 slice whole wheat toast with butter or jelly
Milk

Morning Snack
½ cup cream-style cottage cheese with applesauce
Milk

Lunch
Liverwurst and Swiss cheese sandwich on
pumpernickel bread
Lettuce and tomato salad   Milk

Afternoon Snack
Orange
Whole wheat crackers with butter
Fruit juice

Dinner
Cold Cucumber Soup
Baked Fish with Eggplant   Rice Pilaf
Whole wheat bread and butter
Apple and Pear Compote
Beverage

DAY 13

Breakfast
Freshly squeezed orange juice
¾ cup whole grain cereal with
sliced bananas and milk
Milk

Morning Snack
Corn muffin with butter or jelly
Fruit juice

Lunch
Tuna salad, lettuce, and tomato sandwich on whole
wheat bread
Tangerine   Milk

Afternoon Snack
Apple and Pear Compote
Wedge of Cheddar cheese
Milk

Dinner
Corn Salad on lettuce leaves   Pot Roast
Mashed potatoes   Sautéed String Beans
Hard rolls and butter
Gold-topped Ice Cream   Beverage

DAY 14

Breakfast
Freshly squeezed grapefruit juice
Peanut butter and jelly sandwich on
whole wheat bread
Milk

Morning Snack
1 hard-boiled egg
Cream cheese and chives on whole wheat crackers
Vegetable juice

Lunch
Pot Roast sandwich on hard roll
Lettuce and tomato salad
Coleslaw and pickle   Milk

Afternoon Snack
Grapes with Cheddar cheese   Milk

Dinner
Cottage Cheese Salad and sliced tomatoes on
lettuce leaves
Broccoli and Bean Soup
Bran rolls and butter
Apple and Pear Compote   Beverage

DAY 15

Breakfast
Apple juice
Grilled Cheddar cheese sandwich on rye bread
Milk

Morning Snack
Cream cheese on ½ raisin bagel
Milk

Lunch
Sliced egg, lettuce, and tomato sandwich on
whole grain bread
Carrot sticks, cucumber slices, and pickle
Vegetable juice

Afternoon Snack
Apple and Swiss cheese
Milk

Dinner
Basil Tomatoes with Oil and Vinegar Dressing
Chicken Breasts Florentine   Mashed potatoes
Whole wheat bread and butter
Fresh fruit   Beverage

DAY 16

Breakfast
½ grapefruit   Cinnamon-Cheese Toast
Milk

Morning Snack
1 hard-boiled egg
Tomato wedges and cucumber slices
Milk

Lunch
Sliced turkey and coleslaw sandwich on hard roll
Carrot sticks, green pepper strips, and pickle
Fruit juice

Afternoon Snack
Orange
Peanut butter on 1 slice whole wheat bread
Milk

Dinner
Roast Beef   Wide noodles
Buttered green peas
Hard rolls and butter
Jam Parfait   Beverage

DAY 17

Breakfast
Freshly squeezed orange juice
¾ cup whole grain cereal with
sliced banana and milk
Milk

Morning Snack
Corn muffin with butter or jelly
Milk

Lunch
Boiled ham, Swiss cheese, and lettuce sandwich on
whole wheat bread
Tomato wedges, cucumber slices, and carrot sticks
Vegetable juice

Afternoon Snack
¼ cup raisins and dried fruit   ¼ cup nuts
Milk

Dinner
Cream of Mushroom-Barley Soup
Baked Veal Chops   Steamed broccoli
Bran rolls and butter
Fresh fruit   Beverage

DAY 18

Breakfast
½ grapefruit
Cream cheese and jelly on pumpernickel bread
Milk

Morning Snack
½ cup plain yogurt with sliced fresh fruit
and wheat germ
Fruit juice

Lunch
1 cup cream-style cottage cheese
3 slices fresh pineapple or canned pineapple in juice
1 slice whole grain bread with butter
Milk

Afternoon Snack
Graham crackers with peanut butter
Milk

Dinner
Chick-pea Salad   Spinach Pie
Glazed Carrots
Whole wheat bread and butter
Rice Pudding   Beverage

DAY 19

Breakfast
Freshly squeezed orange juice
1 soft-boiled egg
Toasted English muffin with butter or jelly
Milk

Morning Snack
Bran muffin with butter or jelly
Wedge of cheese   Milk

Lunch
Liverwurst, Swiss cheese, and lettuce sandwich on
hard roll
Coleslaw and pickle   Vegetable juice

Afternoon Snack
Grapes
½ cup cream-style cottage cheese
Milk

Dinner
Lettuce Wedges with Oil and Vinegar Dressing
Pasta with Cauliflower-Veal Sauce
French bread and butter
Fresh fruit   Beverage

DAY 20

Breakfast
Freshly squeezed orange juice
Grilled ham and Swiss cheese sandwich
on rye bread
Milk

Morning Snack
½ cup plain yogurt with sliced fresh fruit
and wheat germ
Fruit juice

Lunch
Spinach Pie
Cucumber slices, carrot sticks, and
green pepper strips
Apple   Milk

Afternoon Snack
Peanut butter and jelly on whole grain crackers
Milk

Dinner
Split Pea Soup   Stuffed Tomato Salad Plate
Pumpernickel rolls and butter
Rice Pudding   Beverage

DAY 21

Breakfast
½ grapefruit
¾ cup whole grain cereal with raisins and milk
Milk

Morning Snack
Corn muffin with butter or jelly
Milk

Lunch
Tuna salad, lettuce, and tomato sandwich on
whole grain bread
Milk

Afternoon Snack
Orange and Swiss cheese
Fruit juice

Dinner
Bean Sprout Fritters   Curried Rice
Bengal Beans   Onion Relish
Sautéed Bananas with Honey
Beverage

DAY 22

Breakfast
½ cantaloupe with ½ cup cream-style cottage cheese
1 slice whole grain toast with butter and jelly
Milk

Morning Snack
1 hard-boiled egg
Tomato wedges and cucumber slices
Milk

Lunch
Roast beef and lettuce sandwich on hard roll
Coleslaw and pickle   Vegetable juice

Afternoon Snack
Graham crackers and jelly
Milk

Dinner
Lentil Salad   Cornish Hen Cacciatore
Linguini   Hard rolls and butter
Ice cream   Beverage

DAY 23

Breakfast
Freshly squeezed orange juice
1 scrambled egg
Toasted English muffin with butter and jelly
Milk

Morning Snack
Cream cheese on 1 slice date-nut bread
Milk

Lunch
Grilled cheeseburger on enriched-flour bun
Lettuce and tomato salad
Coleslaw and pickle   Vegetable juice

Afternoon Snack
Grapes
Peanut butter on whole grain crackers
Milk

Dinner
Egg Flower Soup   Sautéed Flounder Fillets
Victorian Spinach
Whole wheat bread and butter
Fresh fruit   Beverage

DAY 24

Breakfast
¾ cup whole grain cereal with sliced banana
and milk
1 slice toasted enriched bread with butter
Milk

Morning Snack
½ cup cream-style cottage cheese with
shredded carrots
Vegetable juice

Lunch
Boiled ham and Egg Salad sandwich on
whole wheat bread
Lettuce and tomato salad
Orange   Milk

Afternoon Snack
Apple   Ice Milk

Dinner
Mushroom Salad
Pasta and Eggplant Casserole
Hard rolls and butter
Fruit and cheese   Beverage

DAY 25

Breakfast
½ grapefruit
Cream cheese on toasted raisin bread
Milk

Morning Snack
Corn muffin with butter or jelly
Wedge of cheese   Milk

Lunch
Sliced turkey, lettuce, and tomato sandwich
on hard roll
Potato salad and carrot sticks
Fruit juice

Afternoon Snack
Peanut butter and jelly on 1 slice whole wheat bread
Milk

Dinner
Beef Bouillon with Mushrooms and Chives
Broccoli Omelet   Sliced tomatoes
Bran rolls and butter
Bananas and cheese   Beverage

DAY 26

Breakfast
Apple juice
Grilled Cheddar cheese sandwich on rye bread
Milk

Morning Snack
½ cup cream-style cottage cheese with applesauce
Milk

Lunch
Egg Salad, lettuce, and tomato wedges in whole
wheat pita
Coleslaw and pickle
Vegetable juice

Afternoon Snack
Orange
1 bagel with cream cheese
Milk

Dinner
Eggplant Salad   Sautéed Oysters
Cinnamon-Almond Pilaf
Sautéed String Beans
Whole wheat bread and butter
Melon wedges   Beverage

DAY 27

Breakfast
Freshly squeezed grapefruit juice
¾ cup whole grain cereal with raisins and milk
Milk

Morning Snack
Cream cheese on 1 slice raisin bread
Milk

Lunch
Tuna Salad and lettuce sandwich on
whole wheat bread
Tomato wedges, cucumber slices, and green
pepper strips
Vegetable juice

Afternoon Snack
Banana
Peanut butter on whole grain crackers
Milk

Dinner
White Bean Salad   Sautéed Veal Chops
Stewed Cauliflower   Bran rolls and butter
Fruit and cheese   Beverage

DAY 28

Breakfast
Apple juice
Cream cheese and boiled ham sandwich on
pumpernickel bread
Milk

Morning Snack
½ cup plain yogurt with sliced fresh fruit
Fruit juice

Lunch
Swiss cheese and tomato sandwich on hard roll
Coleslaw and pickle
Apple   Milk

Afternoon Snack
Graham crackers with jelly
Milk

Dinner
Corn Salad on lettuce leaves
Chicken in Mustard Sauce
Rice Pilaf   Steamed Spinach
Hard rolls and butter
Fresh fruit   Beverage

DAY 29

Breakfast
½ grapefruit   French toast
Milk

Morning Snack
1 hard-boiled egg   Tomato wedges
1 slice whole grain bread with butter
Milk

Lunch
Liverwurst and lettuce sandwich on
pumpernickel roll
Potato salad and tomato wedges
Vegetable juice

Afternoon Snack
Apple and Cheddar cheese
Whole grain crackers with butter
Milk

Dinner
Egg Flower Soup   Noodle Salad
Sliced tomatoes
Whole wheat bread and butter
Chilled Mandarin orange segments
Beverage

DAY 30

Breakfast
Freshly squeezed grapefruit juice
1 poached egg on toasted whole grain bread
Milk

Morning Snack
½ cup plain yogurt with nuts and raisins
Fruit juice

Lunch
Roast beef and coleslaw sandwich on hard roll
Lettuce and tomato salad
Milk

Afternoon Snack
Apple and Swiss cheese
Milk

Dinner
Lentil Salad   Marinated Haddock
Sautéed Peppers and Potatoes
French bread and butter
Sherbet   Beverage

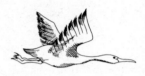 *The Ninth Month*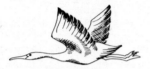

DAY 1

Breakfast
Apple juice
¾ cup whole grain cereal with sliced banana
and milk
Milk

Morning Snack
Cream cheese on 1 slice raisin bread
Milk

Lunch
Salmon Salad, lettuce, and tomato sandwich on
whole wheat bread
Cucumber slices and carrot sticks
Milk

Afternoon Snack
1 slice of pizza   Milk

Dinner
Roast Turkey Breast
Mashed potatoes   Sautéed Zucchini
Cranberry Sauce
Hard rolls and butter
Ice Cream   Beverage

DAY 2

Breakfast
½ grapefruit
Salmon salad on 1 toasted English muffin
Milk

Morning Snack
Bran muffin with cream cheese
Milk

Lunch
Sliced turkey, lettuce, and tomato sandwich on
hard roll
Coleslaw and pickle
Milk

Afternoon Snack
½ cup plain yogurt with raisins
Fruit juice

Dinner
Cucumber and Tomato Salad
Gandules with Rice   Steamed Broccoli
Bran rolls and butter
Stewed fruit   Milk

DAY 3

Breakfast
Stewed Fruit   1 scrambled egg
1 slice whole wheat toast with butter and jelly
Milk

Morning Snack
Butter and jelly on 1 slice raisin bread
Milk

Lunch
Tuna Salad, lettuce, and tomato wedges in
whole wheat pita
Carrot sticks, cucumber slices, and pickle
Freshly squeezed orange juice

Afternoon Snack
Apple
Peanut butter on whole grain crackers
Milk

Dinner
Broccoli and Tomato Salad
Quiche Lorraine   Glazed Carrots
Whole wheat bread and butter
Ice milk with chopped nuts
Beverage

DAY 4

Breakfast
½ grapefruit
¾ cup whole grain cereal with raisins and milk
Milk

Morning Snack
English muffin with toasted cheese
Milk

Lunch
Sliced turkey on hard roll
Lettuce and tomato salad
Coleslaw and pickle   Vegetable juice

Afternoon Snack
Stewed Fruit   Milk

Dinner
Cream of Mushroom-Barley Soup
Beef Liver Sauté   Brown Rice
Sautéed String Beans
Bran rolls and butter
Pears and cheese   Beverage

DAY 5

Breakfast
Freshly squeezed orange juice
Cinnamon-Cheese Toast
Milk

Morning Snack
½ cup plain yogurt sprinkled with
sliced fresh fruit and wheat germ
Fruit juice

Lunch
1 cup cream-style cottage cheese with 3 slices fresh
pineapple or canned pineapple in juice
Pumpernickel roll and butter
Milk

Afternoon Snack
Peanut butter and jelly on whole grain crackers
Milk

Dinner
Lentil Soup   Quiche Lorraine
Sliced tomatoes
Whole wheat bread and butter
Fresh Fruit   Beverage

DAY 6

Breakfast
Freshly squeezed orange juice
Grilled Cheddar cheese sandwich on rye bread
Milk

Morning Snack
1 hard-boiled egg
Bran muffin with butter or jelly
Milk

Lunch
Liverwurst, lettuce, and tomato sandwich on
pumpernickel bread
Coleslaw and pickle   Vegetable juice

Afternoon Snack
¼ cup raisins   ¼ cup nuts
Milk

Dinner
Shrimp with Garlic Sauce
Steamed rice   Sautéed Asparagus
Fresh pineapple slices
Beverage

DAY 7

Breakfast
Freshly squeezed grapefruit juice
¾ cup whole grain cereal with
sliced berries and milk
Milk

Morning Snack
Cream cheese on 1 slice date-nut bread   Milk

Lunch
Sliced egg, lettuce, and tomato sandwich on
whole wheat toast
Carrot sticks, celery sticks, and pickle
Milk

Afternoon Snack
½ cup plain yogurt with raisins and nuts
Fruit juice

Dinner
Lettuce Wedges with Oil and Vinegar Dressing
Sautéed Scallops
Boiled Potatoes with Sour Cream and Chives
Steamed Broccoli   Bran rolls and butter
Ice milk with fruit topping   Beverage

DAY 8

Breakfast
Freshly squeezed orange juice
1 poached egg on whole wheat toast   Milk

Morning Snack
½ cup cream-style cottage cheese with ½ cup sliced,
unsweetened fresh fruit
Milk

Lunch
Roast beef and lettuce on hard roll
Tomato wedges, carrot sticks, and pickle
Fruit juice

Afternoon Snack
Orange
Peanut butter on whole grain crackers
Milk

Dinner
Lentil Soup
Turkey Fricassee with Biscuit Topping
Tossed salad with Oil and Vinegar Dressing
Fresh pineapple slices with vanilla ice cream
Beverage

DAY 9

Breakfast
½ grapefruit
1 English muffin with toasted cheese
Milk

Morning Snack
1 hard-boiled egg
Tomato wedges and cucumber slices
Milk

Lunch
Peanut butter and jelly on whole wheat bread
Tangerine   Milk

Afternoon Snack
½ cup plain yogurt with nuts
Vegetable juice

Dinner
Chick-pea Salad
Spaghetti with Tomato-Caper Sauce
Hard rolls and butter
Fruit and cheese   Beverage

DAY 10

Breakfast
Freshly squeezed orange juice
¾ cup whole grain cereal with raisins and milk
Milk

Morning Snack
Bran muffin with peanut butter and jelly
Milk

Lunch
Tuna Salad and lettuce sandwich on hard roll
Coleslaw and pickle   Vegetable juice

Afternoon Snack
Apple and Swiss cheese
Milk

Dinner
Marinated Chicken Breasts
Rice Salad   String Beans Vinaigrette
Sliced tomatoes
Bran rolls and butter
Melon wedges with ice cream
Beverage

DAY 11

Breakfast
Melon wedge
Tuna Salad on toasted English muffin
Milk

Morning Snack
½ cup plain yogurt sprinkled with wheat germ
Orange segments

Lunch
Sliced turkey and coleslaw sandwich on hard roll
Lettuce and tomato salad
Milk

Afternoon Snack
Peanut butter and jelly on 1 slice whole-wheat bread
Milk

Dinner
Corn Salad on lettuce leaves
Spareribs with Cabbage and Potatoes
Whole wheat bread and butter
Jam Parfait   Beverage

DAY 12

Breakfast
Tangerine
Tuna Salad sandwich on whole wheat toast
Milk

Morning Snack
Cream cheese on 1 slice date-nut bread
Milk

Lunch
Roast beef, lettuce, and tomato sandwich on
rye bread
Coleslaw and pickle   Vegetable juice

Afternoon snack
Graham crackers and jelly
Milk

Dinner
Salmon Salad on lettuce leaves
Rice Salad   Sliced tomatoes
Cucumber Relish
Bran rolls and butter
Fresh fruit with cheese
Beverage

DAY 13

Breakfast
½ grapefruit
¾ cup whole grain cereal with milk
Milk

Morning Snack
1 bagel with cream cheese
Milk

Lunch
Cream cheese and boiled ham sandwich on
pumpernickel bread
Coleslaw, carrot sticks, and green pepper strips
Vegetable juice

Afternoon Snack
¼ cup raisins   ¼ cup nuts
Milk

Dinner
Broccoli and Tomato Salad
Poached Eggs with Stewed Zucchini
Whole wheat bread and butter
Fruit and cheese   Beverage

DAY 14

Breakfast
Freshly squeezed orange juice
1 soft-boiled egg
Toasted English muffin with butter and jelly
Milk

Morning Snack
½ cup plain yogurt with raisins and nuts
Fruit juice

Lunch
Cream-style cottage cheese, lettuce, and tomato
sandwich on whole wheat toast
Apple   Milk

Afternoon Snack
Bran muffin with peanut butter and jelly
Milk

Dinner
Roladen   Wide noodles
Red Cabbage   Applesauce
Pumpernickel bread and butter
Brown Sugar-Banana Custard
Beverage

DAY 15

Breakfast
Freshly squeezed orange juice
Grilled ham and Swiss cheese sandwich on
rye bread
Milk

Morning Snack
Cream cheese on 1 slice date-nut bread
Milk

Lunch
2 hard-boiled eggs
Lettuce and tomato salad
Cucumber slices, carrot sticks, and celery sticks
Hard roll and butter   Vegetable juice

Afternoon Snack
Brown Sugar-Banana Custard
Milk

Dinner
Eggplant Salad   Baked Tile Fish
Stewed Zucchini
Whole wheat bread and butter
Vanilla ice cream topped with Applesauce
Beverage

DAY 16

Breakfast
1 cup Applesauce mixed with 1 cup cream-style
cottage cheese
1 slice toasted whole grain bread with butter
Milk

Morning Snack
Bran muffin with butter or jelly   Milk

Lunch
Liverwurst, lettuce, and Swiss cheese sandwich on
pumpernickel roll
Coleslaw and pickle   Vegetable juice

Afternoon Snack
Grapes
Peanut butter on whole wheat crackers
Milk

Dinner
String Beans Vinaigrette
Eggplant Rollups   Linguini
French bread and butter
Fresh fruit and cheese   Beverage

DAY 17

Breakfast
Freshly squeezed grapefruit juice
¾ cup whole grain cereal with sliced
banana and milk
Milk

Morning Snack
Graham crackers with cream cheese and jelly
Milk

Lunch
Grilled cheeseburger on enriched-flour bun
Lettuce and tomato salad
Coleslaw and pickle   Fruit juice

Afternoon Snack
1 slice of pizza
Milk

Dinner
Pickled Salad   Sautéed Veal Cutlets
Stewed Zucchini
Bran rolls and butter
Rice Pudding   Beverage

DAY 18

Breakfast
Apple juice
1 toasted English muffin with cheese
Milk

Morning Snack
Cream cheese and jelly on 1 slice raisin bread
Milk

Lunch
Egg Salad, lettuce, and tomato sandwich on
whole wheat bread
Cucumber slices, carrot sticks, and celery sticks
Vegetable juice

Afternoon Snack
¼ cup raisins   ¼ cup nuts
Milk

Dinner
Chick-pea Salad   Chicken Gumbo
Steamed rice   Bran rolls and butter
Fresh fruit   Beverage

DAY 19

Breakfast
½ grapefruit
Egg Salad on 1 toasted English muffin
Milk

Morning Snack
Peanut butter and jelly on 1 slice whole wheat bread
Milk

Lunch
Roast beef and coleslaw sandwich on
pumpernickel roll
Apple   Milk

Afternoon Snack
½ cup plain yogurt sprinkled with wheat germ
Vegetable juice

Dinner
Broccoli and Tomato Salad
Linguini with Anchovy and Tomato Sauce
Hard rolls and butter
Fruit and cheese   Beverage

DAY 20

Breakfast
Freshly squeezed orange juice
¾ cup whole grain cereal with raisins and milk
Milk

Morning Snack
Cream cheese on 1 slice date-nut bread
Milk

Lunch
Egg Salad, lettuce, and tomato wedges in
whole wheat pita
Banana   Milk

Afternoon Snack
Apple   ¼ cup nuts
Fruit juice

Dinner
Pickled Salad
Braised Lamb Chops with Lentils Provençale
Whole wheat bread and butter
Rice Pudding   Beverage

DAY 21

Breakfast
Apple juice
Cinnamon-Cheese Toast
Milk

Morning Snack
Corn muffin with butter or jelly
Milk

Lunch
Sliced turkey, lettuce, and tomato sandwich on
hard roll
Coleslaw and pickle
Vegetable juice

Afternoon Snack
Orange
Peanut butter on whole wheat crackers
Milk

Dinner
String Beans Vinaigrette
Eggplant Rollups   Rice Pilaf
Hard rolls and butter
Gold-topped Ice Cream
Beverage

DAY 22

Breakfast
½ grapefruit
1 poached egg on toasted whole wheat bread
Milk

Morning Snack
Cream cheese on 1 slice pumpernickel bread
Milk

Lunch
Boiled ham, Swiss cheese, and lettuce sandwich on
hard roll
Tomato wedges, cucumber slices, and pickle
Vegetable juice

Afternoon Snack
Bran muffin with butter or jelly
Milk

Dinner
White Bean Salad
Chicken Gumbo   Steamed rice
Whole wheat bread and butter
Melon wedges   Beverage

DAY 23

Breakfast
Freshly squeezed orange juice
¾ cup whole grain cereal with
sliced banana and milk
Milk

Morning Snack
Melon wedge with ½ cup cream-style cottage cheese
Fruit juice

Lunch
Salmon Salad, lettuce, and tomato sandwich on
pumpernickel bread
Coleslaw and pickle   Milk

Afternoon Snack
Cheddar cheese on whole wheat crackers
Milk

Dinner
Sliced tomatoes with lemon wedges
Beef Liver and Onions   Mashed potatoes
Asparagus with Butter and Cheese
Hard rolls and butter
Ice milk   Beverage

DAY 24

Breakfast
Apple juice
Salmon Salad on toasted English muffin
Milk

Morning Snack
Corn muffin with butter or jelly   Milk

Lunch
Sliced egg, lettuce, and tomato sandwich on
pumpernickel bread
Cucumber slices, carrot sticks, and
green pepper strips
Milk

Afternoon Snack
½ cup plain yogurt with raisins
Vegetable juice

Dinner
Cold Cucumber Soup
Veal Rolls with Mustard
Steamed Spinach   Glazed Carrots
Whole wheat bread and butter
Ice cream   Beverage

DAY 25

Breakfast
Freshly squeezed grapefruit juice
Grilled ham and Swiss cheese on rye bread
Milk

Morning Snack
Bran muffin with butter or jelly   Milk

Lunch
Tuna salad, lettuce, and tomato wedges in
whole wheat pita
Coleslaw and pickle   Vegetable juice

Afternoon Snack
Pear
Peanut butter on whole grain crackers
Milk

Dinner
Lettuce Wedges with Oil and Vinegar Dressing
Cauliflower Omelet
Lima Beans with Blue Cheese
Bran rolls and butter
Fresh fruit   Beverage

DAY 26

Breakfast
½ grapefruit
¾ cup whole grain cereal with raisins and milk
Milk

Morning Snack
Cream cheese on 1 slice date-nut bread
Milk

Lunch
Sliced turkey, lettuce, and tomato sandwich on
hard roll
Coleslaw and pickle   Fruit juice

Afternoon Snack
½ cup plain yogurt with nuts and raisins
Milk

Dinner
Cold Cucumber Soup
Parmesan Hamburger Patties
Steamed Cabbage and Potatoes
Whole wheat bread and butter
Baked Apples with ice milk
Beverage

DAY 27

Breakfast
Freshly squeezed orange juice
1 scrambled egg
Toasted English muffin with butter and jelly
Milk

Morning Snack
Baked Apple
Milk

Lunch
Liverwurst, lettuce, and tomato sandwich on
pumpernickel roll
Cucumber slices and carrot sticks
Vegetable juice

Afternoon Snack
1 slice of pizza
Milk

Dinner
Marinated Artichokes
Sautéed Veal Cutlets
Macaroncelli with Zucchini Sauce
Hard rolls and butter
Grapes and cheese   Beverage

DAY 28

Breakfast
Apple juice
2 bran muffins with butter or jelly
Milk

Morning Snack
Peanut butter on whole grain crackers
Milk

Lunch
Cream-style cottage cheese, lettuce, and tomato
sandwich on whole wheat bread
Coleslaw and carrot sticks
Fruit juice

Afternoon Snack
Ice cream with chopped nuts

Dinner
Coconut Chicken   Curried Rice
Baked Cauliflower Beignets
Whole grain bread and butter
Fresh fruit and cheese   Beverage

DAY 29

Breakfast
Freshly squeezed orange juice
¾ cup whole grain cereal with sliced
banana and milk
Milk

Morning Snack
½ cup plain yogurt with sliced fresh fruit
and wheat germ
Milk

Lunch
Coconut Chicken   Potato Salad
Lettuce and tomato wedges   Fruit juice

Afternoon Snack
¼ cup raisins   ¼ cup nuts
Milk

Dinner
Basil Tomatoes with Oil and Vinegar Dressing
Pork Chops with Cabbage and Potatoes
Bran rolls and butter
Fresh fruit and cheese   Beverage

DAY 30

Breakfast
Freshly squeezed orange juice
Grilled ham and Cheddar cheese sandwich on
rye bread
Milk

Morning Snack
Corn muffin with butter or jelly
Milk

Lunch
Sliced turkey, lettuce, and tomato sandwich on
whole wheat bread
Carrot sticks and green pepper strips
Apple   Milk

Afternoon Snack
Grapes
Peanut butter on whole grain crackers
Milk

Dinner
Braciole   Spaghetti
Steamed Broccoli with butter
Hard rolls and butter
Fruit and cheese   Beverage

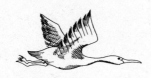 *Breast Feeding*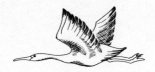

DAY 1

Breakfast
½ grapefruit
¾ cup whole grain cereal with raisins and milk
Milk

Morning Snack
Bran muffin with butter or jelly
Milk

Lunch
Sliced egg, lettuce, and tomato sandwich on
hard roll
Coleslaw, carrot sticks, and green pepper strips
Fruit juice

Afternoon Snack
Cream cheese on 1 slice date-nut bread
Milk

Dinner
Lettuce Wedges with Oil and Vinegar Dressing
Sautéed Flounder Fillets with Tomato-Caper Sauce
Rice Pilaf   Steamed Spinach
Hard rolls and butter   Baked Apples
Milk

DAY 2

Breakfast
Apple juice
Cinnamon-Cheese Toast
Milk

Morning Snack
1 cup plain yogurt with raisins and wheat germ
Fruit juice

Lunch
Roast beef, lettuce and tomato sandwich
on hard roll
Coleslaw and pickle   Milk

Afternoon Snack
Peanut butter and jelly on 1 slice raisin bread
Milk

Dinner
Eggplant Salad   Turkey with Mornay Sauce
Sautéed String Beans
Bran rolls and butter
Fruit and cheese   Milk

DAY 3

Breakfast
Freshly squeezed orange juice
Grilled Swiss cheese sandwich on rye bread
Banana   Milk

Morning Snack
Graham crackers with butter or jelly
Milk

Lunch
Sliced turkey on lettuce leaves
Potato salad, sliced tomato, and cucumber slices
Bran roll and butter
Milk

Afternoon Snack
1 cup cream-style cottage cheese with 2 slices fresh
pineapple or canned pineapple in juice
Fruit juice

Dinner
Egg Flower Soup   Homestyle Beef Liver
Steamed rice   Baked Apples
Milk

DAY 4

Breakfast
½ grapefruit
2 corn muffins with cream cheese and jelly
Milk

Morning Snack
1 cup plain yogurt with sliced, unsweetened
fresh fruit
Fruit juice

Lunch
Grilled hamburger on enriched-flour bun
Coleslaw and lettuce and tomato salad
Milk

Afternoon Snack
Apple and Cheddar cheese
Milk

Dinner
Stuffed Mushrooms
Macaroncelli with Zucchini Sauce
Hard rolls and butter
Vanilla ice cream with sliced bananas
Milk

DAY 5

Breakfast
Freshly squeezed orange juice
¾ cup whole grain cereal with sliced peaches
and milk
Milk

Morning Snack
Cream cheese on 1 slice date-nut bread
Milk

Lunch
Boiled ham, lettuce, and tomato sandwich on
whole wheat bread
Coleslaw and pickle
Fruit juice

Afternoon Snack
Orange
Peanut butter on whole grain crackers
Milk

Dinner
Turkey Patties with Cream Gravy
Sautéed Mushrooms   Glazed Carrots
Whole wheat bread and butter
Rice Pudding   Milk

DAY 6

Breakfast
½ grapefruit   1 scrambled egg
Toasted English muffin with butter and jelly
Milk

Morning Snack
1 cup plain yogurt with raisins and nuts
Milk

Lunch
Tuna Salad, lettuce, and tomato sandwich on
pumpernickel bread
Coleslaw and pickle
Fruit juice

Afternoon Snack
Orange and Swiss cheese
Whole grain crackers with butter
Milk

Dinner
White Bean Salad   Braciole
Spaghetti   Hard rolls and butter
Fresh fruit   Milk

DAY 7

Breakfast
Apple juice
Tuna Salad on toasted English muffin
Milk

Morning Snack
Bran muffin with butter or jelly   Milk

Lunch
Liverwurst, lettuce, and tomato sandwich on
rye bread
Carrot sticks, cucumber slices, and
green pepper strips
Vegetable juice

Afternoon Snack
Cream cheese on 1 slice date-nut bread
Milk

Dinner
Egyptian Pea Soup
Anytime Dinner Salad
Whole wheat bread and butter
Rice Pudding   Milk

DAY 8

Breakfast
Freshly squeezed grapefruit juice
¾ cup whole grain cereal with raisins and milk
Milk

Morning Snack
1 cup cream-style cottage cheese with ½ cup sliced,
unsweetened fresh fruit
Milk

Lunch
Egyptian Pea Soup
Tuna Salad, lettuce, and tomato sandwich on
whole-wheat bread
Vegetable juice

Afternoon Snack
Apple and Cheddar cheese
Whole grain crackers with butter
Milk

Dinner
Marinated Artichokes   Oyster Pilaf
Sautéed Zucchini
French bread and butter
Melon wedge   Milk

DAY 9

Breakfast
Melon wedge   1 soft-boiled egg
1 slice whole grain toast with butter and jelly
Milk

Morning Snack
Peanut butter and jelly on 1 slice whole wheat bread
Milk

Lunch
Swiss cheese, lettuce, and tomato sandwich on
French bread
Coleslaw and pickle   Fruit juice

Afternoon Snack
Orange
Whole grain crackers with butter
Milk

Dinner
Egg Flower Soup
Chicken-Potato Salad on lettuce leaves
Sliced tomatoes   Corn Salad
Bran rolls and butter
Fresh fruit   Milk

DAY 10

Breakfast
Freshly squeezed orange juice
1 cup plain yogurt with wheat germ and raisins
1 slice toasted whole wheat bread with butter
and jelly
Milk

Morning Snack
Corn muffin with butter or jelly   Milk

Lunch
Cream cheese and boiled ham sandwich on
pumpernickel bread
Lettuce and tomato salad   Vegetable juice

Afternoon Snack
Banana
Peanut butter on whole wheat crackers
Milk

Dinner
Beef Bouillon with Mushrooms and Chives
Salmon and Noodle Bake   Ratatouille
Whole wheat bread and butter
Ice milk   Beverage

DAY 11

Breakfast
½ grapefruit
¾ cup whole grain cereal with sliced
banana and milk
Milk

Morning Snack
Cream cheese and jelly on 1 slice raisin bread
Milk

Lunch
Salmon and Noodle Bake
Pumpernickel bread and butter
Cucumber slices, carrot sticks, and green
pepper strips
Vegetable juice

Afternoon Snack
Ice milk with sliced fresh fruit

Dinner
Cottage Cheese Salad   Sautéed Veal Chops
Mashed potatoes   Victorian Spinach
Bran roll and butter
Chocolate-Raisin Bread Pudding
Milk

DAY 12

Breakfast
Apple juice
Grilled Cheddar cheese on English muffin
Milk

Morning Snack
1 hard-boiled egg
½ cup cream-style cottage cheese
Whole grain crackers and butter
Milk

Lunch
Salmon and Noodle Bake
Carrot sticks, celery sticks, and pickle
Bran roll and butter   Vegetable juice

Afternoon Snack
½ cup raisins   ¼ cup nuts   Milk

Dinner
Lettuce Wedges with Oil and Vinegar Dressing
Pork Chops with Chick-peas   Steamed rice
Whole wheat bread and butter
Fresh fruit   Milk

DAY 13

Breakfast
Freshly squeezed orange juice
¾ cup whole grain cereal with raisins and milk
Milk

Morning Snack
Toasted English muffin with cream cheese and jelly
Milk

Lunch
3¼ ounces drained canned tuna
½ cup cream-style cottage cheese
Lettuce wedge, tomato wedges, and cucumber slices
Bran roll and butter
Milk

Afternoon Snack
½ cup plain yogurt with wheat germ and raisins
Vegetable juice

Dinner
Lentil Soup   Spinach Pie
Sliced tomatoes
French bread and butter
Chocolate-Raisin Bread Pudding
Milk

DAY 14

Breakfast
½ grapefruit   1 soft-boiled egg
Toasted English muffin with melted cheese
Milk

Morning Snack
Cream cheese on 1 slice date-nut bread
Milk

Lunch
Spinach Pie   Sliced tomato
Hard roll with butter
Milk

Afternoon Snack
Peanut butter on 1 slice whole wheat bread
Milk

Dinner
Cucumber and Tomato Salad
Sautéed Chicken Livers
Scalloped Potatoes   Steamed Broccoli
Pumpernickel rolls and butter
Jam Parfait   Beverage

DAY 15

Breakfast
½ grapefruit
Grilled ham and Swiss cheese sandwich on
rye bread
Milk

Morning Snack
1 cup plain yogurt with sliced strawberries
Fruit juice

Lunch
Lentil Soup
Sliced chicken, lettuce and tomato sandwich on
pumpernickel roll
Milk

Afternoon Snack
Apple with Cheddar cheese
Whole wheat crackers with butter   Milk

Dinner
Zucchini Soup à la Eve
Haddock with Capers   Stewed Cauliflower
Bran rolls and butter
Fruit and cheese   Beverage

DAY 16

Breakfast
Apple juice
¾ cup whole grain cereal with
sliced banana and milk
Milk

Morning Snack
Cream cheese on 1 slice pumpernickel bread
Milk

Lunch
Lentil Soup
Grilled cheeseburger on enriched-flour bun
Cucumber slices and carrot sticks
Fruit juice

Afternoon Snack
Graham crackers with jelly   Milk

Dinner
Basil Tomatoes with Oil and Vinegar Dressing
Chicken with Lemon Sauce
Fettucine   Sautéed String Beans
Hard rolls and butter   Fresh fruit
Milk

DAY 17

Breakfast
Freshly squeezed orange juice
Cinnamon-Cheese Toast
Milk

Morning Snack
1 cup plain yogurt with sliced,
unsweetened fresh fruit
Milk

Lunch
3¼ ounces drained canned tuna
Coleslaw and pickle
Lettuce and tomato salad
Hard roll with butter
Fruit juice

Afternoon Snack
Apple
Peanut butter on whole wheat crackers
Milk

Dinner
String Beans Vinaigrette
Near-East Chicken Soup
Bran rolls and butter
Brown Sugar-Banana Custard
Milk

DAY 18

Breakfast
½ grapefruit
1 poached egg on whole wheat toast
Milk

Morning Snack
Peanut butter and jelly on 1 slice whole wheat bread
Milk

Lunch
Sliced turkey, lettuce, and tomato sandwich on
hard roll
Coleslaw and pickle   Fruit juice

Afternoon Snack
Brown Sugar-Banana Custard   Milk

Dinner
Broccoli and Tomato Salad
Linguini with White Clam Sauce
Hard rolls and butter   Fruit and cheese
Milk

DAY 19

Breakfast
Freshly squeezed orange juice
¾ cup whole grain cereal with raisins and milk
Milk

Morning Snack
Bran muffin with butter or jelly
Milk

Lunch
Roast beef and lettuce sandwich on rye bread
Lettuce and tomato salad
Cucumber slices and carrot sticks
Vegetable juice

Afternoon Snack
Graham crackers with peanut butter and jelly
Milk

Dinner
Split Pea Soup
Lamb and String Bean Stew
Whole wheat bread and butter
Melon wedges with ice milk
Milk

DAY 20

Breakfast
Freshly squeezed grapefruit juice
2 bran muffins with cream cheese and jelly
Milk

Morning Snack
Banana
Peanut butter on 1 slice whole wheat bread
Milk

Lunch
Lamb and String Bean Stew
Bran roll and butter
Milk

Afternoon Snack
½ cup plain yogurt with raisins and nuts
Fruit juice

Dinner
Mushroom Salad   Artichoke Omelet
Stewed Cauliflower
Pumpernickel bread and butter
Stewed Fruit   Milk

DAY 21

Breakfast
Orange segments   1 scrambled egg
Toasted English muffin with butter and jelly
Milk

Morning Snack
Graham crackers with butter or jelly
Milk

Lunch
Split Pea Soup
Boiled ham, lettuce, and tomato sandwich on
pumpernickel bread
Milk

Afternoon Snack
½ cup plain yogurt with sliced banana
Fruit juice

Dinner
Coleslaw and sliced tomatoes on lettuce leaves
Marinated Steak
Sautéed Peppers and Potatoes
Whole wheat rolls and butter
Ice cream   Milk

DAY 22

Breakfast
½ grapefruit
¾ cup whole grain cereal with milk
Milk

Morning Snack
Corn muffin with butter or jelly
Milk

Lunch
Egg Salad, lettuce, and tomato sandwich on
whole wheat bread
Cucumber slices, carrot sticks, and celery sticks
Milk

Afternoon Snack
Stewed Fruit   Milk

Dinner
Tossed Salad with Oil and Vinegar Dressing
Beef Liver and Onions
Mashed Potatoes   Glazed Carrots
Bran rolls and butter
Stewed Fruit   Milk

DAY 23

Breakfast
Freshly squeezed orange juice
Cinnamon-Cheese Toast
Milk

Morning Snack
Bran muffin with butter or jelly
Milk

Lunch
Split Pea Soup
Boiled ham, Swiss cheese, lettuce, and tomato
sandwich on bran roll
Milk

Afternoon Snack
1 cup plain yogurt with raisins and nuts
Vegetable juice

Dinner
Egg Flower Soup   Shrimp with Garlic Sauce
Steamed rice   Sautéed Asparagus
Sherbet   Milk

DAY 24

Breakfast
Apple juice
Grilled Cheddar cheese sandwich on rye bread
Milk

Morning Snack
1 cup cream-style cottage cheese with ½ cup sliced,
unsweetened fresh fruit
Milk

Lunch
Grilled hamburger in whole wheat pita
Lettuce and tomato salad
Vegetable juice

Afternoon Snack
Peanut butter and jelly on 1 slice whole wheat bread
Milk

Dinner
Marian's Coleslaw and sliced tomatoes on
lettuce leaves
Stuffed Eggplant   Glazed Carrots
Hard rolls and butter
Fresh fruit with cheese
Beverage

DAY 25

Breakfast
Freshly squeezed orange juice
¾ cup whole grain cereal with sliced
banana and milk
Milk

Morning Snack
Corn muffin with butter or jelly
Milk

Lunch
Sliced egg, lettuce, and tomato sandwich on
whole wheat toast
Cucumber slices and carrot sticks
Milk

Afternoon Snack
½ cup raisins   ¼ cup nuts
Milk

Dinner
Pickled Salad
Chicken Parmigiana   Linguini
French bread and butter
Melon wedges   Milk

DAY 26

Breakfast
Melon wedge
1 poached egg on whole wheat toast
Milk

Morning Snack
1 cup plain yogurt with raisins
Vegetable juice

Lunch
Grilled Cheddar cheese sandwich on rye bread
Lettuce and tomato salad
Milk

Afternoon Snack
Graham crackers with jelly
Milk

Dinner
Eggplant-Gumbo Soup
Salmon Salad on lettuce leaves
Sliced tomatoes   Cucumber slices
Green pepper rings
Bran rolls and butter
Fresh fruit   Milk

DAY 27

Breakfast
Freshly squeezed grapefruit juice
2 corn muffins with butter and jelly
Milk

Morning Snack
Cream cheese on 1 slice pumpernickel bread
Milk

Lunch
Eggplant-Gumbo Soup
Grilled hamburger on enriched-flour bun
Fruit juice

Afternoon Snack
Grapes and Cheddar cheese
Whole grain crackers with butter
Milk

Dinner
Chick-pea Salad   Broccoli Omelet
Sautéed Mushrooms
Whole wheat bread and butter
Baked Custard   Beverage

DAY 28

Breakfast
½ grapefruit
¾ cup whole grain cereal with raisins and milk
Milk

Morning Snack
1 cup plain yogurt with ½ cup unsweetened
fresh fruit
Milk

Lunch
Sliced egg, lettuce, and tomato sandwich on
whole wheat toast
Coleslaw and pickle
Vegetable juice

Afternoon Snack
Peanut butter and jelly on whole wheat crackers
Milk

Dinner
Pickled Salad   Sautéed Chicken Breast
Linguini with Marinara Sauce
Asparagus with Butter and Cheese
Hard rolls and butter
Fruit and cheese   Beverage

DAY 29

Breakfast
Freshly squeezed orange juice
Cream cheese and boiled ham sandwich on
pumpernickel bread
Milk

Morning Snack
1 hard-boiled egg
1 slice whole wheat bread with butter
Milk

Lunch
Eggplant-Gumbo Soup
Liverwurst, lettuce, and tomato sandwich on
hard roll
Milk

Afternoon Snack
½ cup cream-style cottage cheese with sliced
banana
Whole wheat crackers   Milk

Dinner
Broccoli and Tomato Salad
Sausages, Peppers, and Potatoes
Whole wheat rolls and butter
Baked Custard   Beverage

DAY 30

Breakfast
½ grapefruit   1 scrambled egg
Toasted English muffin with butter and jelly
Milk

Morning Snack
Cream cheese and jelly on 1 slice
pumpernickel bread
Milk

Lunch
Sausages, Peppers, and Potatoes   Sliced tomatoes
Hard roll and butter   Vegetable juice

Afternoon Snack
Peanut butter on whole grain crackers
Apple   Milk

Dinner
Lentil Salad   Shrimp-stuffed Fillets
Steamed Spinach   Glazed Carrots
Bran rolls and butter
Ice cream   Beverage

Recipes

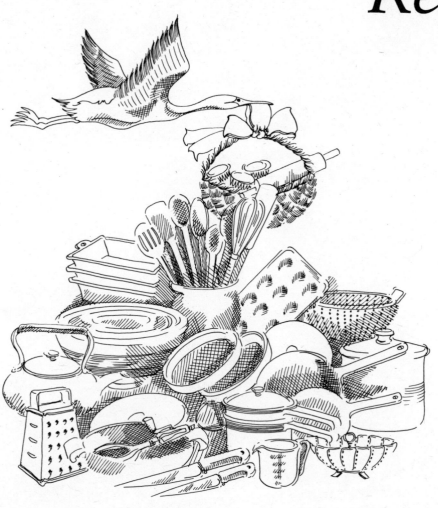

SOUPS

BROCCOLI AND BEAN SOUP

2 servings

½ pound chicken gizzards and hearts, mixed
1 13¾-ounce can chicken broth
1 cup water
1 clove garlic, peeled
1 bay leaf
2 tablespoons vegetable oil
1 medium-sized yellow onion, peeled and chopped
1 clove garlic, peeled and cut in half
1 large stalk broccoli
Salt and freshly ground black pepper
½ cup water
1 cup canned small white beans, drained

1. Wash the chicken gizzards and hearts in cool running water, removing any excess fat. Put them in a saucepan and add the chicken broth, water, whole garlic clove, and bay leaf. Bring to a boil, cover, lower the heat, and simmer for 1¼ hours. Strain and reserve the broth. Discard the garlic and bay leaf. Cut the gristle away from the gizzards and slice the meat into thin slices. Slice the hearts into thin slices. Set the gizzard and heart slices aside.

2. Peel the broccoli stalk and cut it into thin slices. Separate the broccoli head into small flowerets.

3. Heat the vegetable oil in a saucepan and add the onion and halved garlic. Sauté for 5 minutes, stirring occasionally. Add the broccoli stalk slices and sauté for 2 minutes. Lay the broccoli flowerets on top of the vegetables in the saucepan. Sprinkle liberally with salt and pepper. Pour in the water and bring to a boil. Cover and steam for 5 minutes, or until the vegetables are barely tender.

4. Stir the reserved broth and the gizzard and heart slices into the broccoli mixure. Heat over low heat for 5 minutes. Add the drained beans and taste for seasonings. Correct if necessary. Heat just until the beans are hot.

NEAR-EAST CHICKEN SOUP

2 servings

2 chicken quarters
1 15-ounce can chicken broth
3 cups water
1 bay leaf
2 carrots, scraped and cut into julienne strips
1 small white onion, peeled and thinly sliced
2 celery stalks, trimmed and thinly sliced
2 cups finely shredded green cabbage
Pinch of ground cinnamon
Pinch of ground nutmeg
Salt and freshly ground black pepper
1 cup cooked rice

1. Put the chicken, broth, water, and bay leaf into a large saucepan. Bring to a boil, cover,

lower the heat, and simmer for 1 hour. Remove the chicken pieces and allow them to cool. Strain the broth and chill it until you can remove the grease from the top.

2. When the chicken is cool enough to handle, skin and bone it, and cut the meat into ½-inch chunks. Set the chicken aside.

3. Measure the degreased chicken broth into a clean saucepan. You should have 4 cups. If you do not, add water to make up 4 cups. Bring the broth to a boil and add the vegetables and cinnamon, nutmeg, and salt and pepper to taste. Return to a boil, cover, and simmer for 10 minutes, or until the vegetables are just tender. Add the chicken and rice and heat through.

EGGPLANT-GUMBO SOUP

2 to 3 main-dish servings
or 4 first-course servings

2 tablespoons vegetable oil
1 medium-sized yellow onion, peeled and chopped
2 cloves garlic, peeled and minced
1 or 2 dried chili peppers (optional)
1 1-pound eggplant, peeled and cut into ¼-inch cubes
1 8-ounce can stewed tomatoes with liquid
3 cups chicken broth or water
    Salt and freshly ground black pepper
1 10-ounce package frozen cut okra, thawed
1 7-ounce can corn kernels, drained

1. Heat the oil in a large Dutch oven. When the oil is hot, add the onion, garlic, and chili peppers. Sauté over low heat for 5 minutes, stirring occasionally. Raise the heat to medium and add the eggplant cubes. Sauté for 5 minutes,

stirring occasionally. Be sure that the eggplant does not stick to the bottom of the pan.

2. Add the stewed tomatoes and their liquid to the vegetable mixture, breaking up the tomatoes with a wooden spoon as you stir. Add the broth and mix well. Season the soup with salt and pepper to taste and bring to a boil, stirring occasionally. When the soup is boiling, cover the pan, lower the heat, and simmer for 30 minutes, stirring occasionally.

3. Remove the chili peppers and stir the okra into the simmering soup and bring the soup back to a boil. Cover and simmer for 5 minutes, stirring occasionally.

4. Taste the soup for seasonings and add salt and pepper, if necessary. Add the corn to the soup and cook for 1 minute longer.

EGYPTIAN PEA SOUP

8 servings

1 pound dried yellow or green split peas, picked over, washed, and drained
2 medium-sized carrots, scraped and minced
1 celery stalk, minced
1 medium-sized yellow onion, peeled and finely chopped
1 large bay leaf
1 small clove garlic, peeled and minced
4 cups chicken broth
3 cups water
¼ teaspoon salt
⅛ teaspoon freshly ground black pepper
¾ teaspoon ground cumin

1. Put the drained peas in a large heavy pot. Add the carrots, celery, onion, bay leaf, garlic, broth, and water. Bring to a boil over medium-

high heat, stirring occasionally so that the peas do not stick to the bottom of the pot. When boiling, stir in the salt, pepper, and cumin. Cover the pot, lower the heat, and simmer for 1 hour and 15 minutes, stirring occasionally so that the peas do not stick to the bottom of the pot.

2. Remove the bay leaf and cool the soup slightly. Then purée in a blender or through a food mill. Reheat the soup over very low heat, stirring occasionally.

LENTIL SOUP

4 servings

$1/2$ pound dried lentils, picked over, washed, and drained
1 clove garlic, peeled and minced
1 carrot, scraped and minced
1 small onion, peeled and minced
1 small celery stalk, minced
1 bay leaf
1 small smoked ham hock
$1^{1}/2$ cups beef broth
3 cups water
    Salt and freshly ground black pepper

1. Put the drained lentils, garlic, carrot, onion, celery, bay leaf, ham hock, broth, and water in a heavy saucepan. Bring to a boil, lower the heat, cover, and simmer for 1 hour, stirring occasionally, or until the lentils are tender.

2. When the lentils are tender, remove and discard the ham hock and bay leaf. Taste the soup for salt and pepper, and add, if necessary.

SPLIT PEA SOUP

8 servings

1 pound dried green split peas, picked over, washed, and drained
1 1-pound turkey wing, fresh or frozen, defrosted
1 clove garlic, peeled and minced
1 large carrot, scraped and minced
1 celery stalk, minced
1 medium-sized onion, peeled and minced
1 large bay leaf
2 cups chicken broth
4 cups water
    Salt and freshly ground black pepper

1. Put the drained split peas, turkey wing, garlic, carrot, celery, onion, bay leaf, broth, and water in a large heavy saucepan. Bring to a boil, lower the heat, cover, and simmer for 1½ hours, stirring occasionally.

2. When the peas are tender, remove and discard the turkey wing and bay leaf. Pass the soup through a food mill and season with salt and pepper to taste. Reheat over low heat until very hot, stirring occasionally so that the soup does not stick to the pan.

BEEF BOUILLON WITH MUSHROOMS AND CHIVES

2 servings

$1^{1}/2$ cups canned beef bouillon or beef broth
2 large white mushrooms, sliced paper-thin
1 teaspoon minced fresh or freeze-dried chives

1. Heat the bouillon until it just begins to simmer.

2. Put one sliced mushroom in each of 2 soup bowls and pour the hot bouillon over them. Sprinkle the chives over each serving, and serve at once.

EGG FLOWER SOUP

2 servings

2½ cups chicken broth
1   egg, beaten
1   tablespoon soy sauce
4   spinach leaves, stems removed and well washed, shredded
1   scallion, trimmed and minced

1. Put the chicken broth in a small saucepan and bring it just to the simmering point. Pour in the beaten egg in a steady stream, stirring the soup with a fork. Stir in the soy sauce and remove the soup from the heat immediately.

2. Put an equal amount of shredded spinach leaves in 2 soup bowls. Divide the soup equally between the bowls. Garnish the soup with the minced scallion and serve at once.

CREAM OF MUSHROOM-BARLEY SOUP

2 servings

1   10-ounce can condensed beef broth
2   cups water
3   tablespoons barley
2   tablespoons butter or margarine
2   tablespoons finely minced onion
½   pound finely chopped mushrooms
     Salt and freshly ground black pepper
½   cup milk

1. Bring the broth and water to a boil. Add the barley. Stir, return to a boil, cover, and simmer, stirring occasionally, for 30 to 40 minutes, or until the barley is tender.

2. While the barley is cooking, melt the butter in a large frying pan. Add the onion and sauté for 1 minute. Add the mushrooms and sauté, stirring occasionally, for about 10 minutes, or until the mushroom liquid has evaporated and the mixture is quite dry. Season with salt and pepper to taste.

3. Stir the mushrooms into the cooked barley mixture and mix well. Add the milk and mix well. Taste for seasonings, and correct, if necessary.

Note: If you have to reheat the soup, do so over very low heat, stirring often.

ZUCCHINI SOUP À LA EVE

2 servings

2   tablespoons butter or margarine
1   small clove garlic, peeled and minced
1   small white onion, peeled and minced
2   small zucchini (about ½ pound), scraped and diced
¼   to ½ teaspoon curry powder, or to taste
2   cups chicken broth
¼   cup plain yogurt
2   scallions, trimmed and minced

1. Melt the butter in a saucepan. When the butter is completely melted and bubbling, add the garlic and onion and sauté over low heat for 5 minutes, stirring occasionally. Add the zucchini and sauté over low heat for 5 minutes longer. Sprinkle the curry powder over the zucchini-onion mixture and stir it in well. Stir in the

broth and bring the soup to a boil. Cover, lower the heat, and simmer for 15 minutes. Remove the pan from the heat and let the soup cool to room temperature.

2. Purée the soup through a food mill into a bowl. Stir in the yogurt until it is completely blended with the soup. Cover the bowl and refrigerate overnight. Serve cold, topping each serving with 1 minced scallion.

COLD CUCUMBER SOUP

4 servings

2 tablespoons butter or margarine
1 clove garlic, peeled and minced
1 small white onion, peeled and minced
1 celery stalk, minced
1 large cucumber, peeled, seeded, and diced
2 cups chicken broth
    Salt and freshly ground black pepper
¾ cup half-and-half
    Chopped parsley for garnish

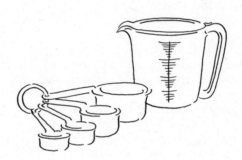

1. Melt the butter in a saucepan. When the butter is completely melted, add the garlic, onion, and celery. Sauté over low heat for 10 minutes, stirring occasionally. Add the cucumber and sauté for 5 minutes longer. Stir in the broth and season with salt and pepper to taste. Bring to a boil, cover, lower the heat, and simmer for 15 minutes, stirring occasionally.

2. Remove the soup from the heat and cool to room temperature. When cool, pass the soup through a food mill into a bowl. Stir in the half-and-half and mix well. Cover the bowl and chill for several hours. Sprinkle each portion with chopped parsley before serving.

SALADS AND CONDIMENTS

HOT SALADE NIÇOISE
2 servings

1   large potato, peeled
2   tomatoes, cored, peeled, seeded, and diced
1   small Spanish onion, peeled and minced
½   teaspoon dried tarragon
½   teaspoon dried basil
2   tablespoons minced parsley
1½ teaspoons salt
⅛   teaspoon freshly ground black pepper
1   7-ounce can tuna fish, drained well
3   tablespoons butter
3   tablespoons unseasoned bread crumbs
½   cup shredded Swiss cheese

1. Cut the potato into quarters and cut the quarters into ¼-inch-thick slices. Steam the potato slices over boiling water until just tender. Remove from the heat immediately and cool.

2. Preheat the oven to 375 degrees.

3. In a large bowl, mix together the potatoes, tomatoes, onion, tarragon, basil, parsley, salt, pepper, and tuna fish. Toss gently with 2 forks.

4. Use 1 tablespoon of the butter to grease the inside of a baking dish large enough to hold the salad. Spoon the salad gently into the baking dish. Sprinkle the bread crumbs evenly over the top and dot with the remaining 2 tablespoons of butter. Bake for 15 to 20 minutes, or until all the ingredients are piping hot. Sprinkle the cheese evenly over the top of the salad and run under the broiler until the cheese melts and browns slightly. Serve hot or at room temperature.

CHICKEN-POTATO SALAD
2 servings

2   pieces skinless and boneless chicken breast
1   cup chicken broth
½   pound potatoes
    Salt
1   hard-boiled egg, peeled and chopped
1   tablespoon drained capers
1   small dill pickle, drained well and chopped
⅓   cup finely minced scallions
⅓   cup plain yogurt
½   cup mayonnaise
    Freshly ground black pepper
    Lettuce leaves and sliced tomatoes

1. Put the chicken and the chicken broth into a small heavy saucepan. Bring to a boil, lower the heat, and simmer, turning the chicken occasionally, for 15 minutes. Drain the chicken, discarding the broth, and cool the chicken to room temperature. When the chicken is cool, cut it into ½-inch cubes. Set aside until needed.

2. Meanwhile, peel the potatoes and cut them into ½-inch cubes. Put them in a saucepan and cover them with cold salted water. Bring to a boil and cook for 8 to 10 minutes, or until they are just tender. Drain well and cool to room temperature.

3. Put the cooled chicken and potato cubes into a salad bowl. Add the chopped egg, capers, chopped pickle, scallions, yogurt, and mayonnaise. Toss gently with two forks to combine the mixture. Taste for seasonings, and add salt and pepper, if necessary. Cover the bowl and refrigerate for at least ½ hour before serving. Serve on lettuce leaves with sliced tomatoes on the side.

PASTA AND SALMON SALAD

3 servings

1   7¾-ounce can salmon
1   small white onion, peeled and minced
½   small green pepper, seeded and minced
1   small carrot, scraped and minced
1   small clove garlic, peeled and minced
1   cup elbow macaroni, cooked al dente, drained, and cooled
½   cup cooked fresh or frozen green peas
2   teaspoons drained capers, chopped
½   cup mayonnaise
2   tablespoons sour cream
    Salt and freshly ground black pepper to taste

1. Drain the salmon and remove the bones and skin.
2. Put the salmon and the remaining ingredients into a salad bowl. Toss with two forks to combine well, making sure that you do not break up the pasta. Cover the bowl and chill for at least ½ hour before serving.

STUFFED TOMATO SALAD PLATE

2 servings

2   large ripe tomatoes, preferably beefsteak (see Note)
    Salt
1   recipe for Cottage Cheese Salad (page 211)
    Freshly ground black pepper
    Lettuce leaves
1   recipe for String Beans Vinaigrette (page 215), without the tomato

1. Wash the tomatoes well in cool running water. Cut a slice off the top of each tomato (which will remove the core completely). Discard this tomato slice. Use a teaspoon to scoop out the inside pulp and seeds of each tomato. Discard the seeds and set the pulp aside for use later. (Be sure that you don't pierce the outer shell and skin of the tomato while you are scooping out the pulp.) Sprinkle the inside of the hollowed-out tomatoes with salt and turn them upside down to drain.
2. Cut the reserved pulp of the tomatoes into very small pieces and combine it with the Cottage Cheese Salad. Taste for seasonings and add salt and pepper, if necessary. Use the mixture to stuff the hollowed-out tomatoes, piling it high.
3. Line two dinner plates with the lettuce leaves. Put one stuffed tomato in the center of each plate. Surround each tomato with an equal portion of String Beans Vinaigrette. Serve at once.
Note: If you can't find good beefsteak tomatoes, use 4 medium-sized ripe tomatoes, treating them the same way you would the beefsteak tomatoes.

ANYTIME DINNER SALAD

2 servings

1   garlic clove, peeled and crushed
2   tablespoons olive oil
1½   tablesoons red wine vinegar
     Pinch of dried thyme
     Pinch of dried basil
     Pinch of red pepper flakes
     Salt and freshly ground black pepper
2   medium-sized potatoes
1   small bunch broccoli
     Lettuce leaves
2   medium-sized tomatoes, cored and sliced
2   hard-boiled eggs, halved
2   scallions, trimmed and cut into 2-inch
     shreds
1   lemon, cut into wedges

1. Put the garlic, oil, vinegar, thyme, basil, and red pepper flakes into a small jar with a tight-fitting lid. Shake to combine well. Taste for seasonings, and add salt and pepper to taste. Set aside, covered, until needed.

2. Peel the potatoes and cut them into ¼-inch-thick slices.

3. Wash the broccoli in cool running water. Cut off about 1 inch from the bottom of the stalks. Peel the stalks right up to the base of the flowers. Cut the stalks (and flowers) in half if they are too thick.

4. Lay the potato slices in a steamer basket and sprinkle them lightly with salt. Steam in a covered pot, over boiling water, for 3 minutes. Lay the broccoli on top of the potatoes and sprinkle it lightly with salt. Cover the pot and steam for 5 to 7 minutes, or until a fork easily pierces the potatoes and broccoli stalks. (Do not overcook the broccoli; it should be bright green

and just *al dente*.) Remove the steamer basket from the pot and let the potatoes and broccoli cool to room temperature.

5. Line a large salad bowl with the lettuce leaves. Pile the cooled broccoli in the center of the bowl. Make a ring of the potato slices around the broccoli. Make an overlapping half circle of the tomato slices on one edge of the bowl, and a half circle of the egg halves on the opposite edge. Scatter the scallion shreds on top of all the ingredients in the bowl. Shake the salad dressing to mix it thoroughly and remove the garlic clove. Dribble the dressing over all the vegetables. Put the lemon wedges in the spaces where the tomato slices and egg halves meet, and serve immediately.

AVOCADO DINNER SALAD

2 servings

     Lettuce leaves
2   lemons
1   large ripe avocado
1   recipe for Egg Salad (page 208)
2   medium-sized ripe tomatoes, cored and sliced
1   small green pepper, seeded and cut into rings
     Salt and freshly ground black pepper

1. Line two dinner plates with lettuce leaves.

2. Squeeze 1 of the lemons and put the juice in a flat soup bowl or small pie plate.

3. Cut the avocado in half lengthwise and remove the pit. Peel each half and then cut it into ¼-inch-thick slices. Dip the avocado slices into the lemon juice, coating both sides. (This will prevent the avocado from darkening while you are assembling the rest of the salad.)

4. Make equal overlapping half circles of the

avocado slices around one half of the lettuce-lined plates. Pile equal portions of the Egg Salad in the center of each plate. Make overlapping quarter circles of the tomato slices and pepper rings opposite the avocado slices on each plate. Sprinkle the vegetables liberally with salt and pepper. Cut the remaining lemon into wedges and add the wedges to each plate. Serve immediately.

NOODLE SALAD

4 servings

3   tablespoons vegetable or peanut oil
1   teaspoon finely minced fresh ginger
2   cloves garlic, finely minced
2   pieces skinless and boneless chicken breast, shredded
2   cups broccoli flowerets
1   medium-sized cucumber, peeled, seeded, and sliced thin
1   celery stalk, sliced thin
½   cup (about 3 large) thinly sliced radishes
4   scallions, chopped
1   cup bean sprouts
3   tablespoons soy sauce
2   tablespoons red wine vinegar
½   pound vermicelli
2   cups shredded Romaine lettuce

1. Put 1 tablespoon of the oil and the ginger and garlic in a small frying pan. Heat over medium heat just until the ginger begins to brown. Add the chicken and cook, stirring constantly, until the chicken turns white and is cooked through (about 3 minutes). Transfer the chicken and spices to a large mixing bowl.

2. Steam the broccoli flowerets until they are just tender and transfer them while they are still warm to the bowl with the chicken. Add the cucumber, celery, radishes, scallions, and bean sprouts to the bowl. Add 1 tablespoon oil, 2 tablespoons soy sauce, and 1 tablespoon vinegar to the bowl and toss the chicken and vegetable mixture with two wooden spoons until it is well blended.

3. Cook the vermicelli in at least 2 quarts of boiling water until it is just *al dente* (about 5 minutes). Drain well, cool under cold running water, and drain well again. Add the drained vermicelli to the bowl with the chicken and vegetables. Add the remaining 1 tablespoon each of oil, soy sauce, and vinegar and toss with two wooden spoons to combine well. Cover the bowl and refrigerate for at least ½ hour.

4. Just before serving add the shredded lettuce to the bowl and toss to combine well.

EGGPLANT AND RICE SALAD

2 servings

1   1-pound eggplant
5   tablespoons olive oil
1   large clove garlic, peeled and crushed
¾   teaspoon ground cumin
1   cup leftover Rice Pilaf (page 282), chilled
2   scallions, trimmed and chopped
2   teaspoons red wine vinegar
¼   teaspoon ground ginger
    Salt and freshly ground black pepper

1. Peel the eggplant and cut it into strips ⅛ inch thick and 2 inches long. Put the eggplant strips into a saucepan and cover them with boiling water. Let stand for 10 minutes. Drain very well and let cool.

2. When the eggplant strips are well drained and cool, heat 4 tablespoons of the oil in a medium-size frying pan. When the oil is hot add the garlic and brown it on all sides. Then add the eggplant strips and sauté over medium heat, tossing and stirring, until the eggplant is tender and light brown. Remove the frying pan from the heat and remove and discard the garlic. Sprinkle the cumin over the eggplant and mix in well. Let the eggplant cool to room temperature.

3. Combine the rice pilaf with the scallions, wine vinegar, ginger, and remaining tablespoon of oil. Add the cooled eggplant strips and any oil remaining in the frying pan. Toss with two forks to mix well. Season with salt and pepper to taste and toss again. Cover and chill for at least ½ hour to blend the flavors.

EGG SALAD

2 main-dish servings
or filling for 4 sandwiches

¼ cup minced Spanish onion
1 small clove garlic, peeled and minced
2 tablespoons minced parsley
  Pinch of cayenne pepper
  Scant ½ cup mayonnaise
4 hard-boiled eggs, finely chopped
  Salt and freshly ground black pepper

Combine the onion, garlic, parsley, cayenne, and mayonnaise in a bowl. Mix very well and then add the eggs and mix again. Season with salt and pepper to taste and mix again. Cover the bowl and refrigerate for 15 minutes before serving.

TUNA SALAD

2 main-dish servings
or filling for 4 sandwiches

¼ cup minced Spanish onion
1 celery stalk, minced
1 small clove garlic, peeled and minced
2 tablespoons minced parsley
  Scant ½ cup mayonnaise
1 6½-ounce can tuna, drained
  Salt and freshly ground black pepper

Combine the onion, celery, garlic, parsley, and mayonnaise in a bowl. Mix very well and then add the tuna and mix again. Season with salt and pepper to taste and mix again. Cover the bowl and refrigerate for 15 minutes before serving.

SALMON SALAD

2 main-dish servings
or filling for 4 sandwiches

¼ cup minced red onion
1 small carrot, scraped and minced
1 celery stalk, minced
1 small clove garlic, peeled and minced
2 tablespoons minced parsley
⅓ cup mayonnaise
1 7¾-ounce can salmon, drained
  Salt and freshly ground black pepper

1. Combine the onion, carrot, celery, garlic, parsley, and mayonnaise in a small bowl. Mix very well.

2. Remove the skin and bones from the drained salmon and add the salmon to the dressing in the bowl. Use a fork to combine the mixture

until it is smooth. Season with salt and pepper to taste and mix well again. Cover the bowl and refrigerate for 15 minutes before serving.

PICKLED SALAD

4 servings

2 cups small cauliflower flowerets
1 large carrot, scraped and sliced ½ inch thick
1 celery stalk, cut into ½-inch-thick slices
1 green pepper, seeded, and cut into 1-inch cubes
1 3-once jar stuffed green olives, drained
½ cup red wine vinegar
¼ cup olive or vegetable oil
2 tablespoons water
½ teaspoon salt
⅛ teaspoon freshly ground black pepper
½ teaspoon dried oregano
   Pinch of dried basil
   Shredded lettuce

1. Combine all the ingredients, except the shredded lettuce, in a large frying pan. Bring to a boil over medium heat, stirring occasionally. Cover, lower the heat, and cook for 3 to 5 minutes, or until the vegetables are just tender.

2. Cool the mixture and pour it into a bowl. Cover tightly and refrigerate overnight.

3. To serve, drain the vegetables from the marinade and put the salade on lettuce-lined plates.

MARINATED ARTICHOKES

2 servings

1 10-ounce package frozen artichoke hearts
   Salt
¼ cup thinly sliced red onion
1 clove garlic, peeled and minced
½ teaspoon dried oregano, crumbled
2 tablespoons olive oil
3 tablespoons red wine vinegar
   Freshly ground black pepper
   Lettuce leaves

1. Cook the artichoke hearts in salted water according to package directions. Drain well. While still warm, put the artichoke hearts in a bowl and add the red onion, garlic, and oregano. Toss to combine well. Let sit until cool.

2. Pour the oil and vinegar over the artichoke hearts and toss. Taste for seasonings, and add salt and pepper. Serve on lettuce leaves.

WHITE BEAN SALAD

2 servings

1 8-ounce can white kidney beans, drained
¼ cup minced red onion
¼ cup minced green pepper
1 tablespoon minced parsley
1 clove garlic, peeled and minced
   Salt and freshly ground black pepper
2 tablespoons olive or vegetable oil
3 tablespoons red wine vinegar
   Shredded lettuce
1 ripe tomato, cored and sliced thin
8 pitted black olives, chopped

1. Combine the beans, onion, green pepper, parsley, and garlic in a bowl. Toss to mix well. Sprinkle liberally with salt and pepper. Pour the oil and vinegar over the salad and toss gently to combine. Let sit at room temperature for at least ½ hour, tossing gently once or twice.

2. To serve, line 2 salad plates with shredded lettuce. Spoon equal portions of the bean mixture onto each plate. Garnish each serving with tomato slices and chopped olives.

BROCCOLI AND TOMATO SALAD

2 servings

1	small bunch broccoli
	Salt
¼	cup thinly sliced red onion
3	tablespoons olive oil
1½	tablespoons red wine vinegar
	Pinch of freshly ground black pepper
¼	teaspoon finely minced garlic
½	teaspoon dried oregano
1	ripe tomato, cored and diced

1. Cut off about 1 inch from the bottom of the broccoli stalks. Cut off the stalks at the base of the flowers. Peel the stalks and cut them into ¼-inch-thick slices. Separate the flowers into flowerets. Wash the broccoli pieces in cool running water. Drain.

2. Lay the broccoli stem slices in layers in a steamer basket and sprinkle lightly with salt. Steam in a covered pot, over boiling water, for 3 minutes. Add the broccoli flowerets to the steamer basket, sprinkle them lightly with salt, and steam for 3 to 5 minutes, or until a fork pierces the stalk pieces easily. (Do not overcook; the broccoli should be bright green and just *al dente.*) Remove the steamer basket from the heat immediately. Let the broccoli cool for a few minutes and then put it in a bowl. Add the red onion.

3. Combine the oil, vinegar, pepper, garlic, and oregano together and mix well. Pour over the still-warm broccoli. Toss to coat the broccoli with the dressing. Let sit at room temperature for 15 minutes before serving. Add the tomato to the broccoli just before serving. Toss, taste for seasonings, and correct, if necessary.

MARIAN'S COLESLAW

6 servings

1	2-pound head green cabbage
1	small yellow onion, peeled
1	small carrot, trimmed and scraped
2	tablespoons white vinegar
1	tablespoon vegetable oil
1	teaspoon granulated sugar
1¼	teaspoons salt
½	teaspoon freshly ground black pepper
⅛	teaspoon celery seeds
½	cup mayonnaise

1. Remove the tough outer leaves from the cabbage and cut off any excess stem at the base of the cabbage. Cut the cabbage into equal quarters, but do not remove the core. Grate the cabbage into a large mixing bowl, using the large holes of a hand grater. (The core will help to keep the cabbage layers together.)

2. Grate the onion and carrot into the bowl with the cabbage, using the small holes of a hand grater. Add the vinegar, oil, and granulated sugar and toss well.

3. Season the vegetable mixture with salt,

pepper, and celery seeds. Add the mayonnaise and mix well. Taste for seasonings, and add more salt and pepper, if necessary.

4. Transfer the coleslaw to the smaller bowl, cover tightly, and refrigerate overnight before serving.

CORN SALAD

2 servings

1/4 cup minced red onion
1/4 cup minced green pepper
1 12-ounce can corn kernels, drained
1/8 teaspoon dry mustard
1 tablespoon red wine vinegar
1 tablespoon vegetable oil
   Lettuce leaves

Combine the onion, green pepper, corn, mustard, vinegar, and oil in a bowl. Mix very well, cover the bowl, and refrigerate for at least 1/2 hour. Serve on lettuce leaves.

COTTAGE CHEESE SALAD

2 servings

1 cup cream-style cottage cheese
1 small carrot, scraped and minced very fine
1 small celery stalk, trimmed and minced very fine
2 scallions, trimmed and minced very fine
1/4 teaspoon salt
1/8 teaspoon freshly ground black pepper
   Pinch of dried basil
   Lettuce leaves

Mix all the ingredients with the exception of the lettuce leaves together in a small bowl. Cover tightly and refrigerate for at least 1/2 hour before serving on the lettuce leaves.

CUCUMBER AND TOMATO SALAD

2 servings

1 large cucumber, trimmed and cut into very thin slices
   Salt
2 ripe tomatoes, cored and diced
2 tablespoons freshly squeezed lemon juice
2 tablespoons olive or vegetable oil
   Pinch of cayenne pepper
   Shredded lettuce

1. Put the cucumber slices in a bowl and sprinkle them liberally with salt. Let sit for 1 hour.

2. Pour off the water that has accumulated around the cucumbers. Add the tomatoes, lemon juice, oil, and cayenne pepper to the cucumbers. Toss to mix well. Season with more salt and pepper, if necessary.

3. Put a bed of shredded lettuce on 2 salad plates and spoon the cucumber salad evenly over the lettuce. Serve at room temperature.

CHICK-PEA SALAD

2 servings

1   8-ounce can chick-peas, drained
1/4 cup chopped red onion
3   tablespoons olive oil
2   tablespoons red wine vinegar
     Salt and freshly ground black pepper
1/2 teaspoon finely minced garlic
1/4 teaspoon dried oregano, crumbled
1   small cucumber, peeled, seeded, and diced
1   ripe tomato, washed, cored, and diced
     Lettuce leaves

1. Combine the chick-peas, onions, oil, vinegar, pepper, garlic and oregano in a salad bowl. Toss to mix well. Let sit for ½ hour, tossing occasionally.

2. Add the diced cucumber and tomato to the chick-pea mixture and toss to mix well. Taste for seasonings, and correct, if necessary. Serve the salad on lettuce leaves.

EGGPLANT SALAD

2 servings

1   1-pound eggplant
2   tablespoons olive oil
1   tablespoon freshly squeezed lemon juice, or more, to taste
1/4 teaspoon salt
1/8 teaspoon freshly ground black pepper
     Pinch of cayenne pepper
1/4 cup minced onion
1/4 cup minced green pepper
2   tablespoons minced black olives
     Lettuce leaves
1   tomato, cored and sliced

1. Preheat the oven to 375 degrees.

2. Put the eggplant on a baking sheet and bake it, turning occasionally, until it is very soft. Remove the eggplant from the oven and let it cool until you can peel off the skin comfortably with your fingers.

3. Put the eggplant flesh in a bowl and mash it with a wooden spoon, until it is almost a paste. Add the oil, lemon juice, salt, black pepper, cayenne pepper, onion, green pepper, and olives to the eggplant. Blend well with a wooden spoon. Taste for seasonings and correct, if necessary.

4. Line a salad bowl with the lettuce leaves and mound the eggplant mixture on the lettuce. Garnish with the tomato slices. Serve at room temperature.

LENTIL SALAD

2 servings

1   small white onion, peeled
4   whole cloves
1   clove garlic, peeled
1/2 cup dried lentils, picked over, washed, and drained
1   bay leaf
     Salt
3   cups water
1/3 cup finely minced red onion
1   small celery stalk, minced
     Freshly ground black pepper
3   tablespoons red wine vinegar
2   tablespoons olive oil
     Lettuce leaves

1. Push the cloves firmly into the onion. Put the onion, garlic, lentils, bay leaf, ½ teaspoon salt, and the water into a saucepan. Bring to a

boil, stirring occasionally. When the water has reached the boiling point, cover the pan, lower the heat, and simmer the lentils, stirring occasionally, for 45 minutes.

2. Remove the pan from the heat, uncover, and let the lentils cool to room temperature.

3. Drain the lentils very well, discarding the onion, garlic, and bay leaf. Put the drained lentils into a small mixing bowl and add the red onion, celery, salt and pepper to taste, vinegar, and oil. Toss with two forks until well combined. Cover the bowl and chill very well. Serve on lettuce leaves.

LETTUCE WEDGES WITH OIL AND VINEGAR DRESSING

2 servings

1/2 head of iceberg lettuce, cut in half and cored
1 tablespoon minced scallion
2 tablespoons olive oil
1 tablespoon red wine vinegar
1/4 teaspoon finely minced garlic
  Pinch of dried basil, crumbled
  Pinch of salt and freshly ground black pepper

1. Put the lettuce quarters in 2 individual salad bowls. Sprinkle the scallions equally over each chunk of lettuce. Refrigerate until ready to serve.

2. Combine the oil, vinegar, garlic, basil, and salt and pepper in a small cup. Stir with a spoon and let sit at room temperature until you spoon it over the lettuce.

MUSHROOM SALAD

2 servings

1/2 pound mushrooms, sliced thin
  Salt and freshly ground black pepper
  Pinch of ground nutmeg
3 tablespoons freshly squeezed lemon juice
1 tablespoon olive oil
1 tablespoon red wine vinegar
1 teaspoon freeze-dried chives
1 teaspoon finely minced parsley
  Pinch of dried thyme
  Pinch of dried oregano
  Lettuce leaves

1. Put the mushrooms in a bowl and season with salt and pepper to taste and the nutmeg. Toss to combine.

2. Mix together the lemon juice, oil, vinegar, chives, parsley, thyme, and oregano. Pour over the mushrooms and toss to combine. Refrigerate the salad for 1/2 hour. Serve on lettuce leaves.

EGYPTIAN POTATO SALAD

6 servings

1 1/2 pounds boiling potatoes, washed well
  Salt
1 large white onion, peeled and minced
1/4 teaspoon ground coriander
1/8 teaspoon cayenne pepper
1/2 cup plain yogurt
1/2 cup mayonnaise
  Freshly ground black pepper

1. Put the potatoes in a large saucepan and add 1 teaspoon salt and water to cover the potatoes by 2 inches. Bring to a boil over medium

heat. Boil uncovered for 15 to 20 minutes, or until the potatoes can be pierced by a skewer. Drain the potatoes and cool briefly.

2. Peel the potatoes while they are still warm and dice them into ½-inch cubes. Put the potatoes in a small bowl. Add the onion, coriander, cayenne, yogurt, and mayonnaise. Use two forks to toss and combine well. Season with salt and pepper to taste and toss again. Cover the bowl and refrigerate for several hours, or until well chilled.

MARINATED POTATO SALAD

2 servings

⅓ cup white vinegar
⅓ cup water
1 bay leaf
1 clove garlic, peeled
    Large pinch of celery seeds
4 whole black peppercorns
2 medium-sized potatoes, peeled and cut into
    ¼-inch-thick slices
    Chicken broth
½ cup thinly sliced Spanish onion
    Salt and freshly ground black pepper
1 tablespoon chopped parsley

1. Combine the vinegar, water, bay leaf, garlic, celery seeds, and peppercorns in a small saucepan. Bring to a boil, lower the heat, and simmer for 5 minutes. Cool to room temperature.

2. Meanwhile, put the sliced potatoes into a small heavy saucepan. Add enough chicken broth to cover the potato slices by about ½ inch. Bring to a boil, cover the pan, and simmer for about 7 minutes, or until the potatoes are just tender.

Drain the potatoes immediately and transfer them to a salad bowl.

3. Add the sliced onion to the potatoes and strain the cooled marinade over the potatoes and onions. Season the mixture with salt and pepper to taste and sprinkle with the chopped parsley. Toss to mix well. Cool the salad to room temperature. Cover the bowl tightly and chill for several hours or overnight. Drain before serving.

RICE SALAD

4 servings

2 cups cold cooked rice
1 small green pepper, seeded and minced
1 celery stalk, minced
1 small carrot, scraped and minced
4 radishes, trimmed and minced
¼ cup minced red onion
2 tablespoons red wine vinegar
1 tablespoon olive or vegetable oil
½ cup mayonnaise
    Salt and freshly ground black pepper to taste

Combine all the ingredients in a salad bowl. Toss with two forks to combine well. Cover and chill for at least ½ hour before serving.

STRING BEANS VINAIGRETTE
2 servings

¾ pound fresh string beans, ends removed
   Salt
¼ cup thinly sliced red onion
3 tablespoons olive oil
1½ tablespoons red wine vinegar
   Pinch of freshly ground black pepper
¼ teaspoon finely minced garlic
   Pinch of dried oregano
1 small ripe tomato, cored and diced
   Lettuce leaves

1. Wash the string beans in cool running water and drain them well.

2. Put the drained beans in a steamer basket and sprinkle them lightly with salt. Steam the beans in a covered pot over boiling water for 5 to 7 minutes, or until they are just tender. Remove the beans immediately and put them in a bowl. Top the warm beans with the onion slices.

3. Combine the olive oil, vinegar, pepper, and garlic with a pinch of salt in a small bowl. Beat with a fork or a small whisk until combined. (You can also shake the ingredients in a small jar with a tight-fitting lid.) Pour the dressing over the warm beans and toss well. Sprinkle the oregano over the beans and toss again. Let the beans marinate for at least ½ hour, tossing occasionally.

4. When ready to serve, add the diced tomato to the beans and toss well. Serve the salad on lettuce leaves.

BASIL TOMATOES WITH OIL AND VINEGAR DRESSING
2 servings

2 large ripe beefsteak tomatoes, washed and cored
2 tablespoons olive oil
1 tablespoon red wine vinegar
   Salt
   Freshly ground black pepper
6 large fresh basil leaves, or ½ teaspoon dried basil

1. Slice the tomatoes and arrange in a circle on 2 flat salad plates.

2. Mix the olive oil and vinegar together with salt and pepper to taste. Pour the dressing over the tomato slices and sprinkle the basil evenly over all. Serve at once.

CRANBERRY SAUCE
12 servings

1 12-ounce bag fresh cranberries
1 cup water
¾ cup sugar
½ cup orange juice

Put the cranberries, water, and sugar into a saucepan. Bring to a boil over medium heat, stirring occasionally. When the cranberries start popping, cook for 5 minutes, stirring occasionally. Add the orange juice and cook for 2 minutes longer. Let cool and store in a covered jar in the refrigerator. The sauce will keep for about a month.

CUCUMBER RELISH

2 servings

1 *large cucumber*
  Salt
2 *tablespoons white vinegar*
1 *teaspoon sugar*

1. Peel, seed, and dice the cucumber. Put the cucumber pieces in a small bowl and sprinkle them liberally with salt. Let stand for ½ hour.

2. Pour the cucumber pieces into a sieve and let drain well. Then transfer the drained cucumber pieces to a small bowl. Add the vinegar and sugar to the bowl and toss all the ingredients together. Let stand at room temperature for at least ½ hour before serving.

ONION RELISH

4 servings

2 *very large yellow onions, peeled and minced*
¼ *cup finely minced green pepper*
1 *large clove garlic, peeled and minced*
1 *small ripe tomato, peeled, seeded, and minced*
2 *tablespoons lemon juice*
1 *teaspoon ground coriander*
⅛ *teaspoon dried oregano*
½ *teaspoon salt*
⅛ *teaspoon freshly ground black pepper*
⅛ *teaspoon chili powder*
⅛ *teaspoon dried red pepper flakes*

Mix all the ingredients together in a bowl. Let stand at room temperature for at least ½ hour before serving.

Note: This relish will keep well in the refrigerator if stored in a jar with a screw-top lid. Remember to bring it to room temperature before serving.

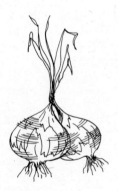

EGGS

ARTICHOKE OMELET

2 servings

4 *artichoke hearts (from a 14-ounce can)*
1 *medium-sized potato*
4 *eggs*
 Salt and freshly ground black pepper
3 *tablespoons butter or margarine*

1. Put the artichoke hearts in a sieve and drain them well.
2. Peel the potato and cut it into ¼-inch cubes. Boil the potato in salted water until it is just tender. Drain well and cool to room temperature.
3. Cut the artichoke hearts into ½-inch pieces.
4. Beat the eggs in a medum-sized mixing bowl until they are frothy. Combine the artichoke and potato pieces with the eggs and season the mixture with salt and pepper to taste.
5. Melt the butter in an 8-inch nonstick frying pan with sloping sides. When the butter is completely melted and bubbling, but not brown, pour in the egg mixture. (You may have to move the vegetables around to distribute them evenly, but do not scramble the eggs.)
6. Let the omelet cook over medium heat until the eggs are just about set. Use a thin spatula to loosen the omelet from the bottom of the pan.
7. Lay a flat inner plate over the frying pan and, holding the plate against the pan, turn the omelet out so that the uncooked side of the omelet is on the dinner plate. Slide the omelet back into the frying pan and cook for 2 to 4 minutes longer, or until the underside is just lightly brown. Divide the omelet in half and serve immediately.

Note: You can use the remaining artichoke hearts from the 14-ounce can to make the Marinated Artichokes on page 209.

ASPARAGUS OMELET

2 servings

6 *cooked asparagus spears, cut into 1-inch lengths*
1 *large potato, peeled, diced, and cooked until just tender and drained*
4 *eggs, beaten*
 Salt and freshly ground black pepper
3 *tablespoons butter or margarine*

1. Combine the asparagus, potato, and eggs in a bowl. Season with salt and pepper to taste.
2. Melt the butter in an 8-inch nonstick frying pan with sloping sides. When the butter is completely melted and bubbling, but not brown, pour in the egg mixture. (You may have to move the vegetables around to distribute them evenly, but do not scramble the eggs.)
3. Let the omelet cook over medium heat until the eggs are just about set. Use a thin spatula to loosen the omelet from the bottom of the pan.
4. Lay a flat dinner plate over the frying pan and, holding the plate against the pan, turn the omelet out so that the uncooked side of the omelet is on the dinner plate. Slide the omelet back

into the frying pan and cook for 2 to 4 minutes longer, or until the underside is just lightly brown. Divide the omelet in half and serve immediately.

BROCCOLI OMELET

2 servings

1½ cups cooked chopped broccoli
1   medium-sized potato, peeled, diced, and
     cooked until just tender, and drained
4   eggs, beaten
     Salt and freshly ground black pepper
2   slices bacon, diced

1. Combine the broccoli, potato, and eggs in a bowl. Season with salt and pepper to taste.
2. Cook the bacon in an 8-inch nonstick frying pan with sloping sides until it is just crisp. Remove the bacon pieces with a slotted spoon and lay on paper towels to drain.
3. Pour off all but 3 tablespoons of the bacon fat from the frying pan. Heat the pan over medium heat.
4. Stir the cooked bacon into the egg mixture and pour the egg mixture into the skillet. (You may have to move the vegetables around to distribute them evenly, but do not scramble the eggs.)
5. Let the omelet cook over medium heat until the eggs are just about set. Use a thin spatula to loosen the omelet from the bottom of the pan.
6. Lay a flat dinner plate over the frying pan and, holding the plate against the pan, turn the omelet out so that the uncooked side of the omelet is on the dinner plate. Slide the omelet back into the frying pan and cook for 2 to 4 minutes longer, or until the underside is just lightly brown. Divide the omelet in half and serve immediately.

CAULIFLOWER OMELET

2 servings

1½ cups cooked chopped cauliflower
1   medium-sized potato, peeled, diced, and
     cooked until just tender, and drained
4   eggs, beaten
     Salt and freshly ground black pepper
3   tablespoons butter or margarine

1. Combine the cauliflower, potato, and eggs in a bowl. Season with salt and pepper to taste.
2. Melt the butter in an 8-inch nonstick frying pan with sloping sides. When the butter is completely melted and bubbling, but not brown, pour in the egg mixture. (You may have to move the vegetables around to distribute them evenly, but do not scramble the eggs.)
3. Let the omelet cook over medium heat until the eggs are just about set. Use a thin spatula to loosen the omelet from the bottom of the pan.
4. Lay a flat dinner plate over the frying pan and, holding the plate against the pan, turn the omelet out so that the uncooked side of the omelet is on the dinner plate. Slide the omelet back into the frying pan and cook for 2 to 4 minutes longer, or until the underside is just lightly brown. Divide the omelet in half and serve immediately.

SPINACH OMELET

2 servings

2 slices bacon, diced
1 small yellow onion, peeled and minced
1 10-ounce package frozen chopped spinach, thawed
4 eggs, beaten
1 medium-sized potato, peeled, diced, and cooked until just tender, and drained
Salt and freshly ground black pepper
3 tablespoons buter or margarine

1. Put the diced bacon in a frying pan and sauté it over medium heat until it is just crisp. Do not let it brown too much. Use a slotted spoon to remove the bacon to paper towels to drain.

2. Pour off all but 1 tablespoon of the bacon fat from the frying pan. Add the onion and sauté for 5 minutes. Add the thawed spinach and steam, covered, over medium heat for 10 minutes, breaking up the spinach with a fork, if necessary. Drain the onion-spinach mixture in a sieve, pressing out any excess water with the back of a wooden spoon. Cool to room temperature.

3. Combine the eggs, potato, cooled spinach mixture, and drained bacon in a bowl. Season with salt and pepper to taste.

4. Melt the butter in an 8-inch nonstick frying pan with sloping sides. When the butter is hot, but not brown, pour in the egg mixture. (You may have to move the vegetables around to distribute them evenly, but do not scramble the eggs.)

5. Let the omelet cook over medium heat until the eggs are just about set. Use a thin spatula to loosen the omelet from the bottom of the pan.

6. Lay a flat dinner plate over the frying pan and, holding the plate against the pan, turn the omelet out so that the uncooked side of the omelet is on the dinner plate. Slide the omelet back into the frying pan and cook for 2 to 4 minutes longer, or until the underside is just lightly brown. Divide the omelet in half and serve immediately.

POACHED EGGS WITH STEWED ZUCCHINI

2 servings

3 cups Stewed Zucchini (page 298)
4 eggs

1. Put the zucchini in a frying pan and bring just to a simmer over medium heat.

2. When the zucchini is simmering, use a wooden spoon to make 4 indentations in it. Break 1 egg into each of the indentations and spoon some of the sauce over each egg. Cover the frying pan and lower the heat slightly. Cook for 5 to 6 minutes, or until the eggs are set. Serve immediately.

QUICHE LORRAINE

4 servings

1 tablespoon butter or margarine
1 medium-sized yellow onion, peeled and minced
3 eggs
2 cups half-and-half
1 cup diced Swiss cheese
¼ pound boiled ham, diced
1 teaspoon salt
⅛ teaspoon freshly ground black pepper
Pinch of ground nutmeg
1 8-ounce cylinder crescent rolls

1. Melt the butter in a small frying pan. When it is hot and bubbling, add the onion. Sauté for 5 minutes, stirring occasionally. Let the onion cool in the frying pan.

2. Put the eggs and half-and-half in a large bowl and beat until well combined. Stir in the Swiss cheese, diced ham, salt, pepper, nutmeg, and cooled onion. Mix well.

3. Preheat the oven to 375 degrees.

4. Break open the cylinder of crescent rolls and lay the pieces of dough out next to one another on a 12- x 14-inch piece of wax paper. Put another piece of wax paper of equal size on top of the dough. Roll the dough out to a 12-inch circle. Fit the dough into a 9-inch deep-dish pie plate, making sure that it fits the bottom snugly. Make a stand-up edge along the top of the pie plate. Pour in the prepared custard, smoothing the top to an even layer. Bake for 45 to 50 minutes, or until the custard is set and the crust is golden. (The custard is set when a knife, inserted about 2 inches from the edge, comes out clean.) Let sit for a few minutes before serving.

Note: This makes 4 generous servings. Serve 2 portions for this meal and cover and refrigerate the remaining half of the quiche for another meal. It can be reheated in a 350-degree oven for about 20 minutes.

SPINACH PIE
4 servings

4   slices thick-sliced bacon, diced
1   medium-sized yellow onion, peeled and minced
1   10-ounce package frozen chopped spinach, thawed
3   eggs
2   cups half-and-half
1   teaspoon salt
1/8   teaspoon freshly ground black pepper
    Pinch of ground nutmeg
1/2 to 2/3 cup diced Swiss cheese
1   8-ounce cylinder crescent rolls

1. Put the diced bacon in a frying pan and sauté it over medium heat until it is just crisp. Do not let it brown too much. Use a slotted spoon to remove the bacon to paper towels to drain.

2. Pour off all but 1 tablespoon of the bacon fat from the frying pan. Add the onion and sauté for 5 minutes. Add the thawed spinach and steam, covered, over medium heat for 10 minutes, breaking up the spinach with a fork, if necessary. Drain the onion-spinach mixture in a sieve, pressing out any excess water with the back of a wooden spoon. Cool to room temperature.

3. Put the eggs and half-and-half in a large bowl and beat until well combined. Stir in the salt, pepper, nutmeg, Swiss cheese, onion-spinach mixture, and the drained bacon. Mix well.

4. Preheat the oven to 375 degrees.

5. Break open the cylinder of crescent rolls and lay the pieces of dough out next to one another on a 12- by 14-inch piece of wax paper. Put another piece of wax paper of equal size on top of the dough. Roll the dough out to a 12-inch circle. Fit the dough into a 9-inch deep-dish pie plate, making sure that it fits the bottom snugly. Make a stand-up edge along the top of the pie plate. Pour in the prepared custard, smoothing the top to an even layer. Bake for 45 to 50 minutes or until the custard is set and the crust is golden. (The custard is set when a knife, inserted about 2 inches from the edge, comes

out clean.) Let sit for a few minutes before serving.

Note: This will make 4 generous servings. Cool the remainder of the pie, wrap it well, and refrigerate for another meal. The pie will keep for about 3 days, and can be reheated in a 350-degree oven for about 20 minutes.

CINNAMON-CHEESE TOAST

2 servings

4 *slices whole wheat bread*
2 *ounces softened cream cheese*
2 *eggs*
1 *tablespoon milk*
   Pinch of ground cinnamon
   Dash of vanilla extract
3 *tablespoons butter or margarine*

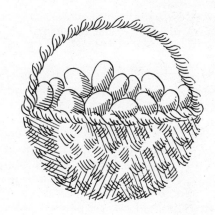

1. Spread each of 2 slices of the bread with 1 ounce of the softened cream cheese. Top each slice with another slice of bread.

2. Beat the eggs until frothy in a flat soup plate or pie plate. Beat in the milk, cinnamon, and vanilla.

3. Melt the butter on a griddle or in a large frying pan. While the butter is melting, soak each of the sandwiches on both sides in the egg mixture until well saturated. Then put the soaked sandwiches on the griddle and cook, turning once, until golden brown on both sides Serve at once sprinkled with additional cinnamon or dribbled with maple syrup.

FISH AND SHELLFISH

SAUTÉED FLOUNDER FILLETS

2 servings

4 small fresh flounder fillets
  Flour for dredging
3 tablespoons butter or margarine
  Salt and freshly ground black pepper
  Lemon wedges

1. Wash the fillets in cool running water, making sure there are no bones left in the fish. If there are, remove them carefully.
2. Coat the fillets completely in the flour.
3. Melt the butter in a frying pan large enough to hold the fillets comfortably. When the butter is hot and bubbling, add the fillets in a single layer. Sauté over medium heat until golden brown. Turn and brown on the second side. Drain the browned fillets briefly on paper towels and serve garnished with lemon wedges.

BAKED ROLLED FLOUNDER

2 servings

2 cups Eggplant Sauce (page 275)
4 small fresh flounder fillets
  Salt and freshly ground black pepper

1. Preheat the oven to 350 degrees.
2. Spread 1 cup of the Eggplant Sauce in the bottom of a small round baking dish.
3. Wash the fillets in cool running water, making sure there are no bones left in the fish. If there are, remove them carefully.
4. Roll the fillets tightly skin side in and put them seam side down in the baking dish. Sprinkle the fillet rolls generously with salt and pepper. Spoon the remaining sauce over the fish rolls and bake for 15 to 20 minutes, or until the sauce is hot and the fish flakes easily.

SHRIMP-STUFFED FILLETS

2 servings

1 7½-ounce can shrimp, drained
1 tablespoon finely minced onion
1 tablespoon finely minced parsley
⅛ teaspoon curry powder
  Pinch of garlic powder
  Salt and freshly ground black pepper
4 small fresh flounder or sole fillets
½ cup clam broth
½ cup water

1. Combine the shrimp, onion, parsley, curry powder, and garlic powder in a small bowl. Use a wooden spoon to work the mixture into a fine paste. Season with salt and pepper to taste.
2. Wash the fillets in cool running water, making sure there are no bones left in the fish. If there are, remove them carefully.
3. Lay the fillets flat, skin side up. Sprinkle them lightly with salt and pepper. Spread an equal amount of the shrimp mixture on each

fillet. Roll the fillets up tightly and put them seam side down in a frying pan just large enough to hold them. Mix the clam broth and water together and pour it around the fillets in the frying pan. Put the frying pan over low heat, cover, and poach the fish rolls for 20 to 25 minutes, or until the fish flakes easily. Carefully remove the fish rolls from the poaching liquid. Serve on a bed of Steamed Spinach (page 297).

HADDOCK WITH CAPERS

2 servings

¾ pound fresh haddock fillet
2 tablespoons butter or margarine
1 tablespoon drained capers
  Salt and freshly ground black pepper
  Lemon wedges

1. Preheat the oven to 350 degrees.
2. Cut the fillet into 2 equal portions. Check to see that there are no bones left in the fish; if there are, remove them carefully. Wash the fish in cool running water and pat the pieces dry with paper towels.
3. Spread the butter over the inside of a baking dish large enough to hold the fish comfortably. Sprinkle an equal amount of capers on each piece of fish. Sprinkle the fish generously with salt and pepper. Bake for 15 to 20 minutes, or until the fish flakes easily. Serve each portion garnished with lemon wedges.

BAKED FISH WITH EGGPLANT

2 servings

1 ¾-pound eggplant
  Salt
  Butter
¾ pound fresh haddock fillet, cut into 2 equal portions
2 large ripe tomatoes, cored, peeled, seeded, and diced
  Freshly ground black pepper
½ cup unseasoned bread crumbs
1 tablespoon finely minced parsley
2 cloves garlic, peeled and finely minced
1 teaspoon dried basil, crumbled
2 tablespoons olive oil

1. Peel the eggplant and cut it into 1-inch cubes. Put the eggplant cubes into a saucepan and sprinkle them with salt. Pour boiling water over the eggplant and let sit for 10 minutes. Drain well, pressing out any excess moisture with the back of a spoon.
2. Butter a baking dish large enough to hold the pieces of fish comfortably.
3. Wash the fillets in cool running water, making sure there are no bones left in the fish. If there are, remove them carefully. Lay the fillets skin side down in the baking dish. Sprinkle lightly with salt.
4. Preheat the oven to 375 degrees.
5. Combine the drained eggplant and tomatoes in a bowl. Sprinkle lightly with salt and pepper. Toss to mix well. Spoon the vegetable mixture over the fillets in the baking dish.
6. In a small bowl, combine the bread crumbs, parsley, garlic, basil, and olive oil. Mix together until moistened completely. Season lightly with salt and pepper. Sprinkle the bread crumb

mixture over the vegetables in the baking dish. Bake for 20 minutes, or until the fish flakes easily. Serve immediately.

MARINATED HADDOCK

2 servings

3/4 *pound fresh haddock fillet*
2 *tablespoons olive oil*
2 *tablespoons lemon juice*
1/2 *teaspoon dry mustard*
1/4 *teaspoon salt*
1/4 *teaspoon freshly ground black pepper*
1/4 *teaspoon dried oregano, crumbled*
1/2 *cup all-purpose flour*
1 *egg*
  Vegetable oil
  Lemon wedges

1. Cut the fillet into 2 equal portions. Check to see that there are no bones left in the fish; if there are, remove them carefully. Wash the fish in cool running water and pat the pieces dry with paper towels.
2. Combine the olive oil, lemon juice, dry mustard, salt, pepper, and oregano together in a bowl large enough to hold the pieces of fish. Add the fish and turn it to coat it completely with the mixture. Let sit for 1/2 hour at room temperature.
3. Spread the flour in a layer on a piece of wax paper.
4. Put the egg in a flat soup plate or pie plate and beat it lightly with a fork.
5. Pour 1/4 inch oil into a frying pan large enough to hold the fish pieces comfortably. Heat the oil over medium heat.
6. Use a fork to remove the fish pieces from

the marinade. Let most of the marinade drip off. Then dip each fillet into the flour, coating it completely. Dip the coated fillet into the beaten egg, coating it completely. Lay the fillet immediately into the hot oil in the frying pan. Fry the fillets until golden brown on both sides. Serve immediately with lemon wedges.

FISH PRIMAVERA

2 servings

2 *medium-sized zucchini*
2 *small potatoes*
2 *large ripe tomatoes, preferably beefsteak*
3 *tablespoons plus 1 teaspoon olive oil*
2 *large cloves garlic, peeled and minced*
  Salt and freshly ground black pepper
  Fresh basil leaves, minced, or dried basil
2 *scallions, trimmed and minced*
3/4 *pound fresh haddock or scrod fillet (any thick, firm, white-fleshed fish will do), cut into 2 portions*

1. Wash the zucchini very well in cool running water. Trim both ends and cut the zucchini into 1 1/2-inch lengths. Cut each length into 1/4-inch-thick slices, lengthwise. Then cut each slice, lengthwise, into 1/4-inch sticks. Bring a small pot of water to a boil and plunge the zucchini sticks into the boiling water. Remove the pot from the heat and let the zucchini sit in the water for 2 minutes, then drain very well.
2. Peel the potatoes and cut them into sticks about the same size as the zucchini. Bring a large pot of water to a boil and plunge the potato sticks into the boiling water. Remove the pot from the heat and let the potato sticks sit in the water for 5 minutes, then drain very well.

3. Core the tomatoes. Bring a large pot of water to a boil and plunge the cored tomatoes into the boiling water. Remove the pot from the heat and let the tomatoes sit in the water for 2 minutes, then drain off the hot water and add cold water to the pot. Let the tomatoes sit in the cold water for 2 to 3 minutes, then peel them and slice them ¼ inch thick.

4. Spread the 3 tablespoons of olive oil over the bottom and sides of a 10-inch deep-dish pie plate. (Most of the oil will end up on the bottom, but don't worry about it.) Make a layer of the tomato slices on the bottom of the dish. Sprinkle one-third of the minced garlic over the tomato slices. Then sprinkle the tomatoes liberally with salt and pepper. Distribute some minced basil and scallions over the tomato layer.

5. Next make a layer of the potatoes on top of the tomatoes. Sprinkle the potato sticks with one-third of the garlic and then liberally with salt and pepper and a few of the scallion pieces.

6. Finally, make a layer of the zucchini sticks. Sprinkle them with the remaining minced garlic, basil, and scallions. Season very well with salt and pepper.

7. Wash the fillets in cool running water, making sure there are no bones left in the fish. If there are, remove them carefully. Lay the fish portions on top of the zucchini and season the fish with salt and pepper. Dribble the remaining teaspoon of oil over the fish and vegetables.

8. Preheat the oven to 375 degrees. Tear off a very long piece of wide, heavy duty aluminum foil. Put the filled baking dish in the center of the foil sheet and bring up the short edges of the foil to meet over the dish. Fold the edges down tightly to enclose the dish securely. Fold over the open sides of the foil until the dish is completely enclosed. (What you are doing is making a papillote with the baking dish.)

9. Put the foil-enclosed baking dish on a baking sheet and transfer both to the middle shelf of the oven. Bake for 30 minutes. At that time, the fish and vegetables should all be tender. Serve each portion with some of the pan juices.

Note: This dish benefits from a lot of basil and freshly ground black pepper, mainly because potatoes and zucchini can be rather bland. So, don't hesitate to be rather heavy handed with these two ingredients.

SPANISH-STYLE COD

2 servings

1 tablespoon olive oil
1 small white onion, peeled and minced
1 clove garlic, peeled and minced
1 medium-sized green pepper, seeded and diced
1 8-ounce can stewed tomatoes
  Salt and freshly ground black pepper
  Pinch of saffron threads
  Pinch of dried oregano
2 fresh cod steaks, cut ½ inch thick
  Bread crumbs

1. Heat the oil in a small saucepan. Add the onion, garlic, and green pepper and sauté over low heat for 5 minutes, stirring occasionally.

2. Drain the stewed tomatoes and reserve the liquid. Cut the tomatoes into very small pieces and add to the sautéed vegetables in the frying pan. Cook and stir for 2 minutes. Add the reserved liquid, salt and pepper to taste, saffron, and oregano to the saucepan. Stir to mix well. Cover and simmer for 10 minutes.

3. Preheat the oven to 350 degrees.

4. Wash the cod steaks under cool running

water. Dip them immediately (while still very damp) into the bread crumbs, coating all sides and pressing the crumbs on with the palm of your hand. Put the cod steaks on a rack in a small baking pan. Bake for 15 to 20 minutes, or until the fish flakes easily. Serve immediately, topping each cod steak with half of the sauce.

SAUTÉED BLUEFISH

2 servings

¾ *pound fresh bluefish fillet*
  Seasoned bread crumbs
1 *tablespoon vegetable oil*
2 *tablespoons butter or margarine*
4 *tablespoons lemon juice*
½ *teaspoon dried oregano, crumbled*
  Salt and freshly ground black pepper

1. Cut the fillet into 2 equal portions. Check to see that there are no bones left in the fish; if there are, remove them carefully. Wash the fish in cool running water. While the fish is still damp, dip it in the bread crumbs, coating all sides and pressing the crumbs on with the palm of your hand. Lay the coated fillets on a flat plate and refrigerate for 10 minutes.

2. Heat the oil and butter in a frying pan large enough to hold the fish comfortably. When the mixture is hot and bubbling, add the fillets flesh side down (the skin will then be up). Cook over medium heat for 5 minutes, or until golden. Turn the fish carefully (using 2 spatulas, if necessary) skin side down, and cook for 5 minutes longer. While the fish is cooking on the second side, sprinkle the lemon juice and oregano over each fillet. Season with a little salt and pepper and serve immediately.

SALMON PATTIES

4 servings

1 *15-ounce can salmon*
2 *slices white bread, trimmed of crusts, soaked in water, and squeezed dry*
1 *egg*
1 *tablespoon finely minced onion*
¼ *teaspoon finely minced garlic*
1 *tablespoon minced parsley*
2 *tablespoons grated Parmesan cheese*
2 *tablespoons bread crumbs*
2 *tablespoons butter or margarine*
1 *tablespoon vegetable oil*

1. Drain the salmon and remove all bones and skin. Put the cleaned salmon into a mixing bowl and add the bread, egg, onion, garlic, parsley, cheese, and bread crumbs. Mix with your hands to combine the ingredients well. Shape the mixture into 4 or 5 equal-sized patties. Put the patties in a single layer on a large plate and refrigerate for at least 10 minutes.

2. Heat the butter and oil together in a large nonstick frying pan. When the mixture is bubbling, add the salmon patties in one layer. Sauté until golden brown on both sides. Drain on paper towels and serve while warm.

POACHED SALMON

2 servings

½   cup chopped carrot
½   cup chopped onion
¼   cup diced celery
4   peppercorns
2   whole cloves
½   teaspoon salt
1   bay leaf
1   tablespoon minced parsley
1½ cup water
2   slices salmon steak, cut about ½ inch thick
    Mayonnaise
    Lemon wedges

1. Combine the carrot, onion, celery, peppercorns, cloves, salt, bay leaf, parsley, and water in a frying pan large enough to hold the salmon in one layer. Bring to a boil and simmer for 5 minutes.

2. Lay the salmon steaks in the poaching liquid, return to a simmer, cover the pan, and poach for 4 minutes. Turn the salmon steaks over carefully and poach 4 to 5 minutes longer, or until the fish flakes easily. Remove the salmon steaks carefully from the poaching liquid and allow them to drain and cool. Serve with mayonnaise and lemon wedges.

SNAPPY RED SNAPPER

2 servings

2   tablespoons olive oil
¼   cup minced green pepper
¼   cup minced red onion
1   clove garlic, peeled and minced

1   teaspoon drained capers
1   14-ounce can peeled Italian tomatoes with liquid
6   chopped fresh basil leaves, or ¼ teaspoon dried basil
¾   teaspoon salt
⅛   teaspoon freshly ground black pepper
    Pinch of dried red pepper flakes
1   1½-pound red snapper, filleted

1. Heat the oil in a large frying pan. When the oil is hot add the green pepper, red onion, and garlic. Sauté over low heat for 5 minutes, stirring occasionally. Add the capers, tomatoes and their liquid, basil, salt, black pepper, and red pepper flakes. Stir to mix well. Bring to a boil, cover the pan, and simmer over low heat for 15 minutes, stirring occasionally.

2. Check to see that there are no bones left in the fish; if there are, remove them carefully. Wash the fillets in cool running water and pat dry with paper towels.

3. Lay the snapper fillets skin side down on the sauce. Spoon some sauce over the top of the fillets. Cover the frying pan and simmer over low heat for 10 minutes. Serve immediately.

BAKED TILE FISH

2 servings

1   fresh tile fish steak, cut ¾ inch thick (about ¾ pound)
1   tablespoon butter or margarine
    Salt and freshly ground black pepper
    Garlic powder
    Onion powder
    Lemon wedges

1. Wash the fish steak under cool running water. Pat dry with paper towels.

2. Preheat the oven to 350 degrees.

3. Spread the butter in a baking dish large enough to hold the fish comfortably. Lay the fish in the buttered dish and sprinkle it generously with salt, pepper, garlic powder, and onion powder. Bake for 20 to 25 minutes, or until the fish flakes easily.

4. To serve, use a fork and spoon to separate the flesh from the central bone. Serve half the steak per portion, garnished with lemon wedges.

SAUTÉED SHRIMP

2 servings

1/2 cup all-purpose flour
Salt and freshly ground black pepper
2 tablespoons butter or margarine
1 tablespoon vegetable oil
1/2 pound shrimp, peeled and deveined
Lemon wedges

1. Combine the flour with salt and pepper to taste on a piece of wax paper.

2. Heat the butter and oil until bubbly in a large frying pan.

3. Dip the shrimp in the flour mixture to coat all sides. Lay the floured shrimp in a single layer in the frying pan and sauté, shaking the pan (to keep the shrimp from sticking) and turning the shrimp once, until they are all pink. Drain on paper towels and serve immediately, garnished with lemon wedges.

SHRIMP IN LOBSTER SAUCE

2 servings

1/4 pound lean ground pork
1 tablespoon dried vegetable flakes
Pinch of salt
Pinch of freshly ground black pepper
2 tablespoons vegetable or peanut oil
1 clove garlic, peeled
1/2 pound shrimp, peeled and deveined
1/4 cup chicken broth
1/2 tablespoon cornstarch
1 tablespoon cold water
2 tablespoons beaten egg
1 scallion, minced

1. Combine the pork, vegetable flakes, salt, and pepper in a small bowl. Mix well with your fingers. Let sit for 10 minutes.

2. Heat the oil in a wok or heavy frying pan. Add the garlic and brown it on both sides over medium heat. Remove and discard the garlic once it has browned.

3. Add the pork to the oil in the frying pan and sauté, stirring, for 2 minutes. Add the shrimp and cook, stirring, for 1 minute, or until the shrimp have turned pink.

4. Add the chicken broth to the wok, lower the heat, and cook for 1 minute.

5. Combine the cornstarch and water and stir it into the shrimp mixture. Stir until the mixture comes to a boil and thickens. Gradually add the egg, stirring constantly, until all the egg is incorporated. Serve immediately, garnishing each portion with some of the minced scallion.

SHRIMP WITH GARLIC SAUCE

2 servings

4 *dried Chinese mushrooms, stems removed*
1 *tablespoon tree ears or black fungus*
2 *teaspoons cornstarch*
½ *cup chicken broth*
2 *teaspoons soy sauce*
1 *teaspoon Hoisin sauce*
2 *tablespoons vegetable or peanut oil*
1 *small white onion, peeled and minced*
1 *teaspoon minced fresh gingerroot*
4 *cloves garlic, peeled and minced*
½ *pound shrimp, peeled and deveined*

1. Put the mushrooms and tree ears in a bowl and cover them with boiling water. Let sit for 20 minutes to soften. Drain and squeeze out all the excess water. Cut the mushrooms into thin strips and dice the tree ears. Set aside for use later.

2. Combine the cornstarch with the chicken broth in a cup. Stir in the soy sauce and Hoisin sauce. Set aside for use later.

3. Heat the oil in a wok or heavy fying pan over medium-high heat. Stir in the onion, gingerroot, and garlic and cook for 1 minute. Add the shrimp and stir and cook until the shrimp have all turned pink. Mix in the mushrooms and tree ears (from step 1). Stir the sauce mixture (from step 2) and pour it over the shrimp and vegetables. Cook, stirring, for 1 minute, or until the sauce has thickened. Serve immediately.

Note: Tree ears and Hoisin sauce can be purchased in Oriental markets.

SAUTÉED SCALLOPS

2 servings

½ *cup all-purpose flour*
  Salt and freshly ground black pepper
½ *pound scallops, washed and drained*
3 *tablespoons butter or margarine*
  Lemon wedges

1. Season the flour with salt and pepper. Toss the scallops in the seasoned flour to coat them lightly.

2. Melt the butter in a frying pan large enough to hold the scallops comfortably. When it is hot and bubbling, add the scallops and cook quickly, for 2 minutes, turning once, or until the scallops are just tender. Serve immediately, garnished with lemon wedges.

SEA SCALLOPS WITH CUCUMBER

2 servings

¾ *pound sea scallops*
1 *tablespoon dry sherry*
¾ *teaspoon salt*
2 *teaspoons cornstarch*
2 *small cucumbers*
3 *tablespoons vegetable or peanut oil*
2 *tablespoons soy sauce*

1. Wash the scallops in cool running water. Pat them dry with paper towels. Cut the scallops into ¼-inch-thick slices and put the slices in a bowl. Add the sherry, ½ teaspoon salt, and the cornstarch to the scallops. Mix with your fingers to coat the scallops well. Set aside until needed.

2. Peel the cucumbers and cut them into quarters lengthwise. Remove the seeds from each quarter and cut each quarter into 1-inch lengths.

3. Heat 1½ tablespoons of the oil in a wok or heavy frying pan. When the oil is hot, add the cucumber pieces and stir them to coat them with the oil. Sprinkle remaining ¼ teaspoon of salt over the cucumber pieces and cook over medium-high heat for 3 minutes, stirring occasionally. Use a slotted spoon to remove the cucumber pieces to a bowl. Set aside until needed.

4. Wipe the wok dry with a paper towel. Return it to medium heat. Pour the remaining 1½ tablespoons of oil into the wok. When the oil is hot, use a slotted spoon to transfer the scallop slices from the marinade to the wok. Stir-fry, tossing the scallops constantly, for 2 to 3 minutes, or until the scallops are just tender. Return the cucumber pieces to the wok and stir to mix well with the scallop slices. Add the soy sauce and mix well, stirring for 1 minute longer. Serve immediately.

STEAMED MUSSELS

2 servings

2 tablespoons olive oil
1 small white onion, peeled and minced
2 cloves garlic, peeled and minced
2 tablespoons finely minced parsley
1 cup clam juice
2 pounds mussels, well washed and bearded

Heat the oil in a Dutch oven. When it is hot, add the onion and garlic and sauté quickly over medium heat for 2 minutes. Add the mussels and cover the pan. Cook over medium-high heat, shaking the pan occasionally, until the mussels have opened wide. Discard any unopened mussels. Serve equal portions of mussels and sauce in deep soup bowls.

Note: For a delicious variation of this dish, add 1 diced ripe tomato to the onion and garlic and spoon the mussels and sauce over cooked linguini.

OYSTER PILAF

2 servings

1 dozen fresh, shucked oysters with their liquor
2 tablespoons vegetable oil
1 small white onion, peeled and minced
1 clove garlic, peeled and minced
2 large ripe tomatoes, peeled, seeded, and diced
  Salt
  Freshly ground black pepper
  Pinch of saffron threads
2 tablespoons finely minced parsley
1 cup chicken broth
½ cup raw rice

1. Put a large sieve over a bowl and add the oysters to the sieve. Allow the oyster liquor to drain into the bowl.

2. Heat the oil in a heavy pot with a cover. When it is hot, add the onion and sauté over medium heat, stirring constantly, for 3 to 4 minutes. Add the garlic and tomatoes and sauté for about 10 minutes, stirring occasionally with a wooden spoon to break up the tomatoes.

3. Season the vegetables with salt and pepper. Add the saffron and parsley and cook for 2 minutes. Add the chicken broth and any oyster liquid in the bowl. Bring to a boil. Use a fork to stir in the rice. Bring back to a boil, cover the

pot, and lower the heat. Cook over low heat for 10 minutes.

4. Add the drained oysters to the rice, mixing them in gently with a fork. (Be sure the oysters are under the surface of the rice.) Cover the pot and cook for 7 minutes longer, or until all the liquid has been absorbed. Let the dish sit, covered, for a few minutes before serving.

SAUTÉED OYSTERS

2 servings

1 *dozen oysters, shucked*
1 *egg*
1½ *cups seasoned bread crumbs*
4 *tablespoons butter or margarine*
 Lemon wedges

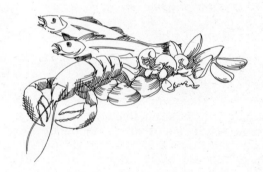

1. Put the oysters in a sieve and let them drain.
2. Beat the egg in a flat soup plate or pie plate.
3. Spread the bread crumbs in a thin layer on a sheet of wax paper.
4. Dip each oyster first in the beaten egg and then in the bread crumbs, coating it completely, and pressing the crumbs on with the palm of your hand. Lay the oysters on a plate as they are coated. Be sure that they do not touch. Separate the layers of coated oysters with sheets of wax paper. Refrigerate the coated oysters for 10 minutes.
5. Melt the butter in a large frying pan. When it is hot and bubbling, add a layer of oysters. Sauté over medium heat for 3 or 4 minutes, or until golden brown. Turn and brown the other side. Drain the browned oysters on paper towels. You may have to add more butter to the pan to finish cooking the oysters. Serve immediately, garnished with lemon wedges.

POULTRY

LEMON-BASTED ROAST CHICKEN

4 servings

1   2½- to 3-pound frying chicken
    Salt and freshly ground black pepper
½   teaspoon finely minced garlic
1   small yellow or white onion, peeled and cut in
    half
1   tablespoon olive oil
2   tablespoons lemon juice
1   large clove garlic, peeled and minced
1   teaspoon dried oregano, crumbled

1. Preheat the oven to 375 degrees.
2. Wash the chicken inside and out in cool running water. Pat it dry with paper towels. Sprinkle the inside of the chicken with salt, pepper, and the finely minced garlic. Put the onion halves in the cavity and close the cavity with skewers or toothpicks. Sprinkle the outside of the chicken with salt and pepper.
3. Put the chicken breast side up on a rack in a roasting pan. Roast for 20 minutes. Turn the chicken breast side down and roast for 20 minutes.
4. Combine the oil, lemon juice, minced garlic, oregano, ¼ teaspoon salt, and a pinch of black pepper in a small cup. Stir to mix well.
5. When the chicken has roasted for 40 minutes, turn it breast side up again and brush it all over with the lemon sauce. Roast for 10 minutes and brush with the remaining sauce. Roast for 10 minutes longer, or until the chicken is tender and golden brown.

6. To serve, quarter the chicken with poultry shears, discarding the onion. Spoon some of the pan juices over each portion.
Note: Let the leftover chicken cool to room temperature. Put it and any remaining pan juices in a glass bowl. Cover tightly with aluminum foil and refrigerate. The leftover chicken makes excellent lunch dishes or it can be reheated in a toaster oven or very low (300-degree) oven for another meal.

CHICKEN GUMBO

4 servings

1   3-pound frying chicken
2   slices bacon
1   large yellow onion, peeled and minced
1   large green pepper, seeded and minced
2   cloves garlic, peeled and minced
1   16-ounce can stewed tomatoes
2   cups chicken broth
    Salt and freshly ground black pepper
1   large bay leaf
    Pinch of dried thyme
1   10-ounce package frozen cut okra
    Steamed rice

1. Wash the chicken well in cold running water and pat it dry, inside and out, with paper towels. Cut the chicken into 8 pieces (2 wings, 2 breast halves, 2 thighs, and 2 drumsticks). Set aside until needed.
2. Put the bacon slices in a large Dutch oven.

Cook the bacon over low heat unil it has given up most of its fat and is crisp and brown. Remove and discard the bacon and add the chicken pieces to the hot fat in one layer (Do not crowd the pieces together, but fry them in two batches, if necessary.) Sauté the chicken pieces over low heat until brown on all sides. Remove the chicken to a plate as it browns.

3. When all the chicken is browned, add the onion, pepper, and garlic to the Dutch oven. Sauté over low heat for 10 minutes, stirring occasionally. Add the stewed tomatoes and chicken broth and mix well. Bring to a boil and season with salt and pepper to taste. Add the bay leaf and thyme and return the chicken to the pan. Cover the pan and simmer for 30 minutes, stirring occasionally and turning the chicken pieces so they cook evenly.

4. After the gumbo has cooked for 30 minutes, add the okra, pushing it down into the sauce with a wooden spoon. Let the gumbo return to a simmer and cook, covered, 10 minutes longer.

5. To serve, put ½ cup steamed rice in the middle of a deep soup plate. Lay two pieces of chicken on either side of the rice and ladle over about 1 cup of the sauce and okra from the pan.

ARROZ CON POLLO

4 servings

1	3½-pound chicken
2	tablespoons vegetable oil
1	large yellow onion, peeled and chopped
1	large green pepper, seeded and chopped
2	celery stalks, minced
2	cloves garlic, peeled and minced
½	cup diced smoked ham, or 2 slices bacon, diced
1	8-ounce can stewed tomatoes
	Pinch of saffron threads
	Large pinch of dried oregano
	Salt and freshly ground black pepper
2	teaspoons drained capers
8	pimiento-stuffed olives
1½	cups chicken broth
1	cup rice

1. Cut the chicken into 8 pieces, reserving any fat that can be pulled away from the skin at the neck and thigh areas. Wash the chicken pieces in cool running water and pat dry with paper towels.

2. Put the chicken fat in a large Dutch oven over low heat and cook it until it has given up most of its liquid fat. Add the 2 tablespoons of vegetable oil and heat them with the chicken fat. When the fat and oil are hot, add the chicken pieces and brown them on all sides. Remove the chicken to a plate as it browns.

3. Pour off all but 2 tablespoons of the fat from the Dutch oven. Add the onion, green pepper, celery, and garlic and sauté over low heat for 10 minutes, stirring occasionally. Add the ham and sauté for 5 minutes.

4. Drain the stewed tomatoes and reserve the liquid. Chop the tomatoes finely and add to the vegetables in the Dutch oven with the saffron, oregano, salt and pepper to taste, capers, and olives. Sauté for 5 minutes. Add the reserved tomato liquid and the chicken broth and simmer for 5 minutes. Return the chicken to the pan and bring to a boil. Cover, lower the heat, and simmer for 25 minutes, stirring occasionally.

5. Remove the chicken from the pan and stir the rice into the sauce. Put the chicken back, on top of the rice, cover the pan, and cook over low heat for 20 minutes, or until the rice is tender

and all the liquid as been absorbed. Remove the pan from the heat and let it sit, covered, for 5 minutes before serving.

Note: I do not recommend freezing the leftovers because the texture of the rice will be affected. Leftovers can be reheated in a toaster oven or in a nonstick frying pan with a cover. Put about 2 tablespoons of chicken broth in the bottom of the pan before you add the Arroz con Pollo.

ROAST CHICKEN WITH CURRY STUFFING

2 servings

1	2½- to 3-pound frying chicken
1½	cups finely chopped peeled apple
¼	cup black raisins
1	medium-sized yellow onion, peeled and minced
¼	cup minced parsley
½	cup cooked rice
1	tablespoon lemon juice
2	teaspoons curry powder
	Salt and freshly ground black pepper

1. Preheat the oven to 375 degrees.
2. Wash the chicken in cool running water and pat dry, inside and out, with paper towels.
3. Combine the apple, raisins, onion, parsley, rice, lemon juice, and curry powder in a bowl. Stir to mix well. Season with salt and pepper to taste.
4. Stuff the body cavity of the bird with the mixture. Close the cavity with skewers or toothpicks. Tie the wings to the body with string. Tie the legs together with string.
5. Put the chicken breast side up on a rack in a roasting pan. Roast for 15 minutes. Turn the chicken on its side and roast for 15 minutes. Turn the chicken breast side down and roast for 15 minutes. Turn the chicken on its other side and roast for 10 minutes. Turn the chicken breast side up and roast for 10 minutes longer, or until the chicken is golden brown and done.
6. Remove the chicken from the oven and remove the strings holding the wings and thighs. Let the chicken rest for 5 minutes before cutting it into quarters with poultry shears.

Note: Serve 2 quarters and all of the stuffing, divided evenly, at this meal. Cool and refrigerate the remaining quarters for the meal with Roast Chicken with Curry Sauce (page 235).

COCONUT CHICKEN

4 servings

2	eggs
¼	cup milk
1	teaspoon salt
1	teaspoon curry powder
1	2½- to 3-pound chicken, cut into serving pieces, washed and dried
	Vegetable oil
1	cup unseasoned bread crumbs
1	cup flaked coconut

1. Combine the eggs, milk, salt, and curry powder in a large bowl and beat well. Add the cut-up chicken to the bowl and stir to coat each piece with the mixture. Let sit for 15 minutes.
2. Preheat the oven to 350 derees. Coat the inside of a 9- by 13-inch baking pan with oil and set it aside.
3. Combine the bread crumbs and coconut on a large sheet of wax paper. Mix them well with

your fingers. Lift the chicken pieces from the marinade one at a time and coat them well with the bread crumb-coconut mixture, pressing it on to the chicken with your hands. Put the coated chicken in the prepared baking pan and bake for 1¼ hours, or until brown and tender.

Note: Leftovers can be wrapped securely and refrigerated; they are good served cold.

ROAST CHICKEN WITH CURRY SAUCE

2 servings

2   *chicken quarters from the recipe for Roast Chicken with Curry Stuffing (page 234)*
2   *tablespoons butter or margarine*
1   *small white onion, peeled and minced*
½   *cup finely chopped peeled apple*
1½   *teaspoons curry powder, or to taste*
¼   *teaspoon ground ginger*
2   *tablespoons all-purpose flour*
1   *cup chicken broth, heated*
¼   *cup milk*
2   *tablespoons chopped Major Grey's chutney*

1. Bring the chicken quarters to room temperature while you make the curry sauce.

2. Melt the butter in a frying pan large enough to hold the chicken comfortably. When it is hot and bubbling, add the onion and apple. Sauté over low heat for 5 minutes, stirring occasionally. Sprinkle the curry powder, ginger, and flour over the onions and apples and mix well. Cook, stirring, for 1 minute. Remove from the heat and let the mixture cool a little.

3. Gradually add the chicken broth, stirring until the sauce is smooth. Stir in the milk and mix well. Cook over low heat for 5 minutes, stirring constantly, or until the sauce has thickened. Stir in the chopped chutney and mix well. Add the chicken quarters to the frying pan and spoon some of the sauce over them. Cover the pan and heat over very low heat for 5 to 10 minutes, or until the chicken is heated through.

SKILLET CHICKEN

2 servings

3   *tablespoons butter or margarine*
2   *chicken quarters, washed and dried*
1   *clove garlic, peeled and minced*
2   *ripe tomatoes, cored, peeled, seeded, and diced*
3   *scallions, trimmed and coarsely chopped*
     Salt and freshly ground black pepper
¾   *cup chicken broth*

1. Melt the butter in a frying pan large enough to hold the chicken comfortably. When it is hot and bubbling, add the chicken skin side down. Sauté over medium heat until golden. Turn the chicken to the other side and add the minced garlic to the oil in the pan. Cook for 3 minutes. Add the tomatoes and scallions, sprinkling them around the chicken. Sprinkle the chicken and vegetables lightly with salt and liberally with pepper. Cover and cook over low heat for 5 minutes.

2. Pour the chicken broth into the frying pan, stirring to mix it well with the vegetables. Cover and cook over low heat for 10 to 15 minutes longer, or until the chicken is tender. Serve immediately.

CHICKEN IN MUSTARD SAUCE

2 servings

3 tablespoons butter or margarine
2 chicken quarters, washed and dried
1 small white onion, peeled and minced
   Salt and freshly ground black pepper
½ cup chicken broth
2 tablespoons Dijon mustard
½ cup heavy cream

1. Melt the butter in a frying pan large enough to hold the chicken comfortably. When it is hot and bubbling, add the chicken skin side down. Sauté until golden brown. Turn and brown on the other side. Remove the browned chicken to a plate. Add the onion to the frying pan and sauté until soft. Return the chicken to the frying pan and sprinkle it liberally with salt and pepper. Pour the chicken broth into the frying pan, stirring it into the onions. Cover the pan and cook over low heat for 15 minutes, stirring occasionally and turning the chicken so that it cooks evenly.

2. Remove the chicken to a plate and keep it warm. Stir the mustard into the liquid in the frying pan, making sure it is all incorporated. Add the cream to the pan juices and cook gently, stirring, until the sauce has thickened slightly. Serve the sauce spooned over the chicken.

CHICKEN VALENCIANA

2 servings

2 chicken quarters, washed and dried
½ teaspoon salt
¼ teaspoon freshly ground black pepper
¼ teaspoon dried marjoram
½ teaspoon finely minced garlic
¼ teaspoon dried thyme
¼ teaspoon dried basil
1 medium-sized yellow onion, peeled and sliced thinly
1 red or green pepper, seeded and cut into rings
1 large tomato, cored, seeded, and diced
1 small navel orange, peeled and sliced

1. Preheat the oven to 350 degrees.
2. Cut 2 12-inch squares of heavy-duty aluminum foil. Put a chicken quarter in the center of each piece of foil. Divide the remaining ingredients equally between the chicken quarters. Bring the edges of the foil together over the chicken and vegetables. Turn down a few times to seal the edges together, being careful not to pull the foil too tightly over the chicken and vegetables. Seal the sides by turning the edges up twice and pressing them together.
3. Put the foil packages in a shallow baking pan and bake for 1½ hours. To serve, remove the chicken and vegetables from the foil packages.

CHICKEN WITH LEMON SAUCE

2 servings

2 chicken quarters
   Salt and freshly ground black pepper
1 large garlic clove, peeled and finely minced
2 tablespoons olive oil
4 tablespoons lemon juice
1½ teaspoons dried oregano
6 ounces fettuccine noodles, cooked al dente, and drained

1. Preheat the oven to 375 degrees.

2. Wash the chicken quarters in cool running water and pat them dry. Lay the skin side up in a 9-inch-square baking pan. Sprinkle them with salt and pepper.

3. Bake in the top half of the oven for 45 minutes.

4. While the chicken is baking, combine the garlic, oil, lemon juice, oregano, ½ teaspoon salt, and ⅛ teaspoon pepper in a cup. Stir to mix well.

5. When the chicken has baked for 45 minutes, stir the lemon sauce to mix the ingredients and brush the chicken pieces on both sides with the sauce. Turn the chicken skin side down and return to the oven for 15 minutes. Brush the pieces with the sauce again, and turn the chicken skin side up. Return to the oven for 15 minutes. Brush the chicken with the remaining sauce and bake for 10 minutes longer.

6. Remove the chicken to warm serving plates and add the cooked fettucine to the baking pan. Toss the pasta with the pan juices until it is well coated. Divide the pasta and sauce equally between the serving plates and serve immediately.

CHICKEN-SAUSAGE COMBO

4 servings

3 medium-sized yellow onions, peeled and thinly sliced
   Salt and freshly ground black pepper
4 medium-sized baking potatoes, peeled and sliced ¼ inch thick
   Garlic powder
4 chicken quarters
4 links good Italian sweet sausage (not the supermarket variety)

1. Preheat the oven to 375 degrees.

2. Line a 9- by 13-inch baking pan with a 18- by 20-inch sheet of heavy-duty aluminum foil. Lay the onion slices in a single layer on the foil. Sprinkle the onions with salt and pepper. Lay the potatoes in a layer over the onion slices. Sprinkle the potatoes with salt, pepper, and garlic powder.

3. Wash the chicken quarters in cool running water and pat them dry. Sprinkle both sides of the chicken with salt and pepper and lay the chicken pieces skin side up on top of the potatoes. Put the sausage links in between the chicken pieces.

4. Bring the extra foil up and over the chicken to enclose it. Make a flap and crease it well to seal the foil. Then roll the foil tightly until it is just over the chicken. Seal the sides by pinching them together and rolling them up against the chicken.

5. Bake in the top half of the oven for 1½ hours. Open the foil and turn the chicken and sausages over. Bake for 15 minutes longer. Drain off and discard most of the pan juices. Turn the chicken skin side up and bake for 15 minutes longer.

MOORISH CHICKEN

2 servings

8   tablespoons butter
2   chicken breast halves with bones, but with wings removed
1   large yellow onion, peeled and sliced thin
¼   cup yellow raisins
¼   cup slivered blanched almonds
1½   cups chicken broth
⅔   cup rice

1. Preheat the oven to 350 degrees.

2. Melt 2 tablespoons of the butter in a frying pan. When it is hot and bubbling, add the chicken breast halves skin side down. Sauté over medium heat for 5 minutes, or until golden brown. Turn and brown on the other side. Remove the browned chicken breasts to an ovenproof casserole with a cover. Pour any remaining butter from the frying pan over the chicken. Cover the casserole and put it in the oven.

3. Melt 2 more tablespoons of the butter in the frying pan. When it is hot and bubbling, add the onion slices. Cook over low heat, stirring to separate the slices, for 10 minutes, or until the onion rings are golden. Remove the cover from the casserole with the chicken. Put a sieve over the casserole and spoon the cooked onion slices and butter from the frying pan into the sieve. Press with the back of a wooden spoon to get as much liquid out as possible. Cover the casserole and return it to the oven. Set the onions aside on a plate.

4. Melt 2 more tablespoons of the butter in the frying pan. When it is hot and bubbling, add the yellow raisins. Sauté over low heat for 3 minutes, stirring constantly. Remove the cover from the casserole. Put a sieve over the casserole and spoon the raisins and butter from the frying pan into the sieve. Press with the back of a wooden spoon to get as much liquid out as possible. Cover the casserole and return it to the oven. Set the raisins aside on the plate with the onions.

5. Melt the remaining 2 tablespoons of butter in the frying pan. When it is hot and bubbling, add the almonds. Sauté over low heat until they are golden brown. Stir constantly so the almonds do not burn (which can happen very quickly). Remove the cover from the casserole. Put a sieve over the casserole and spoon the almonds and butter from the frying pan into the sieve. Press with the back of a wooden spoon to get as much liquid out as possible. Set the almonds aside on the plate with the onions and raisins.

6. Pour ½ cup chicken broth into the casserole with the chicken. Cover the casserole, return it to the oven, and bake for 15 minutes.

7. Uncover the casserole and push the chicken to one side. Add the remaining 1 cup chicken broth to the liquid in the casserole. Stir in the rice and lay the chicken pieces on top of the rice. Cover the casserole again and bake for 20 to 25 minutes, or until the rice is tender and the liquid has been absorbed. Stir the reserved raisins and almonds into the rice. Top the chicken breasts with the reserved onion rings. Cover the casserole and bake for 5 minutes longer. Serve immediately.

SAUTÉED CHICKEN BREASTS

2 servings

2   *pieces skinless and boneless chicken breast*
1   *egg*
1   *cup seasoned bread crumbs*
1½ *tablespoons butter or margarine*
1½ *tablespoons vegetable oil*

1. Lay the chicken breasts on a cutting board and pound them lightly with the flat side of a meat mallet, until they are slightly flattened.

2. Beat the egg in a flat soup plate or pie plate.

3. Spread the bread crumbs in a thin layer on a sheet of wax paper.

4. Dip each piece of chicken first in the beaten egg and then in the bread crumbs, coating it completely, and pressing the crumbs on with

the palm of your hand. Lay the coated chicken pieces on a flat plate (not touching) and refrigerate for 10 minutes.

5. Heat the butter and oil in a frying pan large enough to hold the chicken pieces comfortably. When the mixture is hot and bubbling, add the chicken pieces. Sauté over medium heat for 4 minutes on one side, shaking the pan occasionally. Turn the chicken and sauté for 3 to 4 minutes on the other side, or until the chicken is golden brown, and cooked through. Drain on paper towels and serve immediately.

HONEY-BASTED CHICKEN BREASTS

2 servings

2   pieces skinless and boneless chicken breast
1   tablespoon butter or margarine
     Salt and freshly ground black pepper
1½   cups cooked wild and white rice
1   tablespoon honey
½   tablespoon soy sauce
¼   teaspoon dried tarragon

1. Pound the chicken breasts with the flat side of a meat mallet until they are slightly flattened.

2. Melt the butter in a frying pan. When it is hot and bubbling, add the chicken breasts and sauté over medium heat until they are golden on both sides. Sprinkle the chicken with salt and pepper after you turn it.

3. Preheat the oven to 350 degrees.

4. Butter a small casserole. Spread the rice mixture in the bottom of the casserole. Put the sautéed chicken breasts on top of the rice.

5. Mix the honey and soy sauce together in a small cup. Coat the chicken breasts with the mixture and dribble the rest over the rice. Sprinkle the tarragon over the chicken and rice. Bake for 15 minutes, or until the rice is heated through. Serve with Sautéed String Beans (page 298).

CHICKEN WITH ARTICHOKES

2 servings

4   tablespoons butter or margarine
2   pieces skinless and boneless chicken breast
     Salt and freshly ground black pepper
¼   pound mushrooms, sliced
2   tablespoons all-purpose flour
¾   cup chicken broth, heated
¼   teaspoon dried rosemary, crumbled
     Pinch of ground nutmeg
1   package frozen artichoke hearts, cooked according to package directions and drained

1. Melt 2 tablespoons of the butter in a large frying pan. When hot and bubbling, add the chicken pieces. Sauté over medium heat for 3 minutes on each side, or until golden brown. Remove the chicken to a plate, sprinkle with salt and pepper, and keep warm.

2. Wipe out the frying pan with paper towels and add the remaining 2 tablespoons of butter to the pan. Melt the butter. When it is hot and bubbling, add the mushrooms. Sauté over low heat for 5 minutes, stirring occasionally. Sprinkle the flour over the mushrooms and stir to blend well. Cook for 1 minute and remove from the heat. Let the mushroom-flour mixture cool for a few minutes, then slowly add the heated chicken broth, stirring constantly, until the mixture is smooth. Return to low heat and cook until thickened.

3. Season the sauce with the rosemary and nutmeg. Add more salt and pepper, if necessary. Return the chicken breasts to the sauce and cook over low heat for 15 minutes, stirring occasionally. Add the drained artichoke hearts and cook for 5 minutes. Serve immediately.

CHICKEN PARMIGIANA

2 servings

2   cups Marinara Sauce (page 276)
1   recipe for Sautéed Chicken Breasts (page 238)
1/2 cup grated mozzarella cheese
2   tablespoons grated Parmesan cheese

1. Preheat the oven to 350 degrees.
2. Spread 1 cup of the Marinara Sauce in the bottom of an 8-inch pie plate. Put the sautéed chicken breasts on the sauce. Spread 1/4 cup of the grated mozzarella over each chicken breast. Top the chicken breasts with the remaining sauce. Sprinkle 1 tablespoon of grated Parmesan cheese over each chicken breast. Bake for 15 to 20 minutes, or until the cheese is melted and the chicken and sauce are hot.

CRANBERRY CHICKEN BREASTS

2 servings

2   pieces skinless and boneless chicken breasts
2   tablespoons butter or margarine
    Salt and freshly ground black pepper
1   8-ounce can whole cranberry sauce, or 1 cup
    Cranberry Sauce (page 215)
1/2 cup orange juice
    Pinch of ground allspice

1. Lay the chicken breasts on a cutting board and pound them lightly with the flat side of a meat mallet, until they are slightly flattened.
2. Melt the butter in a frying pan large enough to hold the chicken pieces comfortably. When it is hot and bubbling, add the chicken. Sauté over medium heat for 3 minutes on each side, or until the chicken is golden brown. Sprinkle the chicken with salt and pepper and remove it to a plate.
3. Put the cranberry sauce in the frying pan and stir until it has melted. Add the orange juice and allspice and mix well. Cook over low heat for 2 minutes, stirring occasionally. Return the chicken breasts to the frying pan and spoon some of the sauce over them. Cover the pan and cook over low heat for 15 minutes, stirring occasionally. Serve immediately.

CHICKEN KEBABS

2 servings

2   pieces skinless and boneless chicken breast,
    washed and dried
2   tablespoons olive oil
4   tablespoons lemon juice
1/2 teaspoon salt
1/8 teaspoon freshly ground black pepper
1/2 teaspoon finely minced garlic
1   teaspoon dried oregano, crumbled
2   large green peppers, seeded
12 mushroom caps

1. Cut each of the chicken breast halves into 6 equal-sized cubes.
2. Combine the oil, lemon juice, salt, pepper, garlic, and oregano in a bowl. Add the chicken cubes and stir to mix well. Cover the bowl tightly and refrigerate for at least 8 hours, or overnight.

Toss the mixture occasionally to keep all the chicken cubes moistened.

3. Preheat the broiler.

4. Cut the green peppers into 12 -inch squares.

5. Drain the chicken and reserve the marinade. Thread alternating pieces of chicken, pepper, and mushrooms on 2 long skewers, until all the ingredients have been used. Lay the skewers in the broiling pan and brush with the reserved marinade. Broil about 4 inches from the flame for 5 minutes. Turn the skewers, brush again with the marinade and broil for 5 minutes. Turn the skewers again, brush with the remaining marinade and broil for 5 minutes longer, or until the chicken and vegetables are tender. Remove from the skewer and serve immediately on a bed of Rice Pilaf (page 282).

CHICKEN WITH BROCCOLI

2 servings

2   teaspoons cornstarch
¼ teaspoon ground white pepper
¼ cup chicken broth
2   tablespoons vegetable or peanut oil
1   clove garlic, peeled and minced
1   whole skinless and boneless chicken breast, cut into ½-inch cubes
2   cups broccoli flowerets, parboiled and drained
½ cup sliced bamboo shoots

1. Mix together the cornstarch, pepper, and chicken broth. Set aside.

2. Pour the oil into a wok or frying pan and heat over medium-high heat. When the oil is hot, stir in the garlic. Then add the chicken to the oil and cook, stirring constantly, until the chicken pieces have all turned white.

3. Add the broccoli to the wok and stir to coat it with oil. Cover the wok, lower the heat, and cook for 3 minutes. Add the bamboo shoots to the wok and stir to combine them well with the chicken and broccoli.

4. Stir the sauce (from step 1) well to combine it and pour the sauce over the chicken and vegetables. Cook over low heat, stirring constantly, until the sauce is thickened. Serve immediately.

CHICKEN ROLLUPS

2 servings

2 good plain Italian sweet sausages (not the supermarket variety)
2 medium-sized potatoes, peeled and sliced ½ inch thick
2 tablespoons olive or vegetable oil
1 medium-sized yellow onion, peeled, halved, and sliced thin
2 large green peppers, seeded, and sliced thin
2 pieces skinless and boneless chicken breast
Salt and freshly ground black pepper

1. Put the sausages in a small saucepan. Add water to cover by about 2 inches. Bring to a boil, lower the heat, and simmer the sausages for 10 minutes. While the sausages are cooking, prick them occasionally with a fork.

2. Remove the sausages from the water and set them aside on a plate to drain and cool. Add the sliced potatoes to the water in the saucepan and boil for 5 minutes. Drain the potato slices and set aside.

3. Heat 1 tablespoon of the oil in a small nonstick frying pan. When the oil is hot, add the onion and pepper slices. Sauté over medium heat for 5 minutes, tossing and stirring occasionally. Set aside to cool slightly.

4. Pound the chicken breasts lightly with the flat side of a meat mallet to flatten them and even them out. Put 1 sausage in the center of each chicken breast and roll up the breast around the sausage. Hold closed with toothpicks.

5. Preheat the oven to 375 degrees.

6. Spread the remaining tablespoon of oil over the bottom and sides of a small deep baking dish. Layer the potatoes on the bottom of the baking dish and sprinkle generously with salt and pepper. Spread the onion and pepper slices over the potatoes and sprinkle with salt and pepper. Lay the chicken rolls seam side down on the vegetables. Sprinkle the chicken rolls with salt and pepper. Cover the dish tightly with aluminum foil. Bake for 45 minutes and remove the foil. Return the dish to the oven and bake for 10 to 15 minutes longer, or until the sausages are cooked and the chicken is browned. Serve immediately.

SPICY CHICKEN AND EGGPLANT

2 servings

1   1/2- to 3/4-pound eggplant
2   pieces skinless and boneless chicken breast
1   tablespoon cornstarch
3   tablespoons soy sauce
1   tablespoon rice wine or dry sherry
2   tablespoons vegetable or peanut oil
1   tablespoon chili oil, or 4 dried red chili
    peppers
1   clove garlic, peeled and minced
2   tablespoons minced fresh gingerroot
1/2 cup chicken broth

1. Peel the eggplant and cut it lengthwise into thin slices. Cut the slices into 2-inch long shreds.

Put the eggplant shreds in a large bowl and cover them with boiling water. Let sit for 10 minutes. Drain well, squeezing out any excess water. Set aside until needed.

2. Remove any excess fat from the chicken breasts and cut the breasts into thin shreds. Combine the shredded chicken with the cornstarch, 1 tablespoon of the soy sauce, and the rice wine in a bowl. Let sit for 10 minutes.

3. Put the oils, garlic, and gingerroot into a wok or heavy frying pan. Heat, stirring occasionally, over medium-high heat until the garlic and gingerroot begin to sizzle. Drain the chicken shreds and add them to the wok. Cook, turning and stirring constantly, for 3 minutes, or until the chicken has turned white. Add the drained eggplant shreds and mix well. Pour in the chicken broth and the remaining 2 tablespoons of soy sauce and stir to mix well. Cook for 1 minute, and serve immediately.

Note: If you can't find chili oil in an Oriental market, you can substitute chili peppers when the chili oil is called for in the instructions. Just remember to increase the oil you are using by the amount of chili oil called for in the ingredients list. I sugest that you remove the chili peppers before you serve the dish to avoid shocking your palate.

CHICKEN BREASTS FLORENTINE

2 servings

1 pound fresh spinach
  Salt
  Pinch of ground nutmeg
  Freshly ground black pepper
1 recipe for Sautéed Chicken Breasts (page 238)
  Butter or margarine
¼ cup milk
¼ cup grated Parmesan cheese

1. Pick the spinach over to remove any bruised leaves and the stems. Wash the spinach carefully under cool running water to remove any grit. Drain.

2. Put the spinach in a frying pan with a cover. Do not add water; the spinach will steam with just the water clinging to the leaves. Sprinkle the spinach lightly with salt. Cover the pan and cook over medium-high heat for a few minutes, stirring once or twice, or until the spinach is just wilted. Transfer the cooked spinach to a sieve and let it drain. Press out any excess water with the back of a wooden spoon. When cool enough to handle, chop the spinach coarsley and season it with nutmeg and pepper to taste.

3. While the spinach is cooking, prepare the Sautéed Chicken Breasts. Drain them well.

4. Preheat the oven to 350 degrees.

5. Liberally butter a baking dish large enough to hold the chicken breasts in one layer. Lay the chicken breasts in the baking dish. Top each breast with half the spinach mixture. Combine the milk and Parmesan cheese in a small bowl. Beat to combine well. Pour an equal amount of the mixture over the spinach. Bake for 15 to 20 minutes, or until the spinach is piping hot. Serve immediately.

SLICED CHICKEN WITH SCALLIONS

2 servings

2 tablespoons rice wine or dry sherry
4 tablespoons soy sauce
½ teaspoon freshly ground black pepper
4 tablespoons vegetable or peanut oil
2 pieces skinless and boneless chicken breast, cut into thin slices
2 teaspoons rice vinegar or white vinegar
2 teaspoons sesame oil
2 large cloves garlic, peeled and minced
6 scallions, trimmed and cut into 2-inch pieces

1. Combine the rice wine with 2 tablespoons of the soy sauce, the pepper, and 2 tablespoons of the vegetable oil in a large soup bowl. Add the chicken slices and turn to coat evenly. Marinate, turning occasionally, for at least ½ hour.

2. Combine the remaining 2 tablespoons of soy sauce in a small bowl with the rice vinegar and sesame oil. Mix well and set aside.

3. When you are ready to cook the dish, heat the remaining 2 tablespoons of vegetable oil in a wok or heavy frying pan. When the oil is hot, add the garlic and stir to coat the pieces with oil. Drain the marinating chicken slices and discard the marinade. Stir the drained chicken slices into the hot oil and garlic. Sauté, turning and stirring constantly with a wooden spoon, over medium-high heat, until the chicken has turned white. Stir in the scallions and the sauce (from step 2) and mix well. Cook, stirring constantly, for 2 minutes, and serve immediately.

MARINATED CHICKEN BREASTS

2 servings

½ cup white vinegar
½ cup water
3 whole cloves
6 peppercorns
  Pinch of caraway seeds
2 large bay leaves
1 recipe for Sautéed Chicken Breasts (page 238)
2 thin slices Spanish onion

1. Put the vinegar, water, cloves, peppercorns, caraway seeds, and bay leaves in a nonaluminum saucepan. Bring to a boil, lower the heat, and simmer for 15 minutes. Remove from the heat and cool to room temperature.
2. While the marinade is cooling, prepare the chicken breasts and let them cool to room temperature.
3. Lay the chicken breasts in a single layer in a glass casserole. Top each chicken breast with a slice of onion and a bay leaf (from the marinade). Pour the cool marinade over the chicken breasts. Cover the casserole tightly and refrigerate for 24 hours, turning the breasts once or twice so they are flavored evenly. To serve, drain off the marinade completely, top each piece of chicken with the onion slices, and serve cold.
Note: If you marinate these chicken breasts for more than 24 hours, the marinade will be too strong. But you can drain off the marinade after 24 hours and refrigerate the chicken breasts and onion slices. The flavor will not be harmed.

SAUTÉED CHICKEN LIVERS

2 servings

¾ pound chicken livers
  Flour for dredging
3 tablespoons butter or margarine
1 small white onion, peeled, cut in half, and sliced thin
1 clove garlic, peeled and minced
  Salt and freshly ground black pepper
½ teaspoon dried sage, crumbled

1. Remove any blemished spots and fat from the chicken livers. Dredge the livers in the flour and set them aside on a plate so that they do not touch.
2. Melt the butter over low heat in a large frying pan. When it is hot and bubbling, add the onion and garlic. Sauté over medium heat for 2 minutes, stirring constantly. Add the chicken livers to the frying pan in a single layer. Cook, turning occasionally, for about 5 minutes, or until they are just brown. Sprinkle the livers with salt and pepper to taste. Sprinkle the sage over the livers and turn to season them. Serve immediately.

CHICKEN LIVERS FLORENTINE

2 servings

1 pound fresh spinach
  Salt
5 tablespoons butter or margarine
1 medium-sized onion, peeled and minced
  Freshly ground black pepper
  Pinch of ground nutmeg
¾ pound chicken livers
  Flour for dredging

1. Pick the spinach over to remove any bruised leaves and the stems. Wash the unblemished leaves carefully under cold running water to remove the sand. Drain well.

2. Put the spinach in a frying pan with a cover. Do not add water; the spinach will steam with just the water clinging to the leaves. Sprinkle the spinach lightly with salt. Cover the pan and cook over medium-high heat, stirring once or twice, until the spinach is just wilted. Transfer the cooked spinach to a sieve and let it drain. Press out any excess water with the back of a wooden spoon.

3. Melt 2 tablespoons of the butter in a small frying pan. Add the onion and sauté for 5 minutes, or until the onion is soft. Do not let the onion brown. Mix the drained spinach gently with the onion and season the mixture with salt, pepper, and nutmeg to taste. Cover and keep warm while you prepare the chicken livers.

4. Remove any blemished spots and fat from the chicken livers. Dredge the chicken livers in flour and set them aside on a plate so that they do not touch.

5. Melt the remaining 3 tablespoons of butter in a large frying pan. When it is hot but not brown, add the chicken livers in one layer. Sauté over medium heat for 3 to 4 minutes, or until brown. Turn the livers and brown the other side.

6. Put half the spinach on each of two warm plates. Top each serving with an equal amount of chicken livers and serve at once.

CHICKEN LIVERS WITH LEMON, OIL, AND OREGANO

2 servings

2   tablespoons olive or vegetable oil
1   large clove garlic, crushed and peeled
1   small white onion, peeled and minced
¾   pound chicken livers, picked over, washed, and dried
    Flour for dredging
    Salt and freshly ground black pepper
¼   teaspoon dried oregano
    Juice of 1 lemon

1. Heat the oil in a medium-sized nonstick frying pan. When the oil is hot, add the garlic and sauté until golden brown on both sides. Remove and discard the garlic. Add the onion to the frying pan and cook over medium heat for 3 minutes, stirring occasionally. (Do not let the onion brown.)

2. While the onion is cooking, dredge the chicken livers in the flour. Add the livers to the frying pan and cook until brown on both sides.

3. Sprinkle the livers with salt and pepper to taste. Then sprinkle with the oregano and the lemon juice and toss and stir to distribute the spices evenly. Serve immediately.

ROAST TURKEY BREAST

8 to 10 servings

1   4-pound turkey breast, thawed
    Salt and freshly ground black pepper
    Garlic powder
    Onion powder

1. Preheat the oven to 350 degrees.
2. Wash the turkey breast in cool running water

and pat dry with paper towels. Sprinkle the breast on all sides with salt, pepper, garlic powder, and onion powder. Put the breast skin side up on a rack in a roasting pan and roast for 25 minutes per pound, or until the juices run clear. Let sit for 10 minutes before slicing.

Note: Cooked turkey will keep in the refrigerator for several days if wrapped tightly in foil. For moistness, leave the turkey meat in large chunks when you remove it from the bone. This way you can slice or chop what you need, when you need it, and it will be juicy when you serve it. If you are not going to use the turkey within a few days, it should be wrapped in foil and frozen in portion sizes.

TURKEY PATTIES WITH CREAM GRAVY

2 servings

5 tablespoons butter or margarine
1 small white onion, peeled and minced
1½ cups ground cooked turkey
1 egg
  Salt and freshly ground black pepper
  Pinch of poultry seasoning
  Seasoned bread crumbs
½ cup chicken broth
½ cup heavy cream

1. Melt 2 tablespoons of the butter over low heat in a small frying pan. When the butter is hot and bubbling, add the onion. Sauté over low heat until golden brown. Remove from the heat and cool slightly.

2 Combine the ground turkey, egg, and cooled onion in a bowl. Add salt and pepper to taste and the poultry seasoning. Mix in just enough bread crumbs to make the mixture hold together. Form the mixture into 4 patties. Put the patties on a flat plate and refrigerate them for 10 minutes.

3. Melt the remaining 3 tablespoons of butter in a frying pan large enough to hold the turkey patties comfortably. When the butter is hot and bubbling, add the turkey patties and sauté until golden brown on both sides. Remove the patties to a plate and keep them warm.

4. Add the chicken broth to the frying pan and stir it around with a wooden spoon to pick up any browned-on bits in the pan. Cook over medium heat to reduce the sauce a little. Pour the heavy cream into the frying pan and cook gently, stirring, until the sauce has thickened. Taste for seasonings and add salt and pepper, if necessary. Serve the sauce spooned over the turkey patties.

TURKEY FRICASSEE WITH BISCUIT TOPPING

2 servings

2 carrots, scraped
2 medium-sized potatoes, peeled
  Salt
2 cups chicken broth
2 cups broccoli flowerets
2 tablespoons butter or margarine
1 small white onion, peeled and minced
2 tablespoons all-purpose flour
  Pinch of ground sage
  Freshly ground black pepper
2 cups cubed roast turkey
1 4.5-ounce tube-type package of biscuits (6 biscuits)

1. Cut the carrots into ¼-inch-thick slices. Quarter the potatoes and cut them into ¼-inch-thick slices. Put the carrot and potato slices in a steamer basket. Sprinkle them lightly with salt.

2. Pour the chicken broth into a saucepan and bring to a boil. Put the steamer basket with the carrots and potatoes into the saucepan, cover, and steam over low heat for 5 minutes. Add the broccoli flowerets to the steamer basket and sprinkle lightly with salt. Cover and steam for 5 minutes, or until all the vegetables are crisp-tender. Remove from the heat and take the steamer basket out of the saucepan immediately. Cover the chicken broth to keep it warm.

3. Melt the butter over low heat in a small fryng pan. When it is hot and bubbling, add the onion. Sauté over low heat for 10 minutes, stirring occasionally. Do not let the onion brown. Sprinkle the flour over the onion and mix it in well. Cook, sitrring, for 1 minute. Remove the frying pan from the heat and let the onion-flour mixture cool for a few minutes.

4. Preheat the oven to 450 degrees.

5. Gradually add the warm chicken broth to the frying pan, stirring constantly until the mixture is smooth. Return to low heat and cook, stirring, until the sauce has thickened. Stir in the sage and season the sauce with salt and pepper to taste.

6. Butter a 1-quart soufflé dish liberally. Put the cubed turkey in the bottom of the dish and top it with the steamed vegetables. Pour the sauce over all. Arrange the unbaked biscuits on top of the mixture in the dish and bake for 10 to 15 minutes, or until the biscuits are golden brown and the turkey and vegetables are hot. Serve immediately.

TURKEY WITH MORNAY SAUCE

2 servings

3   tablespoons butter or margarine
2   tablespoons minced onion
3   tablespoons all-purpose flour
½   cup milk
½   cup chicken broth
    Salt and freshly ground black pepper
1   egg yolk
2   tablespoons heavy cream
¼   cup grated Parmesan cheese
4   slices turkey breast
4   spears Steamed Broccoli (page 291)

1. Melt the butter over low heat in a small heavy saucepan. When it is hot and bubbling, add the onion and sauté over low heat for 5 minutes, or until the onion is soft. Sprinkle the flour over the onion and stir to combine well. Remove the saucepan from the heat and let the mixture cool a little.

2. When the onion-flour mixture has cooled, gradually stir in the milk and chicken broth, stirring until the mixture is smooth and creamy. Season the sauce with salt and pepper to taste. Return the sauce to the heat and cook over low heat for 5 to 10 minutes, or until the sauce has thickened.

3. Beat the egg yolk and heavy cream together and add the mixture to the sauce slowly, stirring constantly. Stir in the Parmesan cheese until it melts. Remove the sauce from the heat.

4. Preheat the oven to 350 degrees.

5. Lay the turkey slices in a buttered baking dish that can hold them in one layer. Lay a broccoli spear on top of each turkey slice. Pour the sauce over the broccoli and turkey. Bake for 15 minutes, or until piping hot. Serve immediately.

CORNISH HENS DERBY

2 servings

2   small (¾ to 1 pound) Cornish hens, washed
    and drained
1   6-ounce package long-grain and wild rice mix,
    prepared according to package directions and
    cooled
    Livers from the Cornish hens, sautéed and
    chopped
¼   pound mushrooms, finely chopped, sautéed,
    and drained
    Salt and freshly ground black pepper

1. Preheat the oven to 350 degrees.

2. In a bowl combine 1½ cups of the cooked rice mixture, the sautéed livers, and the sautéed mushrooms. Divide the mixture evenly between the hens, stuffing the cavities of the birds until they are nicely rounded. Close the opening over the stuffing with a skewer.

3. Put the stuffed hens on a rack in a roasting pan and sprinkle generously with salt and pepper.

4. Roast for 1 hour, or until the hens are tender and golden brown.

Note: Use the remaining 1½ cups of cooked rice to make the recipe for Honey-basted Chicken Breasts (page 239).

PAN-FRIED CORNISH HEN

2 servings

1   1½-pound Cornish hen, with giblets and liver
3   tablespoons butter or margarine
    Salt and freshly ground black pepper
1   large yellow onion, peeled, cut in half, and
    sliced very thin
1   bay leaf
⅓   cup chicken broth

1. Split the Cornish hen in half and wash the halves thoroughly in cool running water. Pat them dry with paper towels. Wash the giblets and liver in cool running water and pat them dry.

2. Melt 2 tablespoons of the butter over low heat in a large heavy frying pan. When the butter is completely melted and beginning to sizzle, add the hen halves skin side down. Cook until golden brown, then turn and brown the other side. Remove the hen halves to a plate and keep warm.

3. Add the remaining tablespoon of butter to the frying pan. When the butter is completely melted, add the sliced onion and reserved giblets and liver and sauté over very low heat for 10 minutes, stirring occasionally. Add the bay leaf and chicken broth to the frying pan and mix well. Return the hen halves to the pan and bring to a boil. Cover, lower the heat, and cook for 25 to 30 minutes, or until the Cornish hen halves are tender and cooked through. Turn the hen halves occasionally as they are cooking and stir the onions so they do not stick to the pan. Serve at once.

CORNISH HEN CACCIATORE

2 servings

2 tablespoons olive oil
1 1-pound Cornish hen, cut in half
1/2 cup minced red onion
1 medium-sized green pepper, seeded and minced
1 large clove garlic, peeled and minced
1 1-pound can crushed tomatoes
3/4 cup water
1/8 teaspoon ground allspice
1/4 teaspoon dried thyme
1 teaspoon salt
1/4 teaspoon freshly ground black pepper
1 4-ounce can mushroom stems and pieces, drained, or 4 ounces fresh mushrooms, washed, sliced and sautéed

1. Heat the oil in a large heavy frying pan. When the oil is hot, add the Cornish hen halves skin side down and sauté until golden brown. Turn the pieces over and sauté until brown on the second side. Remove the browned hen halves to a plate until needed.

2. Add the onion, green pepper, and garlic to the frying pan and sauté over low heat, stirring occasionally, for 7 minutes, or until the vegetables are soft but not browned. Add the tomatoes, water, allspice, thyme, salt, and pepper to the frying pan. Mix well and bring to a boil. Return the hen halves to the frying pan skin side down. Spoon some of the sauce over the hen halves. Cover the frying pan, lower the heat, and cook for 45 minutes, turning the hen halves occasionally and stirring the sauce so that it does not stick.

3. Add the drained mushroom stems and pieces to the sauce and mix in well. Cook for 5 minutes longer.

CORNISH HEN WITH SCALLIONS

2 servings

1 1-pound Cornish hen
2 tablespoons rice wine or dry sherry
4 tablespoons soy sauce
1/2 teaspoon freshly ground black pepper
5 tablespoons vegetable or peanut oil
1 heaping tablespoon tree ears or black fungus (optional)
2 large cloves garlic, peeled and minced
6 scallions, trimmed and cut into 2-inch shreds
2 teaspoons rice vinegar or white vinegar
2 teaspoons sesame oil

1. Cut the Cornish hen into 8 pieces (2 breasts, 2 wings, 2 thighs, and 2 drumsticks). Wash the pieces in cool water and pat them dry with paper towels.

2. Combine the rice wine with 2 tablespoons of the soy sauce, the pepper, and 3 tablespoons of the vegetable oil in a large flat bowl. Add the Cornish hen pieces and turn them to coat them evenly with the mixture. Marinate, turning occasionally, for at least 1/2 hour.

3. Put the tree ears in a small deep bowl. Cover them with boiling water and let stand for 20 minutes. Drain well, squeezing out any excess moisture, and chop coarsely. Put the chopped tree ears on a large dinner plate with the minced garlic and shredded scallions.

4. Combine the remaining 2 tablespoons of soy sauce in a small bowl with the rice vinegar and sesame oil. Mix well and set aside.

5. When you are ready to cook the dish, heat

the remaining 2 tablespoons of vegetable oil in a wok or heavy frying pan. When the oil is hot, add the garlic and stir to coat the pieces with oil. Remove the Cornish hen pieces from the marinade and add them skin side down to the wok. Fry over medium heat until they are browned on both sides and cooked through (about 6 minutes). Stir in the scallions, tree ears, and sauce (from step 4) and mix well. Cook for 2 minutes, stirring constantly, and serve immediately.

Note: Rice wine, tree ears, rice vinegar, and sesame oil are available in Oriental markets.

MEATS

ROAST BEEF

6 servings

1 3-pound boneless beef roast, such as an eye
   round, top round, or silver tip
1 large clove garlic, peeled and cut into slivers
   Salt
   Freshly ground black pepper

1. Preheat the oven to 350 degrees.
2. Use a paring knife to make random, small, deep cuts in the roast and insert a garlic sliver in each hole, pushing it down with your fingertip. Sprinkle the roast liberally with salt and pepper.
3. Put the roast on a rack in a baking pan and roast for 20 to 25 minutes per pound for medium-rare. (If you want, you can use a meat thermometer to be sure that the roast is done to your taste.)
4. Let the roast sit for 10 to 15 minutes after you remove it from the oven before you slice it.

Note: Put the leftover portion of the roast in a deep dish and pour the pan juices over it. Wrap in foil and refrigerate. Leftovers make excellent lunch sandwiches and dinner dishes.

POT ROAST

6 servings

1 2½-pound top or bottom round roast
1 clove garlic, peeled and cut into slivers
2 tablespoons vegetable oil
1 medium-sized yellow onion, peeled and
   chopped
1 large carrot, scraped and chopped
1 celery stalk, chopped
1 clove garlic, peeled and minced
1 8-ounce can tomato sauce
1 10½-ounce can condensed onion soup
1½ cups water
½ teaspoon salt
¼ teaspoon freshly ground black pepper
1 bay leaf

1. Use a paring knife to make random, small, deep cuts in the meat. Insert a sliver of garlic in each hole, pushing it down with your fingertip.
2. Heat the oil in a Dutch oven. When hot, brown the meat on all sides. Remove the browned meat to a plate, and add the onion, carrot, celery, and minced garlic to the fat in the pan. Sauté over low heat for 5 minutes, stirring occasionally to loosen any browned-on bits in the bottom of the pan. Add the tomato sauce, onion soup, and water and bring to a boil. Stir in the salt, pepper, and bay leaf.
3. Return the browned roast to the pan. Cover, lower the heat, and simmer for 1½ hours, or until the meat is tender.
4. Remove the meat from the sauce and cool the sauce slightly. Purée the sauce through a food mill or in a blender and warm it slightly before serving.

Note: This freezes well and will keep refrigerated, covered tightly, for several days.

BEEF STEW

4 servings

2 tablespoons vegetable oil
1 pound beef stew meat, cut into 1½-inch cubes
1 clove garlic, peeled and crushed (optional)
1 large onion, peeled and sliced
1 10½-ounce can condensed beef bouillon
1 cup water
  Freshly ground black pepper
1 bay leaf
  Pinch of ground marjoram
3 celery stalks, cut into ½-inch-thick slices
3 carrots, scraped and cut into ½-inch-thick slices
2 large potatoes, peeled and cut into 1-inch cubes
  Salt

1. Heat the oil in a Dutch oven or heavy saucepan. Add the beef cubes and brown on all sides. Remove the beef cubes to a plate as they brown.
2. Add the garlic and onion to the pan and sauté for 5 minutes, stirring to separate the onion rings. Remove and discard the garlic. Add the bouillon and water to the pan and season with the pepper, bay leaf, and marjoram. Bring to a boil and return the meat to the pan. Cover the pan, lower the heat, and simmer the stew for 1 hour, stirring occasionally.
3. Add the celery, carrots, and potatoes. Bring the stew back to a simmer, cover, and cook for 20 minutes, or until the meat and vegetables are tender. Taste and add more pepper and salt, if necessary.

MARINATED STEAK

2 servings

1 1¼-pound bone-in chuck steak
4 tablespoons lemon juice
¼ teaspoon finely minced garlic
1¼ teaspoons grated onion
½ teaspoon dried oregano, crumbled
  Salt and freshly ground black pepper

1. Lay the steak in a glass baking dish large enough to hold it comfortably. Pierce the steak all over with a fork. Pour the lemon juice over the steak. Sprinkle the garlic, onion, and oregano over the steak. Sprinkle on salt and pepper liberally. Cover the baking dish with foil and refrigerate overnight, turning the steak occasionally.
2. When ready to cook, heat the broiler to hot. Broil the steak about 3 inches from the flame for 6 minutes on each side, or until done to your preference. Slice thinly across the grain of the meat to serve.

ROLADEN

2 servings

¾ pound thin-sliced round steak
2 teaspoons Dijon mustard
1 carrot, scraped and cut into julienne strips
1 large celery stalk, cut into julienne strips
1 large dill pickle, quartered
1 small white onion, peeled, halved, and sliced
2 tablespoons butter or margarine
1 10½-ounce can condensed onion soup
1½ cups water
  Salt and freshly ground black pepper
1 tablespoon all-purpose flour
2 tablespoons cold water

1. Cut the meat into 4 equal portions and pound each piece with the flat side of a meat mallet to thin it.

2. Spread one side of each piece of meat with ½ teaspoon mustard. Put 2 pieces of carrot, 1 piece of celery, 1 piece of pickle, and 2 or 3 slices of onion in the center of each piece of meat. Fold the ends of the meat over the vegetables and roll up. Secure the rolls with toothpicks.

3. Melt the butter in a frying pan. When it is hot and bubbling, add the meat rolls and brown them on all sides.

4. While the roladen are browning, chop any remaining carrots, celery, and onions. Remove the browned roladen from the frying pan and add the chopped vegetables. Sauté for 5 minutes. Add the onion soup and water and stir to mix well. Bring to a boil and return the roladen to the pan. Cover and simmer for ½ hour, stirring occasionally.

5. After ½ hour, partially uncover the pan and cook for ½ hour longer. Remove the roladen to a plate and keep them warm. Mix the flour and water to a smooth paste and add it to the sauce in the frying pan, stirring constantly until the sauce has thickened. Return the roladen to the sauce and spoon some sauce over them. Serve immediately.

BRACIOLE

4 servings

1   *pound thin-sliced round steak*
     Olive oil
2   *tablespoons seasoned bread crumbs*
½   *teaspoon dried basil, crumbled*
1   *large onion, peeled and finely minced*
4   *teaspoons grated Parmesan or Romano cheese*
2   *hard-boiled eggs, peeled and quartered*
     Salt and freshly ground black pepper
2   *cloves garlic, peeled and minced*
1   *1-pound can crushed tomatoes*
1   *8-ounce can tomato sauce*
1½ *cups water*
½   *teaspoon dried oregano, crumbled*
1   *bay leaf*

1. Cut the meat into 4 equal portions and pound each piece with the flat side of a meat mallet to thin it.

2. Brush each piece of meat on one side with a little oil. Sprinkle ½ tablespoon bread crumbs down the center of each piece of meat. Sprinkle an equal amount of dried basil over each row of bread crumbs. Spread 1 teaspoon of minced onion over the rows of bread crumbs. Sprinkle 1 teaspoon of grated cheese over the onions on each piece of meat. Lay 2 egg quarters end to end over the grated cheese. Sprinkle the meat slices generously with salt and pepper. Bring the sides of the meat slices up over the filling, then roll to enclose the filling completely. Secure the rolls with toothpicks or tie with string.

3. Heat 2 tablespoons of olive oil in a heavy saucepan. When hot, add the braciole and brown on all sides. Remove the braciole to a plate as they brown. Add the remaining onion and the garlic to the pan. Sauté for 5 minutes, stirring occasionally. Do not let brown. Add the crushed tomatoes, tomato sauce, and water. Stir well and bring to a boil. Season with salt and pepper to taste and add the oregano and bay leaf. Stir well and return the braciole to the pan. Cover and simmer for 1 hour, or until the meat is tender. Stir occasionally while the sauce cooks. Serve the braciole with 3 ounces of cooked spaghetti.

HOME-STYLE BEEF
2 servings

3   tablespoons vegetable or peanut oil
1½ tablespoons chili oil, or 5 dried red chili
    peppers
1   clove garlic, peeled and minced
1   teaspoon minced fresh gingerroot
2   carrots, scraped and cut into julienne strips
1   large green pepper, seeded and cut into thin
    strips
1   cup shredded green or Chinese cabbage
½   pound round steak, cut into thin shreds
2   scallions, trimmed and cut into 1½-inch
    shreds
½   cup julienned bamboo shoots
3   tablespoons soy sauce

1. Put 1½ tablespoons of the vegetable oil, ½ tablespoon of the chili oil, and half the garlic and gingerroot into a wok or heavy frying pan. Heat over medium-high heat, stirring occasionally, until the garlic and gingerroot begin to sizzle. Add the carrots, green pepper, and cabbage. Cook for 3 to 4 minutes, stirring and turning constantly. Use a slotted spoon to remove the vegetables to a bowl. Set aside until needed.

2. Put the remaining oils and garlic and gingerroot in the wok. Heat for 1 minute, stirring occasionally. Add the beef shreds and cook and stir for 2 minutes, or until the beef has lost its red color. Stir in the scallions and cook for 1 minute, stirring constantly. Stir in the bamboo shoots.

3. Return the reserved vegetables to the wok and stir to mix well. Stir in the soy sauce and cook for 1 minute. Serve immediately.

Note: If you can't find chili oil in an Oriental market, you can substitute 2 chili peppers the first time the chili oil is called for and 3 chili peppers the second time the chili oil is called for in the instructions. Just remember to increase the oil you are using each time by the amount of chili oil called for in the ingredients list. I suggest that you remove the chili peppers before you serve the dish to avoid shocking your palate.

PARMESAN HAMBURGER PATTIES
2 servings

½ to ¾ pound ground round
2   tablespoons grated Parmesan cheese
    Salt and freshly ground black pepper
3   tablespoons butter or margarine

1. Mix the ground round with the cheese and salt and pepper to taste. Divide into 4 small patties.

2. Melt the butter in a frying pan large enough to hold the hamburger patties in one layer. When the butter is hot and bubbling, add the patties and sauté over medium heat until done to your preference. Serve immediately.

MEATLOAF
6 servings

2   slices white bread
1   10-ounce package frozen chopped spinach
1   pound ground round
1   small white onion, peeled and minced
1   egg
¼   teaspoon finely minced garlic
½   teaspoon salt
⅛   teaspoon freshly ground black pepper
2   tablespoons grated Parmesan cheese

2   hard-cooked eggs, peeled and cut in half,
    lengthwise
1   15-ounce can tomato sauce
1½ cups water

1. Trim the bread of all crusts and put the trimmed slices in a large mixing bowl. Pour cold water over the bread and let it soak for 10 minutes.

2. Cook the spinach according to package directions and drain well, squeezing out any excess liquid with the back of a wooden spoon.

3. Drain the soaked bread and squeeze out any excess liquid. Return the squeezed-out bread to the mixing bowl and add the ground round, onion, egg, garlic, salt, pepper, and cheese. Mix well with your hands. Add the well-drained spinach and mix well with your hands.

4. Cut off a piece of heavy-duty foil large enough to more than enclose the meatloaf. Line a baking pan with the foil.

5. Preheat the oven to 375 degrees.

6. Divide the meat mixture in half. Form one half into an oval in the bottom of the baking pan. Lay the egg halves in two rows on top of the meat oval. Form the remaining meat mixture into another oval and lay it over the eggs. Pinch and smooth the edges of the meat together so they do not separate while baking. Bring the edges of the foil up over the meatloaf and seal. Seal the sides also. Bake for 45 minutes.

7. Open and turn back the foil. Pour the pan juices into a heat-proof bowl and refrigerate. Combine the tomato sauce and water and pour over the meatloaf. Return the meatloaf to the oven and bake for 45 minutes longer.

8. Scoop the fat from the pan juices and discard it. Stir the degreased pan juices into the sauce in the roasting pan and mix well. To serve, slice the meatloaf thinly and top each portion with a few spoons of sauce.

Note: Refrigerate the remaining meatloaf, covered, and use for lunch sandwiches or another dinner menu.

DOROTHY LYONS' SAVORY MINCE

4 servings

1   heaping teaspoon cornstarch
2   envelopes G. Washington's Rich Brown
    Seasoning and Broth mix
1   teaspoon Kitchen bouquet
1½ cups beef broth
1   tablespoon vegetable oil
1   medium-size yellow onion, peeled and
    minced
1   clove garlic, peeled and minced
2   cups ground cooked roast beef
½   teaspoon curry powder, or to taste
½   teaspoon ground cardamom, or to taste
½   teaspoon celery salt
    Salt and freshly ground black pepper

1. Stir the cornstarch, 1 envelope of the G. Washington mix, and the Kitchen Bouquet into ½ cup of the beef broth. Stir until smooth.

2. Pour the remaining 1 cup of beef broth into a small saucepan or frying pan. Bring just to the simmer and gradually stir in the cornstarch mixture. Cook over low heat, stirring constantly, until the gravy has thickened. Set aside.

3. Heat the oil in a frying pan. When it is hot, add the onion and garlic and sauté over medium heat for 5 minutes. Add the roast beef, curry powder, cardamom, celery salt, and reserved beef gravy. Stir to mix well. Taste for seasonings, and

add salt and pepper, if necessary. Simmer over low heat for 15 to 20 minutes, or until very thick.

Note: Use 2 servings for this meal and, if you want, the rest for Shepherd's Pie (below).

SHEPHERD'S PIE

2 servings

Butter
1/2 recipe for Dorothy Lyons' Savory Mince (see page 255)
2 cups seasoned mashed potatoes
Paprika

1. Preheat the oven to 375 degrees.
2. Butter a 1-quart soufflé dish liberally. Spoon the Savory Mince into the dish. Spread the seasoned mashed potatoes on top of the mince, covering it completely. Sprinkle lightly with paprika and dot with butter.
3. Bake for 20 minutes, or until the potatoes are golden and the mince is hot. Serve immediately.

HOME-STYLE BEEF LIVER

2 servings

4 dried Chinese mushrooms, stems removed
1 pound thin-sliced beef liver
1 small yellow onion
4 tablespoons peanut or vegetable oil
1 teaspoon chili oil, or 2 dried red chili peppers
1 teaspoon minced fresh gingerroot
2 cloves garlic, peeled and minced
1 large green pepper, seeded and julienned
1 large carrot, scraped and julienned
3 tablespoons soy sauce

1. Put the dried mushrooms in a small bowl and cover them with boiling water. Let the mushrooms soak for 20 minutes. Drain them well and squeeze out any excess water. Cut the mushrooms into julienne strips. Set aside until needed.
2. Remove the skin and any gristle from the liver and cut the liver into julienne strips about 1/4 inch thick and 2 inches long. Set aside until needed.
3. Peel the onion and cut it in half. Slice each half into thin slices. Set aside until needed.
4. Put 2 tablespoons of the peanut oil and 1/2 teaspoon of the chili oil with half the ginger and half the garlic into a wok or heavy frying pan. Heat over medium-high heat, stirring occasionally, until the ginger and garlic are light brown. Add the onion, green pepper, and carrot. Sauté, stirring constantly, for 4 minutes. Use a slotted spoon to remove the vegetables to a dish. Set aside until needed.
5. Add the remaining peanut oil, chili oil, ginger, and garlic to the wok. Heat over medium heat, stirring constantly, until the ginger and garlic start to sizzle. Add the liver shreds and sauté, stirring constantly, for 3 to 4 minutes, or until the liver is just cooked. Return the reserved vegetables to the wok and stir in the mushroom shreds. Pour the soy sauce over the liver and vegetables and cook over low heat, stirring constantly, for 1 minute. Serve immediately.

Note: You will probably find it easier to cut the liver into julienne strips if you lay the skinned liver flat on a piece of aluminum foil and freeze it for about 20 minutes. This will make the liver firm enough to slice thinly.

Also, if you can't find chili oil in an Oriental market, you can substitute 2 of the dried chili peppers each time the chili oil is called for in the instructions. Just remember to increase the oil you are using each time by the amount of chili oil called for in the ingredients list. I suggest that you remove the chili peppers before you serve the dish to avoid shocking your palate.

BEEF LIVER AND ONIONS
2 servings

3 *tablespoons butter or margarine*
2 *medium-sized yellow onions, peeled, cut in half, and sliced thin*
   Salt and freshly ground black pepper
½ to ¾ *pound beef liver, cut into 2 portions*
½ *cup all-purpose flour*

1. Melt 2 tablespoons of the butter in a large heavy frying pan. When the butter is completely melted and beginning to sizzle, add the onions. Sauté over very low heat, stirring occasionally, until they are golden brown and very soft. (This may take as long as 15 minutes, but the onions should be cooked slowly so that they retain their sweetness.) Sprinkle the onions with salt and pepper during the last few minutes of cooking. Use a slotted spoon to remove the onions from the frying pan to a plate. Set them aside until needed.

2. While the onions are cooking, remove the skin and any gristle from the liver. Wash the liver in cool running water and pat it dry with paper towels.

3. Put the flour on a piece of wax paper and season it with salt and pepper. Mix thoroughly.

4. When you are ready to cook the liver, add the remaining tablespoon of butter to the frying pan. When the butter has melted completely and is beginning to sizzle, coat the liver on both sides with the seasoned flour. Shake off any excess flour and lay the liver pieces in a single layer in the frying pan. Sauté the liver over medium heat for 3 to 4 minutes on a side, shaking the pan and turning the liver only once while it cooks. The liver should be browned nicely on both sides.

5. When the liver has cooked on the second side, distribute the reserved onions equally over the pieces. Cover the frying pan, lower the heat, and cook for 2 minutes. Serve immediately.

BEEF LIVER SAUTÉ
2 servings

¾ *pound beef liver, cut ¼ inch thick*
2 *tablespoons olive oil*
1 *large clove garlic, peeled and minced very fine*
1 *large green pepper, seeded and cut into ½-inch dice*
1 *large ripe tomato, peeled, seeded, and cut into ½-inch dice*
1 *large white onion, peeled and coarsely chopped*
   Salt and freshly ground black pepper
1 *tablespoon cider vinegar*

1. Remove the skin and any gristle from the liver and cut the liver into ½-inch pieces. Set aside until needed.

2. Heat the oil in a 10-inch nonstick frying pan. When the oil is hot, add the garlic and stir it around for 1 minute. Add the pieces of liver and sauté over medium-low heat, stirring constantly, for 3 minutes.

3. Add the green pepper, tomato, and onion to the frying pan and raise the heat to medium. Sauté the mixture for 3 minutes, stirring occa-

sionally. Sprinkle liberally with salt and pepper. Pour the cider vinegar into the frying pan and stir to mix well. Cover the frying pan, and lower the heat. Cook, covered, for 1 minute and serve immediately.

HERBED VEAL CHOPS

2 servings

3   tablespoons butter or margarine
2   veal chops, cut 1/2 inch thick
1/2 cup all-purpose flour
    Salt and freshly ground black pepper
1   teaspoon dried thyme

1. Melt the butter over low heat in a frying pan large enough to hold the chops comfortably.
2. Dust the chops lightly with the flour. When the butter is hot and bubbling, add the chops and cook over low heat for 5 minutes. Turn the chops and sprinkle liberally with salt, pepper, and thyme. Cook on the second side for 5 minutes, or until the veal is tender. Serve immediately.

SAUTÉED VEAL CHOPS

2 servings

2 veal chops, about 1/2 inch thick
  Salt and freshly ground black pepper
2 tablespoons butter or margarine
1 clove garlic, peeled and crushed

1. Sprinkle the chops on both sides with salt and pepper.
2. Put the butter and garlic in a frying pan large enough to hold the chops comfortably. Melt the butter, over low heat turning the garlic occasionally to flavor the butter. When the butter

is hot and bubbling, remove the garlic and add the chops. Cook over medium heat for about 5 minutes on each side, or until the chops are brown and tender. Serve at once.

BAKED VEAL CHOPS

2 servings

1/2 cup unseasoned bread crumbs
2   tablespoons grated Romano cheese
    Salt and freshly ground black pepper
2   veal chops, cut 1/2 inch thick
2   tablespoons olive oil
2   celery stalks, sliced thin
1   large potato, peeled and sliced thin
1   large white onion, peeled and sliced thin
1/2 cup chicken broth
1/4 pound mushrooms, sliced thin
4   canned artichoke halves, drained

1. Mix the bread crumbs and cheese together with salt and pepper to taste. Coat the veal chops with the bread crumb mixture. Refrigerate the veal chops for 10 minutes.
2. Preheat the oven to 375 degrees.
3. Heat the oil over medium heat in a frying pan large enough to hold the chops comfortably. When it is hot, add the veal chops and brown them quickly on both sides. Put the browned chops in an ovenproof casserole with a cover.
4. Add the celery, potato, and onion slices to the casserole. Sprinkle the vegetables with salt and pepper. Pour in the chicken broth, cover the casserole, and bake for 30 minutes. Add the mushrooms to the casserole, cover, and bake for 15 minutes longer, or until the vegetables and meat are tender. Add the artichoke halves and bake for 5 minutes longer, or until they are warmed through. Serve immediately.

SAUTÉED VEAL CUTLETS

2 servings

4   thin veal cutlets
1   egg
⅔   cup seasoned bread crumbs
1   tablespoon grated Parmesan cheese
     Salt and freshly ground black pepper
3   tablespoons butter or margarine

1. Lay the veal cutlets on a cutting board and pound them lightly with the flat side of a meat mallet to thin them.

2. Beat the egg in a flat soup bowl or pie plate. Add the veal cutlets and mix well. Let sit for 5 minutes.

3. Put the bread crumbs and Parmesan cheese on a large sheet of wax paper. Season with salt and pepper to taste.

4. Lift each veal cutlet out of the beaten egg with a fork. Lay it flat on the bread crumb mixture. Use the excess wax paper to toss bread crumbs on top of the cutlet. Press the crumbs on with the palm of your hand. Turn the cutlet, toss more bread crumbs on top, and press the crumbs on again with the palm of your hand. Put the breaded cutlet on a flat plate. Follow the same procedure with the remaining cutlets. Do not let the cutlets on the plate touch. Separate the layers of cutlets with wax paper. Refrigerate the cutlets for 10 minutes.

5. Melt the butter in a large frying pan. When it is hot and bubbling, add the cutlets. Sauté over medium heat for 3 minutes, or until golden brown. Turn the cutlets and sauté for 3 minutes longer, or until golden brown on the second side. Drain the cutlets on paper towels. Serve immediately.

SPEDINI

2 servings

4   thin slices veal cutlet
     Salt and freshly ground black pepper
1   thin slice boiled ham, cut into 4 strips
1   ½-inch-thick slice mozzarella cheese, cut into 4 long strips
2   scallions, trimmed and chopped
4   teaspoons grated Parmesan cheese
½   cup all-purpose flour
2   tablespoons olive oil
½   cup chicken broth

1. Lay the veal slices on a cutting board and pound them lightly with the flat side of a meat mallet to thin them. Sprinkle the cutlets lightly with salt and pepper.

2. Lay 1 strip of boiled ham in the center of each veal cutlet. Put 1 strip of mozzarella cheese on each piece of ham. Divide the scallions equally among the veal cutlets, sprinkling them next to the strips of mozzarella. Sprinkle 1 teaspoon of Parmesan cheese over each cutlet. Bend the sides of the cutlets up over the filling and roll tightly. Secure the rolls with toothpicks.

3. Spread the flour on a sheet of wax paper and coat the rolls with the flour.

4. Heat the oil over medium heat in a frying pan large enough to hold the rolls comfortably. When hot, add the rolls and brown them on all sides, turning as necessary. Season the veal rolls lightly with salt and pepper and pour the chicken broth into the frying pan. Stir the chicken broth with a wooden spoon to pick up any browned-on bits in the frying pan. Cover the pan and cook over low heat for 10 to 15 minutes, or until the veal is tender. Serve with Rice Milanese (see page 282).

VEAL ROLLS WITH MUSTARD

2 servings

½ pound veal cutlets, about 4 pieces
4   teaspoons Dijon mustard
1   small white onion, peeled, cut in half, and
*   sliced thin*
*   Salt and freshly ground black pepper*
3   tablespoons butter or margarine
½ cup chicken broth

1. Lay the cutlets on a cutting board and pound them lightly with the flat side of a meat mallet to thin them.

2. Spread one side of each piece of veal with 1 teaspoon of mustard. Divide the onion slices equally over the veal slices. Sprinkle the veal with salt and pepper. Roll up the veal slices tightly, leaving the ends open. Secure with toothpicks.

3. Melt the butter over medium heat in a frying pan. When it is hot and bubbling, add the veal rolls. Brown the rolls on all sides. When the rolls are browned, pour the chicken broth into the frying pan, stirring to loosen any browned-on bits in the pan. Cover the pan and cook over low heat for 15 minutes, or until the veal is tender.

VEAL CUTLETS FLORENTINE

2 servings

1   pound fresh spinach
*   Salt*
*   Pinch of ground nutmeg*
*   Freshly ground black pepper*
1   recipe for Sautéed Veal Cutlets (see page 259)
*   Butter or margarine*
4   thin slices mozzarella cheese

1. Pick over the spinach to remove the stems and any bruised leaves. Wash the spinach under cool running water to remove any grit. Drain.

2. Put the spinach in a frying pan with a cover. Do not add water; the spinach will steam with just the water clinging to the leaves. Sprinkle the spinach lightly with salt. Cover the pan and cook over medium-high heat, stirring once or twice, until the spinach is just wilted. Transfer the cooked spinach to a sieve and let it drain. Press out any excess water with the back of a wooden spoon. When cool enough to handle, chop the spinach coarsely and season it with nutmeg and pepper to taste.

3. While the spinach is cooking, prepare the Sautéed Veal Cutlets. Drain them well on paper towels.

4. Preheat the oven to 350 degrees.

5. Liberally butter a baking dish large enough to hold the veal cutlets in one layer. Lay the veal cutlets in the baking dish in a single layer. Top each cutlet with an equal amount of the seasoned chopped spinach. Lay a slice of mozzarella cheese on top of each mound of spinach. Bake for 15 to 20 minutes, or until the cheese has melted and the spinach is warm. Serve immediately.

SICILIAN CUTLETS

2 servings

2 thin slices prosciutto
2 thin slices Genoa salami
2 tablespoons pignoli nuts
2 tablespoons sliced mushrooms
1 1-inch-thick slice Italian bread, cubed
1 clove garlic, peeled
2 tablespoons grated Romano cheese
1 egg
1 tablespoon oil
4 slices veal cutlet
2 cups Marinara Sauce (page 276)

1. Grind together the prosciutto, salami, pignoli, mushrooms, bread, and garlic in a meat grinder. Add the cheese, egg, and oil and mix to a thick paste.
2. Preheat the oven to 350 degrees.
3. Spread the paste evenly over the 4 slices of veal. Pour 1 cup of Marinara Sauce into a baking dish large enough to hold the veal slices. Lay the veal slices in the sauce and spoon the remaining sauce over the cutlets. Bake for 50 minutes, or until the veal is tender.

VEAL STEW

4 servings

2 tablespoons olive or vegetable oil
1 medium-sized white onion, peeled, cut in half, and sliced thin
3 stalks celery, sliced
1 large carrot, scraped and diced
1 clove garlic, peeled and minced
1 pound veal stew meat, cut into 1½-inch cubes
   Salt and freshly ground black pepper
3 cups Marinara Sauce (page 276)
1 4-ounce can mushroom stems and pieces, drained

1. Heat the oil in a Dutch oven or heavy saucepan. Add the onion, celery, carrot, and garlic and sauté for 5 minutes. Push the vegetables to the side and add the veal cubes. Brown the veal cubes on all sides. Sprinkle the vegetables and meat generously with salt and pepper. Stir in the Marinara Sauce and bring to a boil. Cover, lower the heat, and simmer the stew for 50 minutes, stirring occasionally.
2. Add the drained mushrooms and cook until they are heated through.

MEAT BALLS WITH EGGPLANT

4 servings

1 slice white bread, trimmed of crusts
1 pound ground veal
1 egg
¼ cup finely minced onion
   Pinch of dried basil
   Salt and freshly ground black pepper
½ cup unseasoned bread crumbs
   Flour for dredging
6 tablespoons vegetable oil
1 large onion, peeled and minced
2 cloves garlic, peeled and minced
1 1½-pound eggplant, peeled and cut into ½-inch cubes
1 1-pound can crushed tomatoes
¾ cup chicken broth
½ teaspoon dried oregano
⅛ teaspoon ground cinnamon
⅛ teaspoon ground nutmeg

1. Soak the bread in water to cover for 10 minutes. When the bread is soft, squeeze it dry and put it in a small mixing bowl with the veal, egg, minced onion, basil, and salt and pepper to taste. Mix well and add the bread crumbs. Use your hand to combine the bread crumbs with the meat mixture. Form the meat mixture into 24 small balls.

2. Put some flour on a sheet of wax paper and toss the balls in the flour until they are lightly coated.

3. Heat 3 tablespoons of the oil over medium heat in a heavy saucepan. When the oil is hot, add the floured veal balls and brown them on all sides. As the meat balls are browned, remove them to a plate with a slotted spoon.

4. When all the meat balls have been browned, add the remaining 3 tablespoons of oil to the saucepan. When the oil is hot, add the onion and garlic and sauté over low heat, stirring occasionally, for 10 minutes. Add the eggplant cubes to the sautéed onion and garlic and toss to coat the eggplant with the oil. Add the tomatoes, chicken broth, oregano, cinnamon, nutmeg, ½ teaspoon salt, and ⅛ teaspoon pepper to the eggplant mixture. Mix well and bring to a boil. Return the browned meat balls to the pan and stir them into the vegetables. Cover the pan and simmer for 45 minutes.

STUFFED EGGPLANT

2 servings

1 1½-pound eggplant
2 tablespoons olive or vegetable oil
1 small yellow onion, peeled and minced
1 clove garlic, peeled and minced
½ pound ground veal, lamb, or beef
1 4-ounce can mushroom stems and pieces, drained and chopped
½ cup cooked rice
½ teaspoon dried oregano, crumbled
1 tablespoon chopped parsley
⅛ teaspoon ground cinnamon
   Pinch of ground nutmeg
   Salt and freshly ground black pepper
1 8-ounce can tomato sauce
1 egg
½ cup milk
¼ cup grated Parmesan cheese

1. Cut the eggplant in half and scoop out the flesh with a spoon, leaving a ¼-inch shell. Dice the flesh and set it aside.

2. Heat the olive oil in a large frying pan and add the onion and garlic. Sauté over low heat for 5 minutes, stirring occasionally. Add the ground veal and sauté for 2 minutes, breaking up the veal with a wooden spoon. Add the diced eggplant flesh and cook, stirring, for 10 minutes. Remove from the heat.

3. Preheat the oven to 375 degrees.

4. Add the mushrooms, rice, oregano, parsley, cinnamon, nutmeg, pepper, and tomato sauce to the frying pan. Stir to mix well. Divide the mixture evenly between the 2 eggplant shells. Put the eggplant shells in a buttered baking pan and cover tightly with foil. Bake for 30 to 45 minutes, or until the eggplant is tender. Remove foil.

5. Beat the egg, milk, and cheese together until well blended. Pour a little at a time over the eggplant stuffing, using a fork to separate the stuffing so that the custard seeps into the stuffing. Put the baking pan under the broiler, about 4 inches away from the flame, and broil until the tops of the stuffed eggplant halves are lightly browned. Serve immediately.

LAMB CHOPS WITH SAUTÉED MUSHROOMS
2 servings

2   tablespoons butter or margarine
2   round-bone shoulder lamb chops, about ½ inch thick
    Salt
    Freshly ground black pepper
⅛   teaspoon garlic powder
⅛   teaspoon onion powder
½   pound mushrooms, caps and stems, sliced

1. Melt the butter in a large nonstick frying pan. When it is very hot, add the lamb chops. Sauté over medium heat for 6 minutes, browning on one side. Turn the chops and sauté for 5 minutes on the second side, browning again.

2. Sprinkle the chops with salt, pepper, garlic powder, and onion powder to taste. Cover the pan and cook over medium-high heat for 5 minutes. Remove the chops to a plate and keep them warm.

3. Add the mushrooms to the frying pan and sauté over medium-high heat, stirring often, until they give up their liquid. Season the mushrooms slightly with salt and pepper. Continue to sauté, stirring, until almost all of the liquid has evaporated. Return the chops to the pan and cover them with equal amounts of the mushrooms. Cook for 1 minute and serve.

LAMB CHOPS WITH BROWN RICE
4 servings

3   tablespoons butter or margarine
4   shoulder lamb chops, about ½ inch thick
1   cup raw brown rice
    Salt and freshly ground black pepper
1   large yellow onion, peeled and chopped
1   large green pepper, seeded and chopped
2   large ripe tomatoes, peeled, seeded, and chopped
1   large clove garlic, peeled and minced
½   teaspoon dried oregano, crumbled
2   cups chicken broth
½   cup water
1   4-ounce can mushroom stems and pieces, drained

1. Melt 2 tablespoons of the butter in a frying pan. When it is hot and bubbling, add the lamb chops and brown them on both sides.

2. Spread the remaining tablespoon of butter on the inside of an ovenproof casserole with a cover. Make a layer of the brown rice on the bottom of the casserole. Put the browned chops in a layer on top of the rice. Sprinkle the chops liberally with salt and pepper.

3. Preheat the oven to 350 degrees.

4. Mix together the onion, green pepper, tomatoes, garlic, and oregano. Spread the mixture over the chops. Pour the broth and water over the vegetables, cover, and bake for 1½ hours.

5. Stir the drained mushrooms into the rice during the last 5 minutes of baking.

Note: Leftovers can be reheated in a nonstick frying pan with a cover. Put 2 tablespoons of chicken broth into the pan before you add the leftovers.

SPICED LAMB CHOPS

2 servings

2   shoulder lamb chops
½   teaspoon ground cinnamon
½   teaspoon salt
⅛   teaspoon freshly ground black pepper

1. Trim the lamb chops of all excess fat. Make cuts at ½-inch intervals along the outside of the chops so that they will lie flat when they are cooked.
2. Combine the spices and rub the mixture into both sides of the chops. Let sit for 15 minutes.
3. Preheat the broiler. When it is hot, broil the chops 3 inches from the flame, turning once, until they are tender. Serve immediately.

LAMB WITH STEWED ZUCCHINI

2 servings

2   tablespoons butter or margarine
2   shoulder lamb chops
    Salt and freshly ground black pepper
3   cups Stewed Zucchini (page 298)

1. Melt the butter in a large frying pan. When hot and bubbling, add the lamb chops and brown on both sides. Sprinkle the chops with salt and pepper to taste. Cover the pan and cook the chops over medium heat until they are tender, about 15 minutes.
2. When the chops are tender, add the zucchini to the frying pan and cook over low heat until it is warmed through. Serve at once.

HERBED LAMB CHOPS

2 servings

2   shoulder lamb chops
1   hard-cooked egg, peeled and minced
2   tablespoons seasoned bread crumbs
¼   teaspoon finely minced garlic
¼   teaspoon salt
⅛   teaspoon freshly ground black pepper
1   tablespoon minced parsley
2   finely chopped mushroom caps
1   tablespoon minced onion
⅛   teaspoon dried thyme
    Tomato sauce

1. Preheat the oven to 350 degrees.
2. Trim the lamb chops of all excess fat. Make cuts at ½-inch intervals along the outside of the chops so that they will lie flat when they are baked.
3. In a bowl, mix together the egg, bread crumbs, garlic, salt, pepper, parsley, mushrooms, onion, and thyme until well blended. Moisten the mixture with just enough tomato sauce to make it hold together. Spread an equal amount of the mixture in an even layer on top of each of the chops. Put the chops in a buttered baking pan. Cover the pan tightly with foil and bake for 45 to 50 minutes or until the lamb is tender.

LAMB KEBABS

2 servings

2   shoulder lamb chops, about ½ inch thick
3   tablespoons lemon juice
3   tablespoons olive or vegetable oil
    Salt and freshly ground black pepper
½   teaspoon dried thyme
⅛   teaspoon cayenne pepper
½   teaspoon finely minced garlic
⅛   teaspoon ground cumin
2   medium-sized green peppers, seeded
8   mushroom caps

1. Trim the lamb chops of all fat, skin, and bones, and cut the meat into 1-inch cubes. Set aside.

2. Combine the lemon juice, oil, salt, black pepper, thyme, cayenne pepper, garlic, and cumin in a large bowl. Beat to mix well. Add the lamb cubes and toss to coat the lamb with the marinade. Cover the bowl tightly and refrigerate for at least 8 hours, or overnight, tossing the mixture occasionally.

3. Preheat the broiler.

4. Cut the green peppers into 1-inch cubes.

5. Drain the lamb and reserve the marinade. Thread the lamb pieces on 2 long skewers, alternating with the green peppers and mushrooms (lamb, pepper, mushroom), until all the ingredients have been used. Lay the skewers in the broiling pan and brush with the reserved marinade. Broil about 4 inches from the flame for 10 minutes. Turn the skewers, brush again with the marinade and broil for 7 to 10 minutes longer, or until the lamb and vegetables are tender. Remove from the skewer and serve immediately on a bed of Rice Pilaf (see page 282).

HUNAN-STYLE SHREDDED LAMB

2 servings

1   tablespoon tree ears or black fungus
2   dried Chinese mushrooms, stems removed
2   shoulder lamb chops
1   tablespoon cornstarch
2   tablespoons water
3   tablespoons soy sauce
2   tablespoons rice wine or dry sherry
¼   teaspoon salt
2   teaspoons rice vinegar or white vinegar
2   tablespoons vegetable or peanut oil
1   tablespoon chili oil, or 4 dried red chili peppers
1   clove garlic, peeled and minced
2   teaspoons minced fresh gingerroot
6   scallions, trimmed and cut into 2-inch-long shreds
½   cup julienned bamboo shoots

1. Put the tree ears and mushrooms in a bowl and cover them with boiling water. Let sit for 20 minutes to soften. Drain and squeeze out all the excess water. Dice the tree ears and cut the mushrooms into thin strips. Set aside until needed.

2. Trim the lamb chops of all fat, skin, and bones, and cut the meat into 2-inch-long shreds. Combine the lamb shreds with the cornstarch and water in a small bowl. Mix well with your fingers and let sit for 10 minutes.

3. Mix together the soy sauce, rice wine, salt, and rice vinegar in a cup. Set aside until needed.

4. Put the oils, garlic, and gingerroot into a wok or heavy frying pan. Heat, stirring occasionally, over medium-high heat until the garlic and gingerroot begin to sizzle. Drain the lamb shreds and add them to the wok. Cook for 3

minutes, turning and stirring constantly. Add the scallions and cook for 1 minute, stirring constantly. Stir in the bamboo shoots, tree ears, and mushrooms.

5. Stir the sauce mixture (from step 3) and pour it over the meat and vegetables. Cook, stirring, for 2 minutes, or until the sauce has thickened. Serve immediately.

Note: Tree ears, Chinese mushrooms, rice wine, rice vinegar, and chili oil can be purchased in Oriental markets. If you can't find chili oil, you can add the chili peppers when the chili oil is called for in the instructions. Just remember to increase the oil you are using by the amount of chili oil called for in the ingredients list. I suggest that you remove the chili peppers before you serve the dish to avoid shocking your palate.

POTTED LAMB SHANKS

2 servings

2 lamb shanks, about ¾ pound each
2 tablespoons vegetable oil
1 large yellow onion, peeled and chopped
1 large green pepper, seeded and chopped
1 large clove garlic, peeled and minced
1 8-ounce can stewed tomatoes
1 cup chicken broth
½ teaspoon dried rosemary, crumbled
1 teaspoon salt
⅛ teaspoon freshly ground black pepper

1. Wash the lamb shanks in cool water and pat dry with paper towels.

2. Heat the oil in a Dutch oven or heavy saucepan. Add the lamb shanks and brown them on all sides. Remove the browned shanks to a plate.

3. Add the onion, pepper, and garlic to the oil in the pan and sauté over medium heat for 5 minutes.

4. Chop the stewed tomatoes finely, reserving the liquid in the can. Add the tomatoes to the sautéed vegetables and cook and stir for 5 minutes.

5. Add the tomato liquid, chicken broth, rosemary, salt, and pepper to the pan. Stir and bring to a boil. Return the lamb shanks to the pan. Cover and simmer for 1½ hours, stirring and turning the meat occasionally, or until the lamb is tender.

BRAISED LAMB SHANKS WITH LENTILS PROVENÇALE

2 servings

2 ¾-pound lamb shanks
2 tablespoons vegetable oil
1 tablespoon butter or margarine
1 medium-sized onion, peeled and coarsely chopped
1 large carrot, scraped and coarsely chopped
1 celery stalk, coarsely chopped
2 cloves garlic, peeled and minced
2 large ripe tomatoes, peeled, seeded, and chopped
2 cups beef broth
½ cup water
1 bay leaf
½ teaspoon dried thyme
   Salt and freshly ground black pepper
½ cup dried lentils, picked over, washed, and dained

1. Wash the lamb shanks in cool water and pat dry with paper towels.

2. Heat the oil and butter in a heavy saucepan. When the butter is completely melted, add the lamb shanks and brown them on all sides. Remove the browned lamb shanks and set them aside on a plate. Add the onion, carrot, celery, and garlic to the pan and sauté over low heat for 10 minutes, stirring occasionally. When the vegetables have cooked for 10 minutes, add the tomatoes and cook for 5 minutes longer. Add the broth, water, bay leaf, thyme, and salt and pepper to taste. Bring to a boil and return the lamb shanks to the pan. Cover the pan, lower the heat, and simmer for 45 minutes.

3. Add the lentils to the pan and stir them into the vegetable mixture well. Cover the pan and cook over low heat for 1 hour longer, stirring occasionally.

LAMB AND STRING BEAN STEW

4 servings

2   tablespoons vegetable oil
2½   to 3 pounds lamb stew meat with bones (see Note)
2   large yellow onions, peeled and chopped
2   large cloves garlic, peeled and minced
1   2-inch piece cinnamon stick
     Salt and freshly ground black pepper
1   8-ounce can stewed tomatoes with liquid
1   cup chicken broth
1   bay leaf
1   pound fresh string beans
4   medium-sized potatoes

1. Heat the oil in a large heavy frying pan or Dutch oven. When it is hot, add the stew meat in a single layer. Do not crowd the pieces together, but brown the meat in two batches, if necessary. Brown the meat over medium heat, removing the pieces to a plate as they brown.

2. When all the stew meat has browned, add the onions, garlic, and cinnamon stick to the pan. Sauté over low heat for 10 minutes, stirring occasionally to loosen any browned-on bits in the pan. Do not let the onions or garlic brown.

3. Return the stew meat to the pan, laying it in a single layer over the onions. Sprinkle the meat and vegetables with salt and pepper. Cover the pan and cook over low heat for ½ hour, stirring occasionally after 10 minutes.

4. After the lamb has cooked for ½ hour, add the stewed tomatoes and their liquid, the chicken broth, and the bay leaf. Bring the mixture to a boil, breaking up the tomatoes with a wooden spoon. Season with salt and pepper to taste, cover, lower the heat, and simmer for 45 minutes, stirring occasionally.

5. Meanwhile, trim the ends from the string beans and cut the beans into 1½-inch lengths, on the diagonal. Wash the string bean pieces in cool running water and drain them well.

6. Peel the potatoes and cut them into ½-inch-thick slices. Set aside until needed.

7. When the stew mixture has cooked for the additional 45 minutes, add the string bean pieces and potato slices to the pan. Season liberally with salt and pepper and mix well. Bring the stew to a boil over medium heat, cover, lower the heat, and simmer for 35 to 40 minutes, or until the meat and vegetables are tender. Stir the stew occasionally while it is cooking to prevent the potatoes from sticking to the pan.

Note: This dish can also be made using 4 blade lamb shoulder chops instead of the lamb stew meat. Cut the meat into about 1½-inch pieces and leave some meat on the bones, which should be added to the stew.

This dish is good if made the day before it is to be served. If it should be a little greasy, just scoop off the offending grease before heating the dish.

PORK CHOPS WITH CHICK-PEAS

4 servings

Flour for dredging
Salt and freshly ground black pepper
4 thick center-cut pork chops
2 tablespoons olive oil
2 tablespoons butter or margarine
2 large onions, peeled, halved, and cut into thin slices
2 cloves garlic, peeled and minced
1 1-pound can crushed tomatoes
1 cup chicken broth
1/2 teaspoon dried oregano
1 bay leaf
Pinch of ground nutmeg
1 1-pound 4-ounce can chick-peas, drained

1. Season the flour with salt and pepper and dredge the pork chops in it.
2. Heat the oil in a large frying pan and brown the chops on both sides. Remove the chops to a plate as they brown.
3. When you have removed the last chop, add the butter to the frying pan. When it has melted and is bubbling, add the onions and garlic. Sauté over medium heat, stirring occasionally, for 5 minutes. Add the tomatoes, chicken broth, oregano, bay leaf, and nutmeg. Season with salt and pepper to taste. Simmer the sauce for 5 minutes.
4. Add the browned chops to the sauce, turning them to coat them with the sauce. Cover, and simmer for 1 hour, turning the chops occa-sionally, and stirring the sauce so it does not stick.
5. Stir in the drained chick-peas and heat, over very low heat, for 10 minutes. Serve with steamed rice.

PORK CHOPS WITH SAUERKRAUT

2 servings

2 tablespoons butter or margarine
2 1-inch-thick center-cut pork chops
1 large white onion, peeled and chopped
1 pound sauerkraut, rinsed and drained
1/3 cup raisins
Large pinch of caraway seeds
2 1/2 cups water
Salt and freshly ground black pepper

1. Melt the butter in a large heavy frying pan. When the butter is completely melted, add the chops and brown them well on both sides over medium heat. Remove the browned chops to a plate until needed.
2. Add the onion to the fat in the frying pan and sauté over low heat for 5 minutes, stirring occasionally. Add the sauerkraut, raisins, cara-way seeds, and water to the frying pan. Stir to mix well, scraping up all the browned-on bits in the frying pan. Bring the mixture to a boil and lay the chops on top of the sauerkraut mixture. Sprinkle the chops and sauerkraut liberally with salt and pepper. Cover the pan, lower the heat, and cook for 1 hour, turning the chops and stir-ring the sauerkraut occasionally. Taste for seasonings, and add salt and pepper, if necessary.
3. To serve, use a slotted spoon to drain the liquid from the sauerkraut mixture.

PORK CHOPS WITH CABBAGE AND POTATOES

2 servings

2   tablespoons butter or margarine
2   1/2-inch-thick center-cut pork chops
1   small onion, peeled and minced
1   large clove garlic, peeled and minced
2   large ripe tomatoes, peeled, seeded, and
    chopped
1/2 cup chicken broth
    Pinch of dried sage
    Salt and freshly ground black pepper
2   medium-sized potatoes, peeled and cut into
    1/4-inch-thick slices
2   cups thinly sliced green cabbage

1. Melt the butter in a heavy frying pan. When the butter is melted, add the chops and brown them on both sides over medium heat. Remove the chops to a plate and set aside until needed.

2. Add the onion and garlic to the butter remaining in the frying pan. Sauté over low heat for 5 minutes, stirring occasionally. Add the tomatoes and sauté for 5 minutes longer. Pour in the chicken broth and mix well. Bring to a boil and return the browned chops to the frying pan. Sprinkle the chops with the sage and salt and pepper to taste. Lay the potato slices over the chops and sauce in the frying pan. Sprinkle the potato slices with salt and pepper. Cover the frying pan and cook over low heat for 15 minutes.

3. Spread the thinly sliced cabbage in an even layer over the potatoes and chops. Sprinkle the cabbage with salt and lots of black pepper. Cover the frying pan and cook over low heat for 15 minutes. Uncover the frying pan and stir the ingredients thoroughly, turning the chops and mixing the cabbage and potatoes into the sauce.

(Try not to break up the potatoes.) Cover the frying pan and cook for 15 minutes longer, or until all the ingredients are fork-tender. Serve immediately.

SHREDDED PORK WITH SCALLIONS

2 servings

1   tablespoon tree ears or black fungus
1/2 pound boneless pork, shredded
1   tablespoon rice wine or dry sherry
2   tablespoons soy sauce
1/2 teaspoon freshly ground black pepper
4   tablespoons vegetable or peanut oil
1   teaspoon rice vinegar or white vinegar
1   teaspoon sesame oil
2   teaspoons minced garlic
6   scallions, trimmed and cut into 2-inch-long
    shreds

1. Put the tree ears in a bowl and cover them with boiling water. Let soak for 20 minutes. Drain and squeeze out all the excess water. Chop coarsely and set aside until needed.

2. Put the shredded pork in a bowl and mix in the rice wine, 1 tablespoon of the soy sauce, the black pepper, and 2 tablespoons of the vegetable oil. Mix together with your fingers until the pork is well coated. Let sit for 15 minutes.

3. In another small bowl mix the remaining tablespoon of soy sauce with the rice vinegar and the sesame oil. Stir to combine well and set aside until needed.

4. Put the remaining 2 tablespoons of vegetable oil in a wok and heat. When it is hot, add the garlic and stir. Drain the pork and add it to the wok. Cook, stirring, for about 1 minute, or

until the pork shreds are white. Add the scallions, tree ears, and the seasonings (from step 3). Stir to mix well. Cook for 1 minute and serve immediately.

Note: Tree ears, rice wine, rice vinegar, and sesame oil can be purchased in Oriental markets.

SPARERIBS WITH CABBAGE AND POTATOES
2 servings

1½ pounds spareribs
1 tablespoon vegetable oil
    Salt and freshly ground black pepper
    Garlic powder
2 large potatoes, peeled and quartered
3 cups shredded cabbage
1 medium-sized onion, peeled and chopped
1 8-ounce can tomato sauce
1 cup water

1. Cut the spareribs into single rib pieces. Heat the oil in a frying pan and, when it is hot, brown the ribs on all sides over medium heat. Transfer the ribs to an ovenproof casserole as they brown. Sprinkle the ribs liberally with salt, pepper, and garlic powder.

2. Preheat the oven to 350 degrees.

3. Put the potatoes and cabbage in the casserole, sprinkling each vegetable with salt, pepper, and garlic powder. Sprinkle the onions over the cabbage.

4. Mix the tomato sauce ad water together and pour the sauce over the vegetables and meat in the casserole. Cover the casserole and bake for 1 hour and 15 minutes, or until the meat and vegetables are tender. Stir the casserole

occasionally so that the flavors blend. Serve immediately.

PORK HOCKS AND COLLARD GREENS
2 servings

2 tablespoons vegetable oil
1 1-pound fresh pork hock, cut into ½-inch-thick slices
1 small yellow onion, peeled and chopped
1 small green pepper, seeded and chopped
1 8-ounce can stewed tomatoes with liquid
    Pinch of dried thyme leaves
    Salt and freshly ground black pepper
½ cup water
1 10-ounce package chopped collard greens, defrosted

1. Heat the oil in a large frying pan. When the oil is hot, add the pork hock slices in a single layer. Brown the pork hock slices on both sides over medium heat. Remove the browned slices to a plate and keep warm.

2. Add the onion and green pepper to the oil in the frying pan. Sauté over low heat for 10 minutes, stirring occasionally.

3. Meanwhile, drain the stewed tomatoes and reserve the liquid. Cut the tomatoes into small pieces. When the onion and green pepper have cooked for 10 minutes, add the tomato pieces to the frying pan and sauté for 5 minutes over medium heat, stirring occasionally.

4. Add the tomato liquid to the frying pan and mix well. Season the vegetable mixture with salt and pepper to taste and the thyme. Bring to a boil and return the pork hock slices to the frying pan. Spoon a little bit of the sauce over

each slice. Cover the frying pan, lower the heat, and simmer for 1 hour, or until the hocks are tender. Stir the sauce and turn the meat occasionally as it cooks.

5. Remove the pork hock slices from the frying pan and let them cool.

6. Add the water to the frying pan and bring the sauce back to a boil. Add the defrosted collard greens and mix well. Bring the mixture back to a boil, cover the frying pan, and cook over low heat for 20 to 25 minutes, or until the greens are tender. Stir occasionally.

7. Taste the vegetable-sauce mixture for seasonings, and add more salt and pepper, if necessary.

8. Remove the meat from the pork hock slices and discard the bones, skin, and fat. Cut the meat into small pieces and add it to the frying pan. Mix well and heat until the pork is warm. Serve in deep soup bowls over portions of brown rice.

SAUSAGES, PEPPERS, AND POTATOES

3 servings

3 medium-sized baking potatoes, peeled
Salt
2 tablespoons vegetable oil
1 clove garlic, peeled and sliced in half
1 medium-sized yellow onion, cut in half and sliced thin
3 medium-sized green peppers, cut into 1/2-inch cubes
Freshly ground black pepper
1 pound good Italian sweet sausage (not the supermarket variety)

1. Cut the potatoes into quarters and cut the quarters into 1/2-inch-thick slices. Put the potatoes in a pot and add water to barely cover them. Add salt to taste. Bring to a boil, cover, lower the heat, and simmer for 10 minutes, or until the potatoes are just barely tender. Drain well and set aside.

2. Heat the oil in a large nonstick frying pan. Add the garlic and let it brown slightly on both sides over low heat. Remove the garlic and discard it. Add the onion slices to the pan and cook for 1 minute, stirring to separate the onion rings. Add the green peppers and sauté over medium-high heat for 10 minutes, stirring occasionally. Season with salt and pepper to taste. Add the drained cooked potatoes and sauté gently for 3 to 4 minutes. Remove the vegetables to a plate and keep warm.

3. Put the sausages in the frying pan in one layer. Add hot water to half cover the sausages. Bring to a boil, cover, lower the heat to medium, and cook for 10 minutes. Prick the sausages thoroughly with a fork and turn them over. Cover and cook 10 minutes longer. Remove the cover and prick the sausages again.

4. Increase the heat to high and cook the sausages, turning them often, until almost all of the cooking liquid has evaporated and the sausages are browned on all sides. (As the cooking liquid boils down and thickens, spoon about 4 tablespoons of it over the reserved vegetables.)

5. Remove the browned sausages to a plate and cut them into 1/4-inch-thick slices. Pour off all the fat from the frying pan and return the sausages and vegetables to the pan. Mix the ingredients well and heat through over low heat.

JAMBON NORMANDE

2 servings

2 large eating apples
2 tablespoons butter or margarine
1 tablespoon dark brown sugar
⅛ teaspoon ground cinnamon
1 ¾-pound smoked ham steak

1. Peel, core, and quarter the apples. Cut each quarter into four equal slices.

2. Melt the butter in a large nonstick frying pan. When the butter is bubbling add the apple slices in one layer. Cook over medium-high heat for 3 minutes, shaking the pan often. Turn the slices over and cook on the other side for 3 minutes, shaking the pan often.

3. Sprinkle the apple slices with the brown sugar and cinnamon and toss the apple slices for 2 minutes with a spatula to coat them with the cinnamon and sugar. Remove from the pan and set aside.

4. Drain most of the fat from the frying pan. Lay the ham steak in the pan and fry on one side for 4 minutes. Turn and fry for 4 minutes on the other side. After you turn the ham lay the cooked apple slices on the browned side to warm them. Serve immediately.

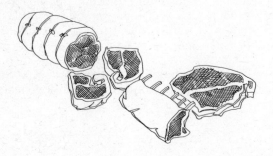

SPAGHETTI SAUCES AND PASTA DISHES

ANCHOVY AND TOMATO SAUCE

2 servings

4 tablespoons olive oil
4 canned anchovy fillets, drained
2 cloves garlic, peeled and minced
1/2 teaspoon dried basil
1 dried red chili pepper
1/2 teaspoon freshly ground black pepper
10 plum tomatoes, peeled, seeded, and diced
1 tablespoon drained capers, chopped
6 to 8 ounces cooked spaghetti

Put the oil and the anchovies into a heavy saucepan and cook over low heat for 3 minutes, mashing the anchovies into the oil with a fork. Add the garlic, basil, chili pepper, black pepper, and tomatoes. Stir well to blend and cook, uncovered, over low heat for 20 minutes, stirring occasionally. Add the capers to the sauce just before you toss the sauce with the cooked spaghetti.

CHICKEN LIVER SPAGHETTI SAUCE

4 servings

2 tablespoons olive oil
1 medium-sized white onion, peeled and minced
1 large clove garlic, peeled and minced

1 celery stalk, minced
1 1/2 pounds fresh plum tomatoes, peeled, seeded, and chopped, or 3 cups canned crushed tomatoes
3/4 cup chicken broth
8 fresh basil leaves, washed, dried, and minced, or 1/2 teaspoon dried basil
1/8 teaspoon dried sage
    Salt and freshly ground black pepper
2 tablespoons butter or margarine
1/2 pound chicken livers, picked over, washed, and cut into 1/4-inch-thick slices
1/2 pound mushrooms, sliced, or 1 4-ounce can mushroom pieces, drained

1. Heat the oil in a heavy frying pan. When the oil is hot, add the onion, garlic, and celery. Sauté over medium heat, stirring occasionally, for 10 minutes. Do not let the onion brown. Stir in the tomatoes and broth and bring to a boil. Add the basil, sage, and salt and pepper to taste. Stir to combine well. Cover and simmer for 20 minutes, stirring and crushing the tomatoes occasionally.

2. Melt the butter in a small frying pan. When the butter is completely melted, add the sliced chicken livers and sauté until cooked through (3 to 4 minutes). Use a slotted spoon to remove the chicken livers and put them on a plate. Add the mushrooms to the frying pan and sauté until the mushrooms give up their liquid and turn

golden brown. (This may take up to 10 minutes.) Use a slotted spoon to remove the mushrooms to the plate with the chicken livers.

3. After the sauce has cooked for 20 minutes, add the chicken livers and mushrooms to the sauce. Cover and cook for 5 minutes longer over low heat.

SAUCE BOLOGNESE

4 servings

2 tablespoons olive oil
1 large white onion peeled and minced
1 small carrot, scraped and minced
1 small stalk celery, trimmed and minced
1 large clove garlic, peeled and minced
1 pound ground round
2 cups beef broth
¼ cup tomato sauce
   Pinch of ground nutmeg
   Salt and freshly ground black pepper
½ pound chopped mushrooms, sautéed and drained

1. Heat the oil in a frying pan or heavy saucepan. Add the vegetables (except for the mushrooms) and sauté them slowly for 10 minutes, stirring often.

2. Add the ground round and cook, breaking up the meat with a wooden spoon, until brown.

3. Add the broth, tomato sauce, nutmeg, and salt and pepper to taste. Stir well. Bring to a boil, lower the heat, cover, and simmer for 20 minutes, stirring occasionally.

4. After 20 minutes, stir the sauce again, partially cover the pan, and simmer for 10 minutes longer.

5. Meanwhile, melt the butter in a medium-sized nonstick frying pan. Add the chopped mushrooms and sauté over medium heat, stirring occasionally, for about 10 minutes, or until the mushrooms give up their liquid and begin to brown. Drain in a sieve and set aside until needed.

6. Stir the mushrooms into the sauce and cook for 2 minutes longer. Serve with small shell macaroni.

WHITE CLAM SAUCE

2 servings

1 10½-ounce can whole baby clams
3 tablespoons olive oil
1 small white onion, peeled and minced
3 cloves garlic, peeled and minced
1 cup clam juice
3 tablespoons minced parsley
   Salt and freshly ground black pepper
6 ounces linguini, cooked al dente and drained

1. Drain the clams and reserve the liquid.

2. Heat the olive oil in a heavy saucepan. When hot, add the onion and garlic. Sauté over low heat for 5 minutes, or until soft but not brown. Add the reserved clam liquid, the clam broth, and the minced parsley. Season with salt and pepper to taste. (Be careful with the salt, as the clam broth is salty.) Bring to a boil, cover, lower the heat, and simmer for 15 minutes. Add the reserved clams just before you turn off the heat under the pot. Toss with the drained linguini and serve immediately.

RED CLAM SAUCE

4 servings

1 10½-ounce can baby clams
2 tablespoons olive oil
1 large yellow onion, peeled and minced
3 cloves garlic, peeled and minced
1 28-ounce can Italian peeled tomatoes with
   liquid
1 8-ounce can tomato sauce
1 cup water
1½ teaspoons salt, or to taste
½ teaspoon freshly ground black pepper
2 dried chili peppers, or ½ teaspoon dried red
   pepper flakes (optional)
½ teaspoon dried basil crumbled
½ teaspoon dried oregano, crumbled

1. Drain the clams well and reserve the juice.
2. Heat the oil in a heavy saucepan. When hot, add the onion and garlic and sauté over low heat for 10 minutes, stirring occasionally. Do not let the onion or garlic brown.
3. Push the tomatoes and their liquid through a food mill, or blend in a blender, and add to the sautéed onion and garlic with the tomato sauce, water, and reserved clam juice. Bring to a boil over medium heat, stirring occasionally. Stir the salt, pepper, chili peppers, and basil into the sauce. Cover and simmer for 20 minutes, stirring occasionally.
4. Sprinkle the oregano over the sauce and stir it in. Cover the pan partially and simmer the sauce for 20 minutes longer. Add the drained clams just before you turn off the heat under the sauce.

EGGPLANT SAUCE

6 servings

2 tablespoons olive or vegetable oil, or 1
   tablespoon of each
1 large yellow onion, peeled and minced
3 cloves garlic, peeled and minced
1 28-ounce can Italian peeled tomatoes with
   liquid
1 8-ounce can tomato sauce
1 cup water
1 1-pound eggplant, peeled and diced
1½ teaspoons salt
¼ teaspoon freshly ground black pepper
½ teaspoon dried basil, crumbled
1½ teaspoons dried oregano, crumbled

1. Heat the oil in a heavy saucepan. When hot, add the onion and garlic and sauté over low heat for 10 minutes, stirring occasionally. Do not let the onion or garlic brown.
2. Push the tomatoes and their liquid through a food mill, or blend in a blender, and add to the sautéed onion and garlic with the tomato sauce, water, and diced eggplant. Bring to a boil over medium heat, stirring occasionally. Stir in the salt, pepper, and basil. Cover and simmer the sauce for 20 minutes, stirring occasionally.
3. Sprinkle the oregano over the sauce and stir it in. Cover the pan partially and simmer the sauce for 20 minutes longer.
4. Cool the sauce slightly and purée it in a food mill or blender. Reheat gently to serve.

MARINARA SAUCE

4 servings

2   tablespoons olive or vegetable oil, or 1
    tablespoon of each
1   large yellow onion, peeled and minced
3   to 4 cloves garlic, peeled and minced
1   35-ounce can Italian peeled tomatoes with
    liquid
1   8-ounce can tomato sauce
1   cup water
1 1/2 teaspoons salt
1/4 teaspoon freshly ground black pepper
1/2 teaspoon dried basil, crumbled
1 1/2 teaspoons dried oregano, crumbled

1. Heat the oil in a heavy saucepan. When hot, add the onion and garlic and sauté over low heat for 10 minutes, stirring occasionally. Do not let the onion or garlic brown.

2. Push the tomatoes and their liquid through a food mill, or blend in a blender, and add to the sautéed onion and garlic with the tomato sauce and water. Bring to a boil over medium heat, stirring occasionally. Stir the salt, pepper, and basil into the sauce. Cover and simmer for 20 minutes, stirring occasionally.

3. Sprinkle the oregano over the sauce and stir it in. Cover the pan partially and simmer the sauce for 20 minutes longer.

MEAT SAUCE

6 servings

3   tablespoons olive or vegetable oil
2   large yellow onions, peeled and minced
4   cloves garlic, peeled and minced
2   pounds ground round or sirloin

2   8-ounce cans tomato sauce
1   6-ounce can tomato paste
1   28-ounce can crushed tomatoes
2 1/2 cups water
2 1/2 to 3 teaspoons salt
1/2 teaspoon freshly ground black pepper
1 1/2 teaspoons dried basil, crumbled
1   teaspoon dried oregano, crumbled

1. Heat the oil in a large Dutch oven. When it is hot, add the onions and garlic. Sauté over low heat for 10 minutes, stirring occasionally. Do not let the onions or garlic brown. Add the ground round and cook, breaking the meat up with a wooden spoon, until all the meat is brown.

2. Stir in the tomato sauce, tomato paste, and crushed tomatoes. Stir well to combine with the meat. Add the water and mix well. Bring to a boil over medium-high heat, stirring occasionally. Add the salt, pepper, basil, and oregano and mix well. Cover the pot, lower the heat, and simmer the sauce for 1 1/2 hours, stirring occasionally so that the meat does not stick to the bottom of the pan.

3. As the sauce cooks you will notice that a foam will form on the top. Use a large tablespoon to scoop off and discard this foam. Scoop off and discard any fat that also rises to the top of the sauce. When the sauce has cooked for 1 1/2 hours, taste for seasonings, and correct, if necessary.

Note: This recipe makes about 3 quarts of sauce. It freezes nicely, so you can put it into 2-cup portions and freeze for later use.

TOMATO-CAPER SAUCE

6 servings

2 tablespoons olive or vegetable oil
1 large yellow onion, peeled and minced
3 cloves garlic, peeled and minced
1 35-ounce can Italian peeled tomatoes with liquid
1 8-ounce can tomato sauce
1 cup water
1 1/2 teaspoons salt
1/4 teaspoon freshly ground black pepper
1/2 teaspoon dried basil, crumbled
1 1/2 teaspoons dried oregano, crumbled
2 tablespoons drained capers

1. Heat the oil in a heavy saucepan. When it is hot, add the onion and garlic and sauté over low heat for 10 minutes, stirring occasionally. Do not let the onion or garlic brown.

2. Push the tomatoes and their liquid through a food mill, or blend in a blender, and add to the sautéed onion and garlic with the tomato sauce and water. Bring to a boil over medium heat, stirring occasionally. Stir the salt, pepper, and basil into the sauce. Cover and simmer for 20 minutes, stirring occasionally.

3. Sprinkle the oregano over the sauce and stir it in. Add the capers and stir again. Cover the pan partially and simmer the sauce for 20 minutes longer.

VEAL SAUCE

4 servings

2 tablespoons olive or vegetable oil
2 cloves garlic, peeled
1/2 pound ground veal
1 28-ounce can Italian peeled tomatoes with liquid
1/2 teaspoon dried basil
Salt and freshly ground black pepper
4 chicken livers, minced
1/2 cup fresh or frozen peas

1. Heat the oil in a heavy saucepan. When the oil is hot, add the garlic and cook over low heat until brown on all sides. (Do not burn.) Remove and discard the garlic. Add the veal to the pan and cook, breaking it up with a wooden spoon, until it has lost its redness.

2. Remove the pan from the heat and fit a food mill directly over the pan. Purée the tomatoes and their liquid through the food mill directly into the pan with the veal. Return the pan to medium heat and bring to a boil. When the sauce is boiling, add the basil and salt and pepper to taste. Cover the pan, lower the heat, and cook for 25 minutes, stirring occasionally. Then add the chicken livers and peas and cook for 10 minutes longer. Check for seasonings, and add more salt and pepper, if necessary.

Note: This sauce can be used in such dishes as the Pasta and Eggplant Casserole (below) or just to sauce spaghetti.

PASTA AND EGGPLANT CASSEROLE

4 servings

1 1 1/2-pound eggplant
Salt
Olive or vegetable oil
1/2 pound macaroncelli or ziti
1 recipe for Veal Sauce (see above) or Marinara Sauce (page 276)
4 ounces mozzarella, diced
1/2 cup grated Romano or Parmesan cheese

1. Peel the eggplant and slice it into ¼-inch-thick round slices. Lay the slices in a colander, sprinkling each layer generously with salt. Put a plate as a weight on top of the eggplant slices and let them drain for ½ hour.

2. Pour ¼ inch olive oil in a frying pan. Heat over medium heat. While the oil is heating, wipe the salt from the eggplant slices with paper towels. Fry the eggplant slices in the oil until golden brown on both sides. Drain well on paper towels. (You may find it necessary to change the paper towels several times. It is important to drain off as much oil as possible from the eggplant.)

3. Coat the bottom and sides of a 2-quart soufflé dish with a film of oil. Make a layer of eggplant slices on the bottom of the dish and stand additional slices around the inside of the dish. (Make sure you have enough eggplant slices left to cover the top of the dish.)

4. Cook the macaroncelli in boiling salted water until it is just *al dente*. Drain the pasta well and mix it with 1 cup of the Veal Sauce and the diced mozzarella. Layer half the pasta mixture on top of the eggplant slices in the soufflé dish. Sprinkle with about 2 tablespoons of the grated cheese. (If you have any extra fried eggplant slices layer them over the cheese at this point.) Spread ½ cup of the Veal Sauce over the eggplant and top with the remaining pasta mixture. Spread another ½ cup of the Veal Sauce over the pasta mixture and sprinkle the pasta with another 2 tablespoons of grated cheese. Top the casserole with the remaining fried eggplant slices.

5. Preheat the oven to 350 degrees. Bake the casserole for about 30 minutes, or until all the ingredients are heated through and the mozzarella is melted. Serve with the additional Veal Sauce and grated cheese.

MACARONCELLI WITH ZUCCHINI SAUCE

4 servings

4   tablespoons olive or vegetable oil
¾   cup finely chopped red onion
1   large clove garlic, peeled and minced
1   28-ounce can peeled Italian tomatoes with liquid
1   teaspoon salt
¼   teaspoon freshly ground black pepper
7   fresh basil leaves, washed, dried, and minced, or ½ teaspoon dried basil
1   pound small zucchini, trimmed, scraped, and cut into julienne strips
¼   teaspoon dried oregano
4   to 6 ounces macaroncelli, cooked al dente and drained

1. Heat 2 tablespoons of the oil in a heavy saucepan. When the oil is hot, add the onion and garlic. Sauté over medium heat for 10 minutes, stirring occasionally. (Do not let the onion or garlic brown.) Remove from the heat and pass the tomatoes through a food mill directly into the pan with the onion and garlic. Return to the heat and bring to a boil over medium heat. Add the salt, pepper, and basil. Stir to mix well, cover, lower the heat, and simmer for 20 minutes.

2. Heat the remaining 2 tablespoons of oil in a small nonstick frying pan. When the oil is hot, add the julienned zucchini. Toss and stir over medium heat for 3 to 5 minutes, or until the

zucchini is barely tender. Pour the zucchini into a sieve and drain well.

3. When the sauce has cooked for 20 minutes, stir it and partially cover the pan. Cook for 10 minutes longer. Add the drained zucchini and cook, partially covered, for 5 minutes longer. Toss half of the sauce with the cooked macaroncelli and serve immediately.

BAKED ZITI

4 servings

2   cups ricotta cheese
2   eggs
4   ounces mozzarella cheese, grated
1/4 cup grated Parmesan cheese
3   cups Meat Sauce (page 276) or Marinara
     Sauce (page 276)
1/2 pound ziti, cooked al dente

1. Combine the ricotta cheese, eggs, mozzarella, and Parmesan cheese in a bowl. Beat with a fork until smooth.

2. Preheat the oven to 350 degrees.

3. Spread a thin layer of the Meat Sauce in the bottom of a 2-quart soufflé dish. Add a layer of cooked ziti. Spread one-third of the ricotta cheese mixture over the ziti. Moisten the layer with about 1/2 cup sauce. Continue making layers in this manner, ending up with a layer of pasta, until all the pasta and cheese are used. Spread a layer of sauce over the top layer of pasta. Cover the soufflé dish tightly with foil.

4. Bake for 30 minutes, or until hot and bubbly. Serve with the remaining sauce.

PASTA WITH CAULIFLOWER-VEAL SAUCE

2 servings

2   tablespoons olive or vegetable oil
1   small white onion, peeled and minced
1/2 cup minced green pepper
1   clove garlic, peeled and minced
1/2 pound ground veal
1   8-ounce can tomato sauce
3/4 cup chicken broth
1 1/2 cups water
     Salt
     Freshly ground black pepper
1   small head cauliflower, broken into small
     flowerets
1/2 pound rotelli or fusilli, cooked al dente

1. Heat the oil in a heavy pot with a cover. Add the onion and green pepper and sauté over low heat for 10 minutes, being careful not to brown the onion. Add the garlic and sauté for 2 minutes longer. Add the ground veal and sauté, stirring constantly and breaking up the veal with a wooden spoon, until the meat loses its raw color (about 10 minutes).

2. Add the tomato sauce, broth, and water to the pot and mix well. Season with salt and pepper to taste. Bring to a boil, lower the heat, and simmer, uncovered, for 15 minutes, stirring occasionally.

3. Add the cauliflower and mix well. Bring back to a boil, lower the heat, and simmer, partially covered for 15 to 20 minutes, or until the cauliflower is just tender. Stir occasionally to prevent the meat and vegetables from sticking to the bottom of the pot.

4. Mix some of the sauce with the hot cooked pasta, and pour the rest equally over each serving.

PASTA WITH STEWED ZUCCHINI

2 servings

1 cup tiny pasta shells
Salt
3 cups Stewed Zucchini (page 298), warmed

1. Cook the pasta in salted water until just tender. Drain well.
2. Return the pasta to the saucepan and add the Stewed Zucchini, stirring to blend well. Serve at once.

CAULIFLOWER WITH PASTA

2 servings

3   cups small cauliflower flowerets
       Salt
1½   cups water
2   tablespoons olive oil
4   large cloves garlic, peeled and minced
1   small white onion, peeled and minced
1½   cups small pasta shells (#22), cooked al
       dente and drained
       Grated Romano or Parmesan cheese

1. Put the cauliflower flowerets in a metal steamer basket. Sprinkle them liberally with salt. Bring 1½ cups of salted water to a boil in a saucepan large enough to hold the steamer basket. When the water is boiling, lower the basket into the pot, cover, and steam for 5 to 7 minutes, or until the cauliflower is just barely tender. Remove the basket from the pot and let the cauliflower cool. Set the steaming liquid aside for use later.
2. Heat the oil in a small frying pan. When the oil is hot, add the garlic and onion. Sauté over very low heat for 10 minutes, stirring occasionally. (The object here is to cook the garlic and onion thoroughly, but not to let them brown at all.) At the end of 10 minutes, add ½ cup of the reserved cauliflower steaming liquid to the frying pan. Simmer, uncovered, for 5 minutes. Add the cauliflower and heat through over low heat.
3. Combine the cauliflower mixture with the hot pasta and mix well. Serve sprinkled with grated cheese.

SPAGHETTI WITH OLIVES AND TOMATOES

2 servings

6   tablespoons olive oil
¼   pound black Greek olives, stoned and
       chopped
1½   tablespoons drained capers, chopped
1   clove garlic, peeled and minced
8   large fresh plum tomatoes, peeled, seeded,
       and diced
½   teaspoon dried basil
1   dried red chili pepper (optional)
       Salt
6   to 8 ounces cooked spaghetti

Combine the oil, olives, capers, garlic, tomatoes, basil, and chili pepper in a heavy saucepan. Cover and marinate at room temperature for 30 minutes. Bring to a boil over medium heat, stirring occasionally. Then simmer over low heat, stirring occasionally, for 15 to 30 minutes, or until the sauce is thick and well blended. Remove from the heat and taste for salt. Toss with the well-drained spaghetti and serve at once.

BAKED STEWED CAULIFLOWER
WITH SHELLS

2 servings

¹/₂ recipe Stewed Cauliflower (page 294)
1 cup pasta shells #22
  Butter or margarine
¹/₄ cup unseasoned bread crumbs
2 tablespoons grated Romano or Parmesan
  cheese

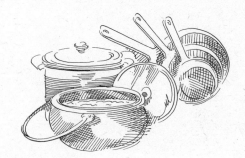

1. Put the cauliflower in a large saucepan and heat it over low heat until it is just bubbling.

2. Meanwhile, cook the pasta shells in boiling salted water until they are just *al dente*. Drain the pasta well, but do not rinse it. Combine the pasta and the heated Stewed Cauliflower.

3. Preheat the oven to 350 degrees. Butter a 1½-quart soufflé dish very well. Transfer the cauliflower and pasta mixture to the soufflé dish. Sprinkle the bread crumbs over the top in an even layer. Then sprinkle on the grated cheese, distributing it evenly. Cover the dish tightly with aluminum foil and bake for 25 to 30 minutes, or until bubbly hot. Serve at once.

RICE AND NOODLES

RICE PILAF

2 servings

2   tablespoons butter or margarine
1   small white onion, peeled and minced
1/2 cup rice
1   cup chicken broth, heated
    Salt and freshly ground black pepper

1. Melt the butter in a small heavy pot with a cover. Add the onion and sauté over low heat for 5 minutes, stirring often. Stir in the rice and move it around with a wooden spoon until the grains are coated with the butter. Add the chicken broth and salt and pepper to taste. (Be careful with the amount of salt you add if the chicken broth is already salted.)

2. Bring to a boil, stir the mixture with a fork, cover, lower the heat, and cook for 15 minutes, or until the liquid has been absorbed and the rice grains are just tender.

3. Let the rice sit, covered, for 5 minutes before serving.

TOMATO-RICE PILAF

2 servings

2   tablespoons butter or margarine
1   small white onion, peeled and minced
1   small garlic clove, peeled and minced
1   8-ounce can stewed tomatoes
    Salt and freshly ground black pepper

3/4 cup chicken broth
1/2 cup rice
2   scallions, chopped

1. Melt the butter in a heavy pot with a lid. Add the onion and garlic and sauté over medium heat for 5 minutes, stirring occasionally.

2. Drain the tomatoes, reserving the liquid. Chop the tomatoes finely, and add to the onion. Sauté for 3 minutes, stirring occasionally. Season with salt and pepper to taste.

3. Add the reserved tomato liquid and chicken broth to the pot and bring to a boil. Stir in the rice, cover, and lower the heat. Steam for 15 to 20 minutes. (After 5 minutes, stir the rice mixture with a *fork* so that the rice doesn't stick. Cover again and continue to cook.) Use a fork to gently add the scallions just before serving.

RICE MILANESE

2 servings

1   cup chicken broth
    Pinch of saffron threads
3   tablespoons butter or margarine
1   small white onion, peeled and minced
1/2 cup rice
    Salt and freshly ground black pepper
3   tablespoons grated Parmesan cheese

1. Put the chicken broth in a small saucepan and add the saffron threads. Heat over low heat until just beginning to simmer.

2. Melt the butter in a small heavy pot with a cover. Add the onion and sauté over low heat for 5 minutes, stirring often. Stir in the rice and move it around with a wooden spoon until the grains are coated with the butter. Add the heated chicken broth and salt and pepper to taste. Bring to a boil, stir the mixture with a fork, cover, lower the heat, and cook for 15 minutes, or until the liquid has been absorbed and the rice is tender.

3. When the rice is cooked, use a fork to gently mix the Parmesan cheese through the rice.

CURRIED RICE

2 servings

2   tablespoons butter or margarine
1   small white onion, peeled and minced
1   small clove garlic, peeled and minced
1/2   cup rice
1 1/2 tablespoons curry powder, or to taste
1/2   teaspoon ground ginger
1/8   teaspoon freshly ground black pepper
1   tablespoon flaked coconut, toasted and
    crushed
1 1/4 cups chicken broth

Melt the butter in a small heavy saucepan. When hot and bubbling, add the onion and garlic. Sauté over low heat for 5 minutes, stirring occasionally. Stir in the rice until it is coated with the butter. Add the curry powder, ginger, pepper, and coconut. Stir to mix well. Pour in the chicken broth and bring to a boil. Stir the mixture with a fork, cover, and lower the heat. Cook for 15 minutes, or until the rice is tender and all of the liquid has been absorbed. Let sit, covered, for a few minutes before serving.

Note: If you stir the rice while it cooks, use a fork. If you use a spoon, the grains will be mashed and stick together.

CINNAMON-ALMOND PILAF

2 servings

2   tablespoons butter or margarine
1/4   cup slivered almonds
1   small white onion, peeled and minced
1/2   cup rice
    Pinch of ground cinnamon
1   cup chicken broth
    Salt and freshly ground black pepper

1. Melt the butter in a small heavy pot with a cover. Add the almonds and sauté, stirring constantly, until they are golden brown. (Be careful that they do not burn or get too brown.) Use a slotted spoon to remove the almonds to a plate. Set them aside until needed.

2. Add the onion to the butter in the pot and sauté over low heat for 5 minutes, stirring occasionally. Do not let the onion brown. Add the rice and move it around with a wooden spoon until the grains are coated with the butter. Stir in the cinnamon and chicken broth. Season with salt and pepper to taste.

3. Bring to a boil and stir the mixture with a fork. Cover the pot, lower the heat, and cook for 15 minutes, or until the broth has been absorbed and the rice is tender.

4. Use a fork to combine the reserved almonds with the rice. Let the rice sit, covered, for 5 minutes before serving.

BROWN RICE

4 servings

2 tablespoons butter or margarine
1 small white onion, peeled and minced
1 cup brown rice
2 cups chicken broth or water
  Salt and freshly ground black pepper
1 4-ounce can mushroom stems and pieces,
  drained

1. Melt the butter in a heavy saucepan. When the butter is completely melted, add the onion and sauté over low heat, stirring occasionally, for 10 minutes. Do not let the onion brown. Add the rice and sauté for 1 minute, stirring constantly. Pour in the chicken broth and bring to a boil over medium heat, stirring once or twice. When the mixture is boiling, cover the pan, lower the heat and cook for 30 minutes. Stir with a fork *only* after 15 minutes.

2. At the end of 30 minutes, stir the rice with a fork again, and taste for doneness. (If it is still crunchy, cook, covered, over very low heat for an additional 10 minutes.) Stir in the drained mushroom stems and pieces with a fork when the rice is done. Cover the pan, and let sit for 5 minutes before serving.

THREE-CHEESE BAKED MACARONI

4 main-dish servings
or 6 side-dish servings

3 tablespoons butter or margarine
3 tablespoons all-purpose flour
1½ cups milk
¼ pound sharp Cheddar cheese, cut into tiny
  pieces
¼ pound Swiss cheese, cut into tiny pieces
  Salt and freshly ground black pepper
1 cup elbow macaroni, cooked al dente (about
  7 minutes) in boiling salted water and
  drained well
1 cup cream-style cottage cheese
  Paprika

1. Melt the butter in a small heavy saucepan over low heat. When the butter is completely melted and just beginning to sizzle, add the flour all at once, stirring it into the butter with a wooden spoon. Cook the mixture over very low heat for 2 minutes, stirring constantly with a wooden spoon. Remove the *roux* from the heat and let it cool for 5 minutes.

2. When the *roux* has cooled for 5 minutes, gradually stir in the milk with a wooden spoon, stirring the mixture constantly until it is smooth. Return the pan to low heat, and cook, stirring constantly, until the mixture begins to thicken. (This may take as long as 15 minutes, but do not be tempted to raise the heat just to cut down on the time.) When the cream sauce has begun to thicken add all the cheese pieces and stir constantly until the Cheddar has melted completely. Remove from the heat and taste for seasonings, adding salt and pepper, if necessary.

3. Combine the drained macaroni with the cottage cheese. Pour in the warm cheese sauce and mix well. Taste the mixture for seasonings, adding salt and pepper, if necessary.

4. Preheat the oven to 350 degrees. Butter a 1-quart soufflé dish very well. Pour the macaroni-cheese sauce mixture into the prepared dish. Sprinkle paprika lightly over the top and bake for 20 to 25 minutes, or until piping hot.

SALMON AND NOODLE BAKE

4 servings

4   tablespoons butter or margarine
4   tablespoons all-purpose flour
2½   cups milk
¼   pound Swiss cheese, cut into tiny pieces
1   7¾-ounce can salmon, drained, skin and
     bones removed, and flaked
     Salt and freshly ground black pepper
½   pound broad egg noodles, cooked for 5
     minutes in boiling salted water and drained
     well

1. Melt the butter in a small heavy saucepan over low heat. When the butter is completely melted and just beginning to sizzle, add the flour all at once, stirring it into the butter with a wooden spoon. Cook the mixture over very low heat for 2 minutes, stirring constantly with a wooden spoon. Remove the *roux* from the heat and let it cool for 5 minutes.

2. When the *roux* has cooled for 5 minutes, gradually stir in the milk with a wooden spoon, stirring the mixture constantly until it is smooth. Return the pan to low heat, and cook, stirring constantly, until the mixture begins to thicken. (This may take as long as 15 minutes, but do not be tempted to raise the heat just to cut down on the time.) When the cream sauce has begun to thicken add all the cheese and stir constantly for 5 minutes. Add the flaked salmon and mix it in well. Remove the sauce from the heat and taste for seasonings, adding salt and pepper, if necessary.

3. Preheat the oven to 350 degrees. Butter a 1-quart soufflé dish very well.

4. Combine the drained noodles with the salmon-cream sauce and mix well. Taste for seasonings, adding salt and pepper, if necessary. Pour the mixture into the prepared dish and cover tightly with aluminum foil. Bake for 20 minutes.

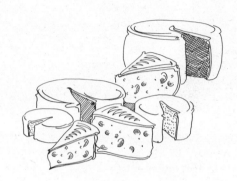

VEGETABLES AND LEGUMES

EGGPLANT PARMIGIANA

4 servings

1   1-pound eggplant
2   eggs
2   cups seasoned bread crumbs
    Vegetable oil for frying
2   cups Meat Sauce (page 276) or Marinara
    Sauce (page 276)
4   ounces mozzarella cheese, grated
¼   cup grated Parmesan cheese

1. Trim the eggplant, but do not peel it. Slice it into ¼-inch-thick round slices.

2. Beat the eggs in a flat soup plate or pie plate.

3. Spread the bread crumbs in a layer on a sheet of wax paper.

4. Dip each eggplant slice first into the beaten eggs, and then into the bread crumbs, coating well on all sides. Press the crumbs on with the palm of your hand. As the eggplant slices are coated lay them on a flat plate so that they do not touch. Separate the layers with wax paper. Refrigerate the coated eggplant for 10 minutes.

5. Pour ¼ inch oil into a large frying pan. When hot, add the eggplant slices in a single layer. Sauté over medium heat until golden brown on both sides, turning once. Drain the browned eggplant on paper towels.

6. Preheat the oven to 350 degrees.

7. Spread ¾ cup of the Meat Sauce in the bottom of a square baking dish. Put a layer of eggplant slices over the sauce. Sprinkle each piece of eggplant with some of each of the cheeses. Pour 2 tablespoons of sauce over the cheese. Continue making layers in this manner until all of the ingredients are used. Bake for 20 minutes, or until the cheese has melted and the dish is piping hot.

EGGPLANT ROLLUPS

4 servings

1   1-pound eggplant
3   eggs
    Seasoned bread crumbs
1   cup ricotta cheese
2   ounces mozzarella cheese, grated
2   tablespoons Parmesan or Romano cheese
3   cups Marinara Sauce (page 276)

1. Preheat the oven to 375 degrees.

2. Peel the eggplant and cut it lengthwise into 8 thin slices.

3. Beat 2 of the eggs in a flat soup plate or pie plate. Spread the bread crumbs on a large piece of wax paper.

4. Dip each eggplant slice first in the beaten eggs and then coat them with the bread crumbs, pressing the crumbs on with the palm of your hand. As each slice is coated, lay it on an ungreased baking sheet. Bake the eggplant slices for 25 minutes. Let cool to room temperature. Do not turn off the oven.

5. Mix together the ricotta, mozzarella, Parmesan, with the remaining egg. Beat to combine well.

6. Put an equal portion of the cheese mixture on each slice of eggplant, spreading it almost to the edges of each slice.

7. Spread 6 tablespoons of Marinara Sauce in the bottom of each of 2 aluminum baking pans. Roll the eggplant slices up and put them seam side down in the baking pans, 4 rolls to each pan. Spoon the remaining Marinara Sauce equally over the eggplant rolls.

8. Lower the oven temperature to 350 degrees and bake the rolls for 25 to 30 minutes.

Note: The servings are very filling, so if you serve this dish with linguini or another pasta, don't overdo it.

ZUCCHINI LASAGNE

4 servings

1   *pound zucchini*
3   *eggs*
     Seasoned bread crumbs for coating
     Vegetable oil
1   *cup ricotta cheese*
4   *ounces mozzarella cheese, shredded*
¼   *cup grated Romano or Parmesan cheese*
     Salt and freshly ground black pepper
½   *recipe for Marinara Sauce (page 276)*

1. Trim the zucchini and wash them well. Cut each zucchini into 1½-inch lengths. Then cut each length into julienne strips.

2. Beat 2 of the eggs in a large flat soup plate or pie plate. Add the julienned zucchini and toss with two forks to coat the zucchini with the beaten eggs.

3. Spread the bread crumbs out on a sheet of wax paper. Spread vegetable oil liberally over the bottom and sides of a jelly roll pan. Preheat the oven to 400 degrees.

4. Use two forks to scoop up portions of the egg-coated zucchini and transfer them to the bread crumbs. Toss the zucchini with the bread crumbs until they are lightly coated. Then lay the coated zucchini in a single layer in the bottom of the jelly roll pan. Continue coating the zucchini and laying them in the jelly roll pan until all are used.

5. Place the jelly roll pan on the middle rack of the oven and bake for 15 minutes. Use a spatula to turn the zucchini over. Bake for 10 minutes longer and remove from the oven. Do not turn the oven off.

6. Combine the ricotta, shredded mozzarella, and the remaining egg in a small mixing bowl. Mix with a fork until the egg is completely incorporated. Beat in the grated cheese and salt and pepper to taste.

7. Spread ½ cup of Marinara Sauce in the bottom of a 2-quart soufflé dish. Layer half the breaded zucchini over the sauce. Spread half the ricotta mixture over the zucchini. Dribble ¼ cup of the Marinara Sauce over the ricotta mixture. Make another layer of the remaining zucchini and top it with the remaining ricotta mixture. Pour ¾ cup of Marinara Sauce over the top of the ricotta mixture, spreading it out evenly. Cover the dish tightly with aluminum foil and bake for 30 to 40 minutes, or until the cheese is bubbly. Let stand, covered, for 10 minutes before serving with the remaining sauce.

RATATOUILLE WITH POACHED EGGS

2 servings

1 recipe for Ratatouille (page 294)
4 large eggs
2 tablespoons grated Parmesan cheese

1. Put the Ratatouille in a large nonstick frying pan. Heat over low heat until it just begins to simmer.

2. Use a wooden spoon to make four depressions in the vegetable mixture. Break an egg into each of the depressions. Cover the frying pan tightly and cook over very low heat for 3 to 5 minutes, or until the eggs are done to your preference.

3. Sprinkle the grated cheese equally over the four eggs. Use a spatula to transfer the eggs and vegetable mixture to two serving plates.

EGGPLANT PATTIES

2 servings

1   1-pound eggplant
1½ teaspoons salt
1   egg
1   small clove garlic, peeled and minced fine
2   scallions, trimmed and minced fine
⅛   teaspoon dried basil
1   tablespoon minced parsley
⅛   teaspoon freshly ground black pepper
     Pinch of ground nutmeg
1   tablespoon grated Romano or Parmesan cheese
½   to ¾ cup seasoned bread crumbs
     Unseasoned bread crumbs for coating

3   tablespoons butter or margarine
3   tablespoons vegetable oil

1. Peel the eggplant and cut it into ½-inch cubes. Put the eggplant into a large saucepan and add enough cold water to cover the eggplant by ½ inch. Bring to a boil over medium heat, stirring occasionally. When the water is boiling, add the salt, lower the heat, and cook, uncovered, for 10 minutes, stirring occasionally. Drain the eggplant in a sieve and cool in the sieve for 15 minutes.

2. Transfer the cooled eggplant to a food mill placed over a mixing bowl. Purée the eggplant until only the seeds are left in the food mill.

3. Add the egg, garlic, scallions, basil, parsley, pepper, nutmeg, and grated cheese to the eggplant purée and mix well with a wooden spoon. Mix in enough seasoned bread crumbs so that the mixture holds together when you form the patties.

4. Make a layer of unseasoned bread crumbs on a sheet of wax paper. Divide the eggplant mixture into eight equal portions. Form each portion into a thin pattie and coat it on all sides with the unseasoned bread crumbs. Lay each of the coated patties on a flat dinner plate, making sure that they do not touch. Separate the layers of patties with wax paper. Refrigerate the patties for 10 minutes.

5. Heat the butter and oil together in a 10-inch nonstick frying pan. When the butter is completely melted, add the eggplant patties in a single layer, making sure that they do not touch. Fry over medium heat until golden brown on both sides, turning them carefully with a spatula and fork. Drain the browned patties on paper towels and serve immediately.

BEAN SPROUT FRITTERS

2 servings

2   eggs
¾   cup cold water
½   teaspoon baking powder
1   teaspoon salt
⅛   teaspoon cayenne
½   teaspoon ground coriander
1   tablespoon soy sauce
½   teaspoon mustard powder
1   cup all-purpose flour
½   pound fresh bean sprouts
2   scallions, trimmed and cut into 1-inch shreds
1   carrot, scraped and cut into 1-inch shreds
1   medium-sized green pepper, seeded and cut into 1-inch shreds
1   celery stalk, sliced paper thin
1   large clove garlic, peeled
    Vegetable or peanut oil for frying

1. Beat the eggs with the water in a mixing bowl until frothy. Then add the baking powder, salt, cayenne, coriander, soy sauce, mustard powder, and flour. Mix well until a soft paste forms. Let stand for 10 minutes.

2. Add the bean sprouts, scallions, carrot shreds, green pepper shreds, and celery slices to the dough. Mix the vegetables into the dough with a fork.

3. Put the garlic and ¼ inch of oil in a large frying pan. Heat over medium heat until the garlic is golden brown on all sides. Remove and discard the garlic.

4. Use a large metal spoon to scoop up 6 portions of the fritter mixture and ease them into the hot oil in the frying pan. (Do not crowd the portions together.) Cook the fritters until golden on one side, then turn and cook until golden on the other side. Drain on paper towels and serve at once.

GANDULES WITH RICE

4 servings

1   8-ounce can stewed tomatoes
2   tablespoons olive or vegetable oil
1   medium-sized onion, peeled and chopped
1   medium-sized green pepper, seeded and chopped
1   cup rice
    Pinch of dried oregano
1   teaspoon salt
⅛   teaspoon freshly ground black pepper
1¾ cups water
1   16-ounce can pigeon peas, drained
½   cup shredded Monterey Jack cheese (with or without jalapeño peppers)

1. Drain the stewed tomatoes well, reserving the liquid. Chop the drained tomatoes and set aside until needed.

2. Heat the oil in a heavy saucepan. When the oil is hot, add the onion and green pepper and sauté over low heat for 5 minutes, stirring occasionally. Add the tomatoes and sauté for 5 minutes longer, stirring occasionally.

3. Stir the rice, oregano, salt, and pepper into the vegetable mixture in the saucepan. Add the reserved tomato liquid and the water. Stir to mix well and bring to a boil. Cover the pan, lower the heat, and simmer for 5 minutes. Stir the rice mixture with a fork, cover again, and cook for 10 minutes longer. (At this time most of the liquid will have been absorbed.)

4. Use a fork to gently mix the drained pigeon peas through the cooked rice. Sprinkle the

shredded cheese over the top of the rice mixture. Cover the pan again and remove from the heat. Let stand, covered, for 5 minutes before serving.

Note: I like to use the cheese with the jalapeño peppers. But the plain cheese will do just as well.

CHILI BEANS AND TOFU

4 servings

3½ tablespoons vegetable oil
1   pound yellow onions, peeled and chopped
3   large cloves garlic, peeled and minced
¼   teaspoon ground cumin
1   to 2 teaspoons chili powder
1   to 1½ teaspoons cayenne pepper
¼   teaspoon crushed red pepper
½   teaspoon dried oregano
1   1-pound can stewed tomatoes with liquid
1   8-ounce can tomato sauce
1½   cups water
1½   teaspoons salt
¼   teaspoon freshly ground black pepper
2   1-pound cans pinto beans with liquid
½   pound firm tofu (bean curd), cut into ¼-inch dice

1. Heat 2 tablespoons of the oil in a large Dutch oven. When the oil is hot, add the onions and garlic and sauté over very low heat for 10 minutes, stirring occasionally. Do not let the onions or garlic brown. Then add the cumin, chili powder, cayenne pepper, red pepper, and oregano. Stir to mix well and sauté for 5 minutes, stirring occasionally.

2. Drain the tomatoes and reserve the liquid. Cut the tomatoes into small pieces. Add them with the liquid, tomato sauce, and water to the onion and spice mixture. Season with the salt and pepper and bring to a boil. Cover the pan, lower the heat, and simmer for 20 minutes, stirring occasionally.

3. Add the pinto beans and their liquid to the pan. Mix well and taste for seasonings, adding more salt and pepper, if necessary. Cover the pan and cook over low heat for 15 minutes, stirring occasionally.

4. Meanwhile, heat the remaining 1½ tablespoons of oil in a medium-sized frying pan. When the oil is hot, add the diced tofu and sauté over medium heat, tossing and turning, until the tofu cubes are brown on all sides. Drain the tofu carefully and add to the bean mixture after it has cooked for 15 minutes. Mix well and cook for 15 minutes longer, stirring occasionally.

TWICE-COOKED TOFU AND VEGETABLES

2 servings

6   dried Chinese mushrooms, stems removed
1   large stalk broccoli
1   tablespoon minced fresh gingerroot
2   large cloves garlic, peeled and minced
3   tablespoons vegetable or peanut oil
4   dried red chili peppers (optional)
½   pound tofu, cut into ½-inch cubes
2   medium-sized carrots, scraped and cut into julienne strips
2   cups shredded green or Chinese cabbage
⅓   cup hot water
1   cup bean sprouts
2   scallions, trimmed and chopped
2   tablespoons soy sauce

1. Put the mushrooms into a small bowl and cover them with boiling water. Let sit for 20 minutes. Drain well and squeeze out any excess water. Cut the mushrooms into thin shreds and set aside until needed.

2. Cut off about 1 inch from the bottom of the broccoli stalk. Peel the stalk right up to the flowerets. Cut the stalk into ¼-inch-thick slices. Separate the flowerets into small flowerets. Put the flowerets and the slices of the broccoli stalk into a bowl and cover them with boiling water. Let sit for 10 minutes. Drain well and set aside until needed.

3. Put half the ginger and half the garlic in a wok or heavy frying pan with 2 tablespoons of the oil and 2 of the chili peppers. Heat over medium heat until the ginger and garlic begin to sizzle and the oil is very hot. Add the tofu cubes and cook, tossing and turning, until they are lightly browned. Use a slotted spoon to remove the tofu to a plate. Set aside until needed.

4. Add the remaining ginger, garlic, oil, and chili peppers to the wok. Heat until the ginger and garlic begin to sizzle. Add the broccoli, carrots, and cabbage to the wok and cook for 2 minutes, stirring constantly. Add the hot water, cover the wok, and steam over medium heat for 3 minutes.

5. Uncover the wok and stir the bean sprouts, scallions, mushrooms, and soy sauce into the vegetable mixture. Gently add the tofu cubes, mixing them in lightly so they don't break up. Cover the wok and cook over low heat for 2 minutes. Serve immediately.

SAUTÉED ASPARAGUS

2 servings

6 *asparagus spears*
1 *tablespoon vegetable or peanut oil*
¼ *teaspoon minced garlic*
¼ *teaspoon minced gingerroot*
2 *tablespoons water*

1. Break the woody ends off the asparagus spears. Wash the spears under cool running water. Drain. Slice the spears on the diagonal into 1-inch lengths.

2. Heat the oil in a wok or heavy frying pan. Stir in the garlic and gingerroot. Add the asparagus and stir-fry for 2 minutes, moving the asparagus constantly. Add the water to the wok and cover. Lower the heat and steam for 2 minutes, or until the asparagus are just tender. Serve immediately.

STEAMED BROCCOLI

2 servings

1 *small bunch broccoli*
   Salt
   Lemon wedges

1. Wash the broccoli in cool running water. Cut off about 1 inch from the bottom of the broccoli stalks. Peel the stalks right up to the base of the flowerets. Cut the stalks (and flowerets) in half if they are too thick.

2. Lay the broccoli in a steamer basket and sprinkle it lightly with salt. Steam in a covered pot, over boiling water, for 5 to 7 minutes, or until a fork pierces the stalk easily. (Do not overcook: The broccoli should be bright green and just *al dente*.) Serve with the lemon wedges.

ASPARAGUS WITH BUTTER AND CHEESE

2 servings

8 ½-inch-thick asparagus spears
  Salt
2 tablespoons butter or margarine
2 tablespoons grated Parmesan or Romano
  cheese
  Freshly ground black pepper

1. Break the woody ends off the asparagus spears. Put the asparagus spears in a bowl of cold water and let soak for 15 minutes. Lift from the water and let drain.
2. Put the drained asparagus spears in a steamer basket. Sprinkle them lightly with salt. Steam in a covered pot, over boiling salted water, for 5 to 7 minutes, or until a fork just pierces the asparagus stems. (The asparagus should be bright green and *al dente,* not gray-green and limp.) Remove the steamer basket from the pot as soon as the asparagus are cooked.
3. Melt the butter in a nonstick frying pan large enough to hold the asparagus in a single layer. When the butter is melted, slide the asparagus from the steamer basket into the frying pan. Shake the frying pan so that the asparagus roll around and get coated with the butter. Transfer to 2 dinner plates and sprinkle each portion with 1 tablespoon of grated cheese. Add some freshly ground black pepper and serve at once.

STEAMED CABBAGE

2 servings

½ pound cabbage, cut into thick slices
  Salt and freshly ground black pepper
  Butter or margarine

Put the sliced cabbage in a steamer basket. Sprinkle the cabbage lightly with salt. Steam the cabbage in a covered pot over boiling water, for about 10 minutes, or until very tender. Season with more salt, if necessary, and pepper, and toss with a little butter to moisten it.

Note: A delicious variation of this recipe is Steamed Cabbage and Potatoes. Peel 2 medium-sized potatoes and cut them into ¼-inch-thick slices. Put the potato slices in the bottom of the steamer basket and sprinkle them lightly with salt. Then proceed with the cabbage.

STEWED CABBAGE

2 servings

2 tablespoons butter or margarine
1 small white onion, peeled and minced
1 clove garlic, peeled and minced
2 cups finely shredded cabbage
2 small ripe tomatoes, cored, peeled, seeded, and
  diced
  Salt and freshly ground black pepper
  Pinch of celery seeds

1. Melt the butter in a heavy saucepan or frying pan. When it is hot and bubbling, add the onion and garlic. Sauté over low heat for 5 minutes stirring occasionally. Add the cabbage and sauté, stirring occasionally, for 5 minutes longer. Cover

the saucepan and let the vegetables steam over low heat for 5 minutes.

2. Add the diced tomatoes to the cabbage mixture and stir well. Season the vegetables with salt and pepper to taste and the celery seeds. Cover the saucepan and cook over low heat for 5 to 10 minutes, stirring occasionally, or until the cabbage is tender.

RED CABBAGE

6 servings

3   tablespoons butter or margarine
1   large yellow onion, peeled and minced
1   1½-pound red cabbage, cored and sliced
     thin
1   red Delicious apple, peeled, cored, and
     coarsely chopped
1½   teaspoons salt
⅛   teaspoon caraway seeds
⅛   teaspoon ground cloves
⅛   teaspoon celery seeds
3   tablespoons cider vinegar
2   cups boiling water

1. Melt the butter in a heavy frying pan or large heavy saucepan. When the butter is completely melted, add the onion and sauté over low heat for 10 minutes, stirring occasionally. Add the cabbage, apple, salt, caraway seeds, ground cloves, celery seeds, and cider vinegar and toss to mix well.

2. Pour the boiling water over the cabbage mixture and bring to a boil. When the mixture is boiling, stir to mix well, cover the pan, lower the heat, and cook for 30 minutes, stirring occasionally. At the end of 30 minutes, cover the pan partially and simmer the cabbage mixture for

20 minutes longer, stirring occasionally. At this point, the cabbage should be tender. Taste for seasonings, and add more salt and pepper, if necessary.

GLAZED CARROTS

2 servings

3   medium-sized carrots, scraped and cut into
     ½-inch thick slices
1   tablespoon butter or margarine
⅓   cup water
     Salt and freshly ground black pepper
1   tablespoon dark brown sugar

1. Put the carrots, butter, and water into a small heavy saucepan. Sprinkle lightly with salt and pepper. Bring to a boil, cover the pan, and cook over medium-high heat for 3 minutes. Uncover the pot and raise the heat. Boil until almost all of the liquid has evaporated.

2. Sprinkle the brown sugar over the carrots and cook over low heat, shaking the pan until the carrots are nicely glazed.

BAKED CAULIFLOWER BEIGNETS

2 servings

6 large cauliflower flowerets
1 egg
  Seasoned bread crumbs
1 tablespoon grated Parmesan cheese
  Salt and freshly ground black pepper

1. Put the flowerets in a steamer basket and steam in a covered pot, over boiling water, for 3

minutes. Remove from the pot immediately and let cool.

2. Preheat the oven to 350 degrees.

3. Beat the egg in a deep bowl. Add the cooled cauliflower flowerets and toss to coat them well with the egg.

4. Combine the bread crumbs with the grated cheese and salt and pepper to taste. Spread the bread crumb mixture on a sheet of wax paper.

5. Dip the egg-coated flowerets into the bread crumb mixture and coat completely. Put the coated flowerets in a buttered baking dish and bake for 10 minutes, or until they are just tender.

STEWED CAULIFLOWER

4 servings

2   tablespoons olive or vegetable oil
1   large yellow onion, peeled and minced
2   cloves garlic, peeled and minced
1   1-pound can crushed tomatoes
1   8-ounce can tomato sauce
3/4 cup water
1/2 teaspoon dried basil, or 5 large fresh basil leaves, minced
1   teaspoon salt
1/8 teaspoon freshly ground black pepper
1   teaspoon drained capers, chopped
1   1-pound head cauliflower, broken into small flowerets

1. Heat the oil in a large heavy frying pan or Dutch oven. When the oil is hot, add the onion and garlic and sauté over low heat for 10 minutes, stirring occasionally. Do not let the onion or garlic brown.

2. Add the crushed tomatoes, tomato sauce, water, basil, salt, pepper, and capers to the pan.

Stir to mix well. Bring to a boil over medium heat, cover the pan, lower the heat, and simmer, stirring occasionally, for 20 minutes.

3. Add the cauliflower to the sauce and bring the sauce back to a boil. When the sauce is boiling, cover the pan, lower the heat, and simmer, stirring occasionally, for 10 to 12 minutes, or until the cauliflower is just fork-tender. Serve immediately.

RATATOUILLE

4 servings

1   1-pound eggplant
1   pound small zucchini
1   pound fresh tomatoes
4   tablespoons olive or vegetable oil, or 2 tablespoons of each
1   large yellow onion, peeled and minced
1   large clove garlic, peeled and minced
1   small green pepper, seeded and minced
3/4 teaspoon salt
1/8 teaspoon freshly ground black pepper
1/4 teaspoon dried oregano

1. Peel the eggplant and cut it into 1/2-inch cubes. Set aside until needed.

2. Trim the zucchini top and bottom and wash them well. Cut each zucchini into quarters lengthwise. Then cut each quarter into 1/8-inch-thick slices. Set aside until needed.

3. Peel and seed the tomatoes and cut them into small cubes. Set aside until needed.

4. Heat the oil in a large frying pan. When the oil is hot add the onion, garlic, and green pepper. Sauté over low heat for 5 minutes, stirring occasionally. Then add the reserved eggplant, zucchini, and tomatoes. Stir well and sprinkle

on the salt, pepper, and oregano. Stir again to mix in the spices. Cover the frying pan and cook over low heat, stirring occasionally, for 35 to 40 minutes, or until the eggplant and zucchini are tender. Taste for seasonings, and add more salt and pepper, if necessary.

Note: This dish is very good cold, at room temperature, or hot.

SAUTÉED MUSHROOMS

2 servings

½ pound mushroom caps with stems
2 tablespoons butter or margarine
1 small clove garlic, peeled and minced
Salt and freshly ground black pepper

1. Wash the mushrooms in cool water, rubbing them gently to remove any dirt. Drain briefly.

2. Slice the mushroom stems into ¼-inch-thick pieces, right down to the cap. Then slice the caps into ¼-inch-thick slices.

3. Melt the butter in a frying pan large enough to hold the sliced mushrooms. When it is hot and bubbling, add the minced garlic. Sauté the garlic over low heat for 1 minute and add all the sliced mushrooms. Sauté over medium-high heat until the mushrooms give off their liquid. (This may take a little time, so don't worry.) Stir the mushrooms occasionally while they are cooking. Cook and stir until the mushroom liquid evaporates and the mushrooms begin to turn golden brown. Season them with salt and pepper to taste and serve immediately.

STUFFED MUSHROOMS

2 servings

6 large mushroom caps (stems removed)
3 tablespoons seasoned bread crumbs
1 tablespoon grated Parmesan cheese
⅛ teaspoon finely minced garlic
1 teaspoon grated onion
Salt and freshly ground black pepper
Pinch of ground nutmeg
Vegetable or olive oil

1. Preheat the oven to 350 degrees.

2. Wipe the mushroom caps with a damp paper towel to remove any surface dirt.

3. Combine the bread crumbs, Parmesan cheese, garlic, onion, salt and pepper to taste, and the nutmeg in a small bowl. Stir to mix well. Add just enough oil to moisten the mixture so that it will hold together when pressed into a spoon. Divide the bread crumb mixture evenly among the mushroom caps, smoothing the stuffing into a dome shape on top.

4. Coat the inside of a small baking pan with oil and put the stuffed mushrooms into the pan. Bake for 15 minutes, or until the mushrooms are tender. Serve immediately.

SAUTÉED PEPPERS AND POTATOES

2 servings

1 large potato
2 large green peppers
1 medium-sized yellow onion
3 tablespoons vegetable oil
Salt and freshly ground black pepper

1. Peel the potato and cut it into quarters. Slice each quarter into ⅛-inch-thick slices. Dry the slices on paper towels.

2. Cut the green peppers in half and seed them. Cut the peppers into ½-inch pieces.

3. Peel the onion and cut it in half. Slice each half into very thin slices.

4. Heat the oil in a nonstick frying pan. Add the potato slices and cook until they are browned on both sides. Shake the frying pan occasionally so that the potatoes do not stick. When the potatoes are browned, use a slotted spoon to remove them to a plate.

5. Add the peppers to the frying pan and cook over high heat for 1 minute. Add the onion slices to the peppers and stir and cook for 1 minute longer. Return the potato slices to the frying pan and season the vegetables with salt and pepper. Toss the vegetables to distribute the spices and serve immediately.

BOILED POTATOES WITH OIL AND PARSLEY

2 servings

4 small red potatoes, scrubbed
  Salt
3 tablespoons olive oil
  Freshly ground black pepper
4 tablespoons finely minced parsley

1. Put the potatoes in a saucepan and cover them with water. Season with a little salt. Bring to a boil, lower the heat, cover the pan, and simmer the potatoes for 8 to 10 minutes, or until they are just tender. Drain immediately.

2. To serve, split the potatoes in half and drizzle the olive oil over them. Season with salt and

lots of pepper. Toss to coat the potatoes well. Sprinkle on the parsley and serve warm.

BOILED POTATOES WITH SOUR CREAM AND CHIVES

2 servings

2 medium-sized potatoes, peeled and quartered
  Salt
2 tablespoons butter or margarine
  Freshly ground black pepper
2 tablespoons sour cream
1 tablespoon fresh or freeze-dried snipped chives

1. Put the potatoes in a saucepan and add water just to cover and salt to taste. Bring to a boil, cover, lower the heat, and boil for 12 to 15 minutes, or until the potatoes are tender but still firm.

2. Drain the potatoes well and put them in a serving bowl. Toss with the butter and salt and pepper to taste. Add the sour cream and chives and toss again until the potatoes are coated completely.

SCALLOPED POTATOES

2 servings

3 medium-sized baking potatoes, peeled
1 small white onion, peeled
  Butter or margarine
  Salt and freshly ground black pepper
  Flour
1½ cups milk, approximately

1. Preheat the oven to 350 degrees.

2. Cut the potatoes into ⅛-inch-thick slices and set aside.

3. Cut the onion in half and slice each half thinly. Set aside.

4. Butter a 1-quart soufflé dish liberally. Put a layer of sliced potatoes in the bottom of the dish, using any small potato pieces to fill in gaps. Sprinkle about one-third of the onion slices over the potatoes. Sprinkle the potatoes and onions liberally with salt and pepper and dot with small pieces of butter. Sprinkle the layer with about 1 teaspoon of flour. Make 2 more layers in this same manner, reserving enough potato slices to make a plain layer on top. Sprinkle the top layer with salt and pepper only and dot it with butter.

5. Heat the milk until small bubbles appear around the edges of the pan. Pour the hot milk over the potatoes to just cover them. Bake for about 1¾ hours, or until the potatoes are tender and the top is golden brown.

STEAMED SPINACH

2 servings

1 *pound fresh spinach*
2 *tablespoons butter or margarine*
1 *small white onion, peeled and minced*
1 *small clove garlic, peeled and minced*
  Salt and freshly ground black pepper

1. Pick the spinach over to remove the stems and any bruised leaves. Wash the unblemished leaves carefully under cold running water to remove the sand. Drain well.

2. Melt the butter in a frying pan large enough to hold the spinach. When it is hot and bubbling, add the onion and garlic. Sauté over low heat for 5 minutes, stirring constantly. Do not let the onion or garlic brown. Add the spinach with just the water clinging to its leaves. Cover the pan

and cook over medium-high heat, stirring once or twice, until the spinach is just wilted. Season with salt and pepper to taste. Drain well before serving, pressing out excess liquid with the back of a wooden spoon.

VICTORIAN SPINACH

2 servings

1 *10-ounce package fresh spinach*
  Salt
3 *tablespoons butter or margarine*
1 *small white onion, peeled and minced*
2 *tablespoons all-purpose flour*
½ *cup milk*
½ *cup shredded sharp Cheddar cheese*

1. Pick over the spinach, removing the stems and any bruised leaves. Wash the spinach very well in cool water to remove any grit. Put the spinach into a heavy saucepan or frying pan with just the water clinging to the leaves. Sprinkle lightly with salt. Cover the pan and cook the spinach over medium-high heat until it is just wilted. Drain in a sieve and press with a wooden spoon to remove any excess water.

2. Melt the butter in a frying pan. When it is hot and bubbling, add the onion. Sauté over low heat for 5 minutes, stirring occasionally. Sprinkle the flour over the onion and cook, stirring, for 1 minute. Remove the pan from the heat and let the mixture cool a little. Gradually stir in the milk, stirring constantly, until the mixture is creamy. Return to a low flame and cook, stirring, for 2 minutes. Add the Cheddar cheese and stir until it melts and is incorporated into the sauce. Add the drained spinach to the sauce and mix well. Cook until the spinach is piping hot. Serve immediately.

SAUTÉED STRING BEANS

2 servings

¾ pound fresh string beans, ends removed
    Salt
2 tablespoons butter or margarine
    Freshly ground black pepper

1. Wash the string beans in cool running water and drain them well.

2. Put the drained beans in a steamer basket and sprinkle them lightly with salt. Steam the beans in a covered pot, over boiling water, for 5 to 7 minutes, or until they are just tender. Remove the beans immediately and run cold water over them to stop the cooking process. Drain very well.

3. Melt the butter in a large frying pan. When it is hot and bubbling, add the drained beans and sauté them quickly over medium-high heat until they are heated through and glazed with the butter. Sprinkle lightly with salt and liberally with pepper. Serve at once.

STEWED ZUCCHINI

4 servings

2   tablespoons olive oil
1   large medium-sized onion, peeled and
       minced
1   clove garlic, peeled and minced
1   8-ounce can tomato sauce
1¼ cups water
1   medium-sized potato, peeled and diced
1   pound zucchini, trimmed, scraped, and cut
       into ½-inch cubes
1   teaspoon salt

¼   teaspoon freshly ground black pepper
½   heaping teaspoon dried basil, crumbled

1. Heat the oil in a large saucepan. When it is hot, add the onion and garlic and sauté over low heat for 5 minutes, stirring occasionally.

2. Add the tomato sauce and water and bring to a boil. Add the potato, zucchini, salt, pepper, and basil and bring to a boil. Cover and simmer for 15 to 20 minutes, or until the vegetables are just tender.

SAUTÉED ZUCCHINI

2 servings

2 medium-sized zucchini
2 tablespoons butter or margarine
1 large clove garlic, peeled and crushed
    Salt and freshly ground black pepper
½ teaspoon dried basil or dried oregano

1. Wash the zucchini very well in cool running water. Trim both ends and cut the zucchini into 1½-inch lengths. Cut each length into ¼-inch thick slices, lengthwise. Then cut each slice, lengthwise, into ¼-inch sticks.

2. Melt the butter in a medium-sized nonstick frying pan over medium heat. When the butter is partially melted, add the garlic and turn it in the melting butter until it is golden brown on all sides and the butter is sizzling. Remove and discard the garlic. Add the zucchini to the frying pan and sauté, tossing and stirring, for 3 to 4 minutes, or until just tender. Sprinkle generously with the salt and pepper and the basil, and toss again to distribute the seasonings. Serve at once.

LIMA BEANS WITH BLUE CHEESE

2 servings

Butter or margarine
1 10-ounce package frozen lima beans, cooked
according to package directions and drained
Salt and freshly ground black pepper
2 ounces blue cheese, crumbled
2 tablespoons unseasoned bread crumbs

1. Preheat the oven to 300 degrees.
2. Butter a small casserole generously. Make layers of the drained lima beans in the casserole, sprinkling each layer with salt, pepper, and blue cheese. Sprinkle the bread crumbs on top of the casserole and dot the bread crumbs with butter. Bake for 15 minutes, or until warmed through.

BENGAL BEANS

2 servings

1   *medium-sized onion*
1   *8-ounce can stewed tomatoes*
2   *tablespoons vegetable oil*
1   *clove garlic, peeled and minced*
¼   *teaspoon ground coriander*
⅛   *teaspoon ground cumin*
⅛   *teaspoon ground ginger*
⅛   *teaspoon chili powder*
½   *teaspoon salt*
⅛   *teaspoon freshly ground black pepper*
1   *10½-ounce can chick-peas, drained*

1. Peel the onion and slice it in half lengthwise. Slice each half into thin slices and set aside until needed.
2. Drain the stewed tomatoes, reserving the liquid. Chop the tomatoes coarsely. Set the chopped tomatoes and liquid aside separately.
3. Heat the oil in a medium-sized frying pan. When the oil is hot, add the garlic and sliced onion. Sauté over medium heat for 10 minutes, stirring occasionally. Do not let the garlic brown. Add the drained chopped tomatoes, coriander, cumin, ginger, chili powder, salt, and pepper to the frying pan. Sauté for 5 minutes, stirring occasionally.
4. Add the drained chick-peas and the reserved tomato liquid to the frying pan. Mix well and cook over low heat for 5 minutes.

CARIBBEAN RED BEANS

2 servings

1   *tablespoon vegetable oil*
1   *small yellow onion, peeled and minced*
1   *large clove garlic, peeled and minced*
1   *small green pepper, seeded and minced*
1   *large ripe tomato, peeled, seeded, and minced*
¼   *teaspoon dried oregano*
    Salt and freshly ground black pepper
1   *10½-ounce can red kidney beans, drained*
¼   *teaspoon drained capers*
4   *stuffed olives, sliced*

1. Heat the oil in an 8-inch nonstick frying pan. When the oil is hot, add the onion, garlic, and green pepper. Sauté over very low heat for 10 minutes, stirring occasionally. Do not let the vegetables brown. Add the tomato and sauté for 5 minutes longer. Season the mixture with the oregano and salt and pepper to taste, and cook over very low heat for 10 minutes, stirring occasionally.
2. Add the beans, capers, and sliced olives, mixing them in gently with a wooden spoon. Cook for 5 minutes longer and serve immediately.

DESSERTS

APPLE AND PEAR COMPOTE

6 servings

2 *red or yellow apples, peeled and cored*
2 *almost ripe pears, peeled and cored*
1 *1-inch piece cinnamon stick*
½ *cup water*
   Sugar (optional)

1. Quarter the apples and pears and cut them into ½-inch-thick slices. Put the slices into a small heavy pot with a cover. Add the cinnamon stick and the water.
2. Bring to a boil, cover, and lower the heat. Cook for about 10 minutes, stirring occasionally. The pears should be just tender and the apples beginning to break up.
3. Pour into a bowl and sweeten, if necessary. Cool, cover, and chill. Remove the cinnamon stick before serving.

BAKED APPLES

4 servings

4 *large baking apples*
4 *tablespoons brown sugar*
4 *1-inch pieces cinnamon stick*

1. Preheat the oven to 375 degrees.
2. Wash and core the apples, making sure that you do not cut through the bottom of the apples. Pour 1 tablespoon of the sugar into the cavity of each apple. Insert a piece of cinnamon stick into the cavity of each apple.
3. Put the apples in a square baking pan and pour in boiling water to come halfway up the apples. Cover the pan tightly with foil and bake for about 45 minutes, or until the apples are tender to the touch. Remove from the cooking liquid and allow the apples to cool to room temperature before serving.

APPLESAUCE

6 servings

2 *pounds Macintosh apples*
1 *2-inch piece cinnamon stick*
1 *cup water*
   Granulated sugar

1. Wash the apples and cut them into quarters. Remove the cores and peel the quarters. Wash the apple pieces thoroughly in cool water and let them drain.
2. Put the cinnamon stick and water into a saucepan. Slice the apple quarters coarsely and add them to the pan. Bring to a boil over medium heat. Cover the pan, lower the heat, and cook, stirring occasionally, for 5 to 10 minutes, or until the apples are tender. (You will find that the apples will break up nicely as you stir them.) Mix in sugar to taste while the applesauce is still warm.
3. Cool the applesauce to room temperature and then transfer the sauce and cinnamon stick

to a glass jar. Cover tightly and refrigerate until needed. The applesauce will keep for almost 2 weeks tightly covered in the refrigerator.

Note: If you like raisins, you can add about ⅓ cup raisins to the applesauce while it is still warm.

APPLE-FIG CREAM
4 servings

1   cup water
2   tablespoons granulated sugar
1   1-inch piece cinnamon stick
¼   teaspoon light mustard seeds
1   pound Macintosh apples, peeled, cored, and
    quartered
5   dried figs, stems removed, finely minced

1. Put the water, sugar, cinnamon stick, and mustard seeds into a small heavy saucepan. Bring to a boil, lower the heat, and simmer, uncovered, for 10 minutes, stirring occasionally. Strain the syrup to remove the cinnamon stick and mustard seeds and return it to the saucepan.

2. Bring the syrup back to a boil and add the apple quarters and minced figs. Stir to mix well. Cover the pan and cook over low heat for 10 minutes, stirring occasionally to break up the apples and to prevent the mixture from sticking. Cool to room temperature and transfer the cream to a glass or crockery bowl. Cover tightly and refrigerate overnight before serving.

SAUTÉED BANANAS WITH HONEY
2 servings

2 ripe bananas
2 tablespoons butter or margarine
2 tablespoons honey
2 tablespoons shredded coconut, toasted

1. Peel the bananas and cut them in half lengthwise.

2. Melt the butter in a frying pan large enough to hold the bananas comfortably. When it is hot and bubbling, add the bananas. Sauté over medium heat for 1 minute. Turn carefully and sauté for 1 minute longer. Spoon the honey equally over the banana halves. Cook for 30 seconds longer. Remove the bananas to 2 serving plates. Sprinkle 1 tablespoon of the toasted coconut over each serving. Serve immediately.

STEWED FRUIT
6 servings

1 pound mixed dried fruit, such as pitted prunes,
   apples, apricots, peaches, pears, etc.
3 cups cold water
2 whole cloves
1 2-inch piece cinnamon stick
1 tablespoon honey (optional)

1. Put the dried fruit in a large saucepan with the cold water, cloves, and cinnamon stick. Bring to a boil, lower the heat, and simmer, uncovered, for 20 minutes, stirring occasionally.

2. Remove the pan from the heat and taste the fruit mixture. If desired, sweeten it with the honey. Let the mixture cool to room temperature, then transfer it to a glass jar with a tight lid. Refrigerate overnight before serving.

JAM PARFAIT

1   cup ricotta cheese
1   tablespoon confectioners' sugar
¼   teaspoon vanilla extract
1   tablespoon slivered almonds (optional)
2   tablespoons cherry or strawberry preserves
    Ground cinnamon

1. Put the ricotta into a small mixing bowl. Use a fork to beat the ricotta until it is smooth and very creamy.

2. Put the confectioners' sugar into a small sieve and press the sugar through the sieve with the back of a spoon over the top of the beaten ricotta. Again, use the fork to combine the sugar and ricotta. Beat in the vanilla and stir in the almonds. Swirl the preserves lightly through the beaten ricotta mixture with a small spoon (don't mix in too thoroughly). Divide the cream between two stemmed wine glasses (probably the only time you'll be using wineglasses during your pregnancy), cover the glasses tightly with foil, and refrigerate for at least ½ hour before serving. Sprinkle a little ground cinnamon over the top of the parfait just before serving.

Note: I've found that the cherry preserves hold together better than the strawberry preserves when combined with the ricotta. But they both taste equally good. Do not make this dessert too far in advance of serving. It is a good, last-minute dish.

GOLD-TOPPED ICE CREAM
2 servings

3   tablespoons honey
4   small scoops good vanilla ice cream
2   tablespoons toasted coconut or toasted sliced almonds

1. Put the honey into a very small saucepan and heat it over very low heat until it is runny and warm.

2. Put 2 scoops of vanilla ice cream into individual serving dishes. Pour the warm honey equally over each serving. Top with the coconut or almonds and serve immediately.

FROZEN YOGURT CREAM
2 servings

1   cup plain yogurt
2   tablespoons heavy cream
1½ tablespoons honey
2   tablespoons plus 2 teaspoons strawberry preserves

1. Combine the yogurt, heavy cream, honey, and 2 tablespoons of the strawberry preserves in a small mixing bowl. Stir to mix well.

2. Put 1 teaspoon of strawberry preserves in the bottom of two heavy custard cups. Divide the yogurt cream equally between the two custard cups. Cover tightly with aluminum foil and freeze for 1 hour *only.* (Any more time in the freezer and the cream will be almost too hard to get a spoon into.)

Note: This is a dessert that you can make at the last minute, so that it will set while you are eating the first courses of your dinner.

CHOCOLATE-RAISIN BREAD PUDDING

4 servings

2   cups milk
1/2 cup chocolate chips
2   eggs
1/4 cup sugar
2   cups pumpernickel bread cubes, cut 1/4 inch
     square
1/3 cup raisins
1/4 teaspoon vanilla extract
     Butter

1. Pour the milk into a small saucepan and heat it over low heat until small bubbles appear around the sides of the pan. Do not let the milk come to a boil. Remove the pan from the heat and stir in the chocolate chips. Stir continuously until the chocolate has melted completely.

2. Break the eggs into a medium-sized mixing bowl. Beat the eggs with a wire whisk until they are frothy. Gradually beat in the warm chocolate-milk mixture until well combined.

3. Stir in the sugar, bread cubes, raisins, and vanilla extract, and mix well. Let sit for 5 minutes.

4. Preheat the oven to 350 degrees. Lightly butter a 1-quart soufflé dish. Bring a large saucepan of water to a boil.

5. Pour the pudding mixture into the prepared soufflé dish. Place the dish in the center of a 9- x 13-inch roasting pan. Pour 1 to 1½ inches of boiling water into the roasting pan. Bake in the middle of the oven for 1 hour, or until the pudding is set. (You can test the pudding for doneness by inserting a knife about 1 inch from the edge. If the knife comes out clean, the pudding is done.) Remove the soufflé dish from the roasting pan as soon as you take it out of the oven. Let the pudding cool to room temperature before serving.

Note: This pudding is also good cold. Be sure to trim the crusts from the bread before you cut it into cubes. Just a word about the pumpernickel: I know it sounds strange, but you can't tell it's pumpernickel bread—really!

BROWN SUGAR-BANANA CUSTARD

6 servings

2½ cups milk
1   1-inch piece cinnamon stick
4   eggs
1/4 cup granulated sugar
1/4 cup dark brown sugar
1/2 teaspoon vanilla extract
1   medium-sized banana, mashed (about 1/2
     cup)
     Butter

1. Put the milk and cinnamon stick into a small saucepan and heat over low heat until small bubbles appear around the sides of the pan. Do not let the milk come to a boil. Remove the pan from the heat and let the milk cool for 15 minutes.

2. Put the eggs, sugars, and vanilla into a medium-sized mixing bowl. Use a wire whisk to beat the eggs and flavorings together until they are frothy. Add the mashed banana and beat until the mixture is well combined.

3. Preheat the oven to 375 degrees. Generously butter the inside of a 1-quart soufflé dish. Bring a large saucepan of water to a boil.

4. Remove the cinnamon stick from the milk and slowly beat the warm milk into the egg

mixture until it is well combined. Pour the custard mixture into the prepared soufflé dish. Place the dish in the center of a 9- x 13-inch roasting pan. Pour 1 to 1½ inches of boiling water into the roasting pan. Bake in the middle of the oven for 1½ hours, or until a knife inserted near the outside edge of the dish comes out clean. Remove the soufflé dish from the roasting pan as soon as you take it out of the oven. Let the custard cool to room temperature before serving.

Note: This dish is also good served cold, and makes an excellent snack as well as dessert.

BAKED CUSTARD

4 servings

2   cups milk
3   eggs
⅓   cup sugar
1   teaspoon vanilla extract
    Pinch of ground nutmeg
    Butter

1. Pour the milk into a small saucepan and heat it over low heat until small bubbles appear around the sides of the pan. Do not let the milk come to a boil. Remove the pan from the heat and let the milk cool for 15 minutes.

2. Put the eggs, sugar, vanilla, and nutmeg into a medium-sized mixing bowl. Use a wire whisk to beat the eggs and flavorings together until they are frothy.

3. Preheat the oven to 375 degrees. Generously butter the inside of a ¾-quart soufflé dish. Bring a large saucepan of water to a boil.

4. Slowly beat the warm milk into the egg mixture until it is well combined. Pour the custard mixture into the prepared soufflé dish.

Place the dish in the center of a 9- x 13-inch roasting pan. Pour 1 to 1½ inches of boiling water into the roasting pan. Bake in the middle of the oven for 1 hour, or until a knife inserted near the outside edge of the dish comes out clean. Remove the soufflé dish from the roasting pan as soon as you take it out of the oven. Let the custard cool to room temperature before serving.

Note: This dish is also good served cold, and makes an excellent snack as well as dessert.

RICE PUDDING

¼   cup long-grain rice
2   cups milk
2   tablespoons plus 1 teaspoon sugar
1   1-inch piece cinnamon stick
1   egg
⅓   cup raisins
¼   teaspoon vanilla extract
¼   cup heavy cream

1. Put the rice, milk, 2 tablespoons of sugar, and cinnamon stick into a 1-quart heavy saucepan. Stir with a wooden spoon to combine well. Put the saucepan on a Flame-tamer or asbestos pad over medium heat. Cover the saucepan and cook, stirring occasionally for 2 hours. (Do not let the rice stick to the bottom of the pan and do not let the milk boil. The idea is to have the milk absorbed very slowly while the rice becomes very, very soft.)

2. When the mixture has cooked for 2 hours, beat the egg with a fork in a small bowl. When the egg is well beaten, add about 4 tablespoons of the milk from the rice mixture to the beaten egg and beat it in well. (Don't worry, there will be enough excess milk there for you to do it, if your flame was low enough.) Pour the egg

mixture slowly into the saucepan, stirring constantly with a wooden spoon. Cover the pan and cook for 15 minutes longer.

3. Remove the rice pudding from the heat and stir in the raisins and vanilla. Cover the pan again and let the pudding cool to room temperature.

4. When the pudding has cooled, transfer it to a glass bowl, cover tightly with aluminum foil, and refrigerate for 8 hours or overnight.

5. About 2 hours before you serve the pudding for the first time, chill a small bowl and a wire whisk. When they are completely cold, pour the heavy cream into the bowl and beat until the cream is stiff. Sprinkle the remaining teaspoon of sugar over the cream and beat it in well.

6. Remove the cinnamon stick from the cold rice pudding and combine the sweetened whipped cream with the cold rice pudding, mixing it in very well with a wooden spoon. Cover tightly with aluminum foil and refrigerate until needed.

Note: This is an extremely creamy pudding, which I like much better than the baked versions. If you prefer a more solid rice pudding, you can dispense with the sweetened heavy cream. Also, I find that this is sweet enough for me, but you might like it a little sweeter. If you do, add 3 tablespoons of sugar to the rice and milk instead of 2.

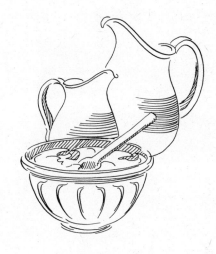

Bibliography

Preparing for Pregnancy

Abbasi, Ali A., et al. "Experimental Zinc Deficiency in Man." *J. Lab. Clin. Med.* 96 (Sept. 1980): 544.

Amelar, Richard, Lawrence Dubin, and Patrick Walsh. *Male Infertility.* Philadelphia: W. B. Saunders, 1977.

Brody, Jane E. "An Eating Disorder of Binges and Purges Reported Widespread." *New York Times*, 20 Oct. 1981.

Chernin, Kim. *The Obsession: Reflections on the Tyrany of Slenderness.* New York: Harper & Row, 1981.

Churchill, John A. "Factors in Intrauterine Impoverishment." In *Nutritional Impacts on Women*, edited by K. Moghissi and T. Evans. New York: Harper & Row, 1977.

Crosby, Warren M. et al. "Fetal Malnutrition: An Appraisal of Correlated Factors." *Amer. J. Obst. & Gyn.* 128 (1 May 1977): 22.

Diebel, Patricia. "Effects of Cigarette Smoking on Maternal Nutrition and the Fetus." *JOG Nurs.* 9 (Dec. 1980).

Edwards, L. E. et al. "Pregnancy in the Underweight Woman: Course, Outcome, and Growth Patterns of the Infant." *Amer. J. Obst. & Gyn.* 135 (1979): 297.

"Fathers' Smoking May Harm Fetuses." *New York Times*, 20 Jan. 1983.

FDA Drug Bulletin, Nov. 1980.

———— , July 1981.

Food and Nutrition Board. National Research Council, 1980. *Recommended Dietary Allowances.* 9th rev. ed. Washington: National Academy of Sciences.

Guttmacher, Alan. *The Fetus, Pregnancy, Birth, and Family Planning.* New York: Viking, 1973.

Hurley, Lucille S., and H. Swenerton. "Congenital Malformations Resulting from Zinc Deficiency in Rats." *Proc. Soc. Exp. Biol. Med.* 123 (1966): 692.

McGarry, John M., and Joan Andrews. "Smoking in Pregnancy and Vitamin B_{12} Metabolism." *Br. Med. J.* 2 (1972): 74.

Mahan, Charles S. "Revolution in Obstetrics: Pregnancy Nutrition." *J. Fla. Med. Assoc.* 66 (Apr. 1979): 367.

March of Dimes Birth Defects Foundation. "Birth Defects: Tragedy and Hope." New York, Jan. 1979.

———— . "Drugs, Alcohol, Tobacco Abuse During Pregnancy." New York, Oct. 1980.

———— . "Caffeine and Pregnancy: Answers to Common Questions." *J. Pract. Nurs.* 31 (Jan. 1981).

Morris, Merri B., and Louis Weinstein. "Caffeine and the Fetus: Is Trouble Brewing?" *Amer. J. Obst. & Gyn.* 140 (15 July 1981).

Oullette, Eileen M., and Henry L. Rosett. "The Effect of Maternal Alcohol Ingestion During Pregnancy in Offspring." In *Nutritional Impacts on Women*, edited by K. Moghissi and T. Evans. New York: Harper & Row, 1977.

Pitkin, Roy M. "Nutrition During Pregnancy." In *Nutritional Disorders of American Women*, edited by M. Winick. New York: Wiley, 1977.

————. et al. "Maternal Nutrition." *Amer. J. Obst. & Gyn.* 40 (Dec. 1972): 773.

Ryan, Kenneth J., and Steven Schoenbaum. "No Association Between Coffee Consumption and Adverse Outcome of Pregnancy." *New Eng. J. Med.* 306 (Jan. 1982): 141.

Stewart, Bruce H. "Drugs That Cause and Cure Male Infertility." *Drug Therapy.* (Dec. 1975): 420.

Weathersbee, Paul, Larry Olsen, and J. Robert Lodge. "Caffeine and Pregnancy: A Retrospective Survey." *Postgrad. Med.* 62 (Sept. 1977): 64.

Winick, Myron M. "Eating Habits Called Factor in Life-Span." *Newsday,* Sept. 16, 1981.

The First Month

Brody, Jane E. *Jane Brody's Nutrition Book*. New York: Norton, 1981.

Burros, Marian. "Feeding Programs Reported at Risk." *New York Times,* 23 Sept. 1981.

Flanagan, Geraldine L. *The First Nine Months of Life*. New York: Simon & Schuster, 1962.

Food and Nutrition Board. National Research Council, 1980. *Recommended Dietary Allowances*. 9th rev. ed. Washington: National Academy of Sciences.

Guttmacher, Alan. *The Fetus, Pregnancy, Birth, and Family Planning*. New York: Viking, 1973.

Habicht, Jean-Pierre et al. "Relation of Maternal Supplementary Feeding to Birth Weight." In *Nutrition and Fetal Development*, edited by M. Winick, vol. 2. New York: Wiley, 1974.

Lechtig, Aaron et al. "Effect of Moderate Maternal Malnutrition on the Placenta." *Amer. J. Obst. & Gyn.* 123 (15 Sept. 1975): 191.

March of Dimes Birth Defects Foundation. "Be Good to Your Baby Before It Is Born." New York, Jan. 1979.

————. "Drugs, Alcohol, Tobacco Abuse During Pregnancy." New York, Oct. 1980.

Nisander, Kenneth, and Esther Jackson. "Physical Characteristics of the Gravida and Their Association with Birth and Perinatal Death." *Amer. J. Obst. & Gyn.* 119 (1 June 1974): 306.

Pitkin, Roy M. "Nutritional Support in Obstetrics and Gynecology." *Clin. Obst. & Gyn.* 19 (Sept. 1976): 489.

Rosso, Pedro. "Placental Growth, Development, and Function in Relation to Maternal Nutrition." *Fed. Proc.* 39 (Feb. 1980): 250.

————. "Prenatal Nutrition and Fetal Growth Development." *Pediatrics Annals* 10 (Nov. 1981): 21.

Rugh, Robert, and Landrum B. Shettles. *From Conception to Birth*. New York: Harper & Row, 1971.

Rush, David. "Examination of the Relationship Between Birthweight, Cigarette Smoking During Pregnancy, and Maternal Weight Gain." *J. Obst. Gyn. Br. Commonw.* 81 (Oct. 1974): 746.

Stewart, Felicia et al. *My Body, My Health: The Concerned Woman's Guide to Gynecology*. New York: Wiley, 1979.

Vermeersch, Joyce. "Physiological Basis of Nutritional Needs." In *Nutrition in Pregnancy and Lactation*. Saint Louis: C. V. Mosby, 1977.

Williams, Roger J. *Nutrition Against Disease*. New York: Pitman, 1971.

Williams, Sue R. "Nutritional Guidance in Prenatal

Care." In *Nutrition in Pregnancy and Lactation*. Saint Louis: C. V. Mosby, 1977.

Zlatnick, Frank J. "Dietary Protein and Human Pregnancy Performance." *J. Reprod. Med.* 22 (April 1979): 193.

The Second Month

Boston Women's Health Collective. *Our Bodies, Our Selves*. New York: Simon & Schuster, 1979.

Burton, Benjamin T. *Human Nutrition*. 3d ed. New York: McGraw-Hill, 1976.

Carter, C. O. "Clues to the Aetiology of Neural Tube Malformation." *Div. Med. Chil. Neurol.* 16 (1974): 3.

Flanagan, Geraldine L. *The First Nine Months of Life*. New York: Simon & Schuster, 1962.

Food and Nutrition Board. National Research Council, 1980. *Recommended Dietary Allowances*. 9th rev. ed. Washington: National Academy of Sciences.

Laurence, K. M. et al. "Increased Risk of Recurrence of Pregnancies Complicated By Fetal Neural Tube Defects in Mothers Receiving Poor Diets and Possible Benefits of Dietary Counseling." *Br. Med. J.* 281 (Dec. 1980): 1952.

Moghissi, Kamran S. "Maternal Nutrition in Pregnancy." *Clin. Obst. Gyn.* 21 (June 1978): 297.

Pitkin, Roy M. "Nutritional Support in Obstetrics and Gynecology." *Clin. Obst. & Gyn.* 19 (Sept. 1976): 489.

————. "Nutrition During Pregnancy." In *Nutritional Disorders of American Women*, edited by M. Winick. New York: Wiley, 1977.

————. et al. "Maternal Nutrition: A Selective Review of Clinical Topics." *J. Obst. & Gyn.* 40 (Dec. 1972): 773.

Rosso, Pedro. "Prenatal Nutrition and Fetal Growth Development." *Pediatric Annals* 10 (21 Nov. 1981).

Rugh, Robert, and Landrum B. Shettles. *From Conception to Birth*. New York: Harper & Row, 1971.

Smithells, R. W., S. Sheppard, and C. J. Schorah. "Vitamin Deficiencies and Neural Tube Defects." *Arch. Dis. Child.* 51 (1976): 944.

Stone, Martin et al. "Folic Acid Deficiency in Pregnancy." *Amer. J. Obst. & Gyn.* 99 (Nov. 1967): 638.

Vermeersch, Joyce. "Physiological Basis of Nutritional Needs." In *Nutrition in Pregnancy and Lactation*. Saint Louis: C. V. Mosby, 1977.

Williams, Roger J. *Nutrition Against Disease*. New York: Pitman, 1971.

Williams, Sue R. "Nutritional Therapy in Special Conditions of Pregnancy and Lactation." In *Nutrition in Pregnancy and Lactation*. Saint Louis: C. V. Mosby, 1977.

Winick, Myron M. *Growing Up Healthy: A Parent's Guide to Good Nutrition*. New York: Morrow, 1982.

The Third Month

Barrett, David E., Marian Yarrow-Radke, and Robert E. Klein. "Chronic Malnutrition and Child Behavior: Effects of Early Calorie Supplementation on Social and Emotional Functioning at School Age." *Developmental Psychology*. 18 (July 1982): 541.

Boston Women's Health Collective. *Our Bodies, Our Selves*. New York: Simon & Schuster, 1979.

Burton, Benjamin T. *Human Nutrition*. 3d. ed. New York: McGraw-Hill, 1976.

Edwards, L. E. et al. "Pregnancy in the Underweight Woman: Course, Outcome, and Growth

Patterns of the Infant." *Obst. & Gyn.* 135 (Oct. 1979): 297.

Flanagan, Geraldine L. *The First Nine Months of Life.* New York: Simon & Schuster, 1962.

Food and Nutrition Board. National Research Council, 1980. *Recommended Dietary Allowances.* 9th rev. ed. Washington: National Academy of Sciences.

Robinson, Margaret. "Salt in Pregnancy." *Lancet* (25 Jan. 1958): 178.

Rosso, Pedro. "Effects of Maternal Dietary Restrictions During Pregnancy." In *Nutritional Impacts on Women*, edited by K. Moghissi and T. Evans. New York: Harper & Row, 1977.

Vermeersch, Joyce. "Physiological Basis of Nutritional Needs." In *Nutrition in Pregnancy and Lactation.* Saint Louis. C. V. Mosby, 1977.

Williams, Roger J. *Nutrition Against Disease.* New York: Pitman, 1971.

Williams, S. *Handbook of Maternal and Infant Nutrition.* Berkeley, Calif.: S.R.W. Productions, 1976.

Winick, Myron M. "Malnutrition and Mental Development." In *Malnutrition and Brain Development.* New York: Oxford University Press, 1976.

The Fourth Month

Boston Women's Health Collective. *Our Bodies, Our Selves.* New York: Simon & Schuster, 1979.

Brewer, Gayle S., and Thomas Brewer. *What Every Pregnant Woman Should Know: The Truth About Pregnancy.* New York: Random House, 1977.

Brewer, Thomas H. "Human Maternal-Fetal Nutrition." *Obst. & Gyn.* (Dec. 1972): 868.

Brody, Jane E. *Jane Brody's Nutrition Book.* New York: Norton, 1981.

Drayer, Jan I., and Michael A. Weber. "Mild and Moderate Hypertension During Pregnancy." *Drug Therapy* (Sept. 1981): 77.

Flanagan, Geraldine L. *The First Nine Months of Life.* New York: Simon & Schuster, 1962.

Food and Nutriton Board. National Research Council, 1980. *Recommended Dietary Allowances.* 9th rev. ed. Washington: National Academy of Sciences.

Kaminetzky, Harold. "Sodium in Pregnancy." Part 1. *Obst. & Gyn.* 35 (April 1978): 255.

————— . "Sodium in Pregnancy." Part 2. *Obst. & Gyn.* 35 (June 1978): 401.

Lindberg, Bo S. "Salt, Diuretics, and Pregnancy." *Gynecol. Obst. Invest.* 10 (June 1979): 145.

Metcoff, Jack. "Biochemical Markers of Intrauterine Malnutrition." In *Nutrition and Fetal Development*, edited by M. Winick. New York: Wiley, 1974.

Moghissi, Kamran S. *Clinical Obstetrics and Gynecology.* New York: Harper & Row, 1978.

Pike, Ruth L., and Helen Smiciklas. "A Reappraisal of Sodium Restriction During Pregnancy." *Int. J. Gyn. & Obstet.* 10 (Jan. 1972): 1.

Pitkin, Roy M. "Nutritional Support in Obstetrics and Gynecology." *Clin. Obst. & Gyn.* 19 (Sept. 1976): 489.

Robinson, Margaret. "Salt in Pregnancy." *Lancet* (Jan. 1958): 178.

Rosso, Pedro. "Placental Growth, Development, and Function in Relation to Maternal Nutrition." *Fed. Proc.* 39 (Feb. 1980): 250.

Rugh, Robert, and Landrum B. Shettles. *From Conception to Birth.* New York: Harper & Row, 1971.

Schewitz, Lionel J. "Hypertension and Renal Disease in Pregnancy." *Med. Clin. N. A.* 55 (Jan. 1971): 47.

Winick, Myron. *Malnutrition and Brain Development.* New York: Oxford University Press, 1976.

Worthington, Bonnie S., Joyce Vermeersch, and Sue R. Williams. *Nutrition in Pregnancy and Lactation.* Saint Louis: C. V. Mosby, 1977.

The Fifth Month

Boston Women's Health Collective. *Our Bodies, Our Selves.* New York: Simon & Schuster, 1979.

Bourne, Gordon, and David N. Danforth. *Pregnancy.* London: Harper & Row, 1975.

Brewer, Thomas, and Gayle S. Brewer. *What Every Pregnant Woman Should Know: The Truth About Pregnancy.* New York: Random House, 1977.

Brody, Jane E. *Jane Brody's Nutrition Book.* New York: Norton, 1981.

Burton, Benjamin T. *Human Nutrition.* 3d ed. New York: McGraw-Hill, 1976.

Flanagan, Geraldine L. *The First Nine Months of Life.* New York: Simon & Schuster, 1962.

Kaminetzky, Harold. "Sodium in Pregnancy." Part 1. *Obst. & Gyn.* 35 (April 1978): 255.

Lindberg, Bo A. "Salt, Diuretics, and Pregnancy." *Gyn. Obst. Invest.* 10 (June 1979): 145.

McFee, John G. "Anemia: A High Risk Complication of Pregnancy." *Clin. Obst. & Gyn.* 16 (1973): 153.

Mahan, Charles S. "Revolution in Obstetrics: Pregnancy Nutrition." *J. Fla. Med. Assoc.* 66 (April 1979): 367.

Pitkin, Roy M. "Nutritional Support in Obstetrics and Gynecology." *Clin. Obst. & Gyn.* 19 (Sept. 1976): 489.

——— . "Nutrition During Pregnancy: The Clinical Approach." In *Nutritional Disorders of American Women*, edited by M. Winick. New York: Wiley, 1977.

——— . et al. "Maternal Nutrition: A Selective Review of Clinical Topics." *Jour. Obst. & Gyn.* 40 (Dec. 1972): 6.

Rugh, Robert, and Landrum B. Shettles. *From Conception to Birth.* New York: Harper & Row, 1971.

Williams, Roger J. *Nutrition Against Disease.* New York: Pitman, 1971.

Worthington, Bonnie S., Joyce Vermeersch, and Sue R. Williams. *Nutrition in Pregnancy and Lactation.* Saint Louis: C. V. Mosby, 1977.

The Sixth Month

Boston Women's Health Collective. *Our Bodies, Our Selves.* New York: Simon & Schuster, 1979.

Brody, Jane E. *Jane Brody's Nutrition Book.* New York: Norton, 1981.

Burton, Benjamin T. *Human Nutrition.* 3d ed. New York: McGraw-Hill, 1976.

Collipp, Jack P. "Cardiomyopathy and Selenium Deficiency in a Two Year Old Girl on L. I." *New Eng. J. Med.* 304 (21 May 1981): 1304.

Flanagan, Geraldine L. *The First Nine Months of Life.* New York: Simon & Schuster, 1962.

Food and Nutrition Board. National Research Council, 1980. *Recommended Dietary Allowances.* 9th rev. ed. Washington: National Academy of Sciences.

Hambidge, K. M. "Trace-Element Nutrition." *Pediatric Annals* 10 (Nov. 1981): 53.

March of Dimes Birth Defects Foundation. "Drugs, Alcohol, Tobacco Abuse During Pregnancy." New York, Oct. 1980.

Moghissi, Kamran S. "Maternal Nutrition in Pregnancy." *Clin. Obst. & Gyn.* 21 (June 1978): 297.

Rosso, Pedro. "Prenatal Nutrition and Fetal Growth Development." *Pediatric Annals.* 10 (21 Nov. 1981): 21.

Rugh, Robert, and Landrum B. Shettles. *From Conception to Birth.* New York: Harper & Row, 1971.

U.S. Department of Health, Education, and Welfare. Public Health Service. National Institute on Drug Abuse. *What you Need to Know About Marijuana.* Washington: Government Printing Office, 1980.

Williams, S. *Handbook of Maternal and Infant Nutrition.* Berkeley, Calif.: S.R.W. Productions, 1976.

Williams, Sue Rodwell. "Nutritional Therapy in Special Conditions of Pregnancy." In *Nutrition in Pregnancy and Lactation.* Saint Louis: C. V. Mosby, 1977.

The Seventh Month

Boston Women's Health Collective. *Our Bodies, Our Selves.* New York: Simon & Schuster, 1977.

Brasel, Jo Anne. "Cellular Changes in Intrauterine Malnutrition." In *Nutrition and Fetal Development,* edited by M. Winick, vol. 2. New York: Wiley, 1974.

Brewer, Gayle, and Tom Brewer. *What Every Pregnant Woman Should Know: The Truth About Pregnancy.* New York: Random House, 1977.

Flanagan, Geraldine L. *The First Nine Months of Life.* New York: Simon & Schuster, 1962.

Food and Nutrition Board. National Research Council, 1980. *Recommended Dietary Allowances.* 9th rev. ed. Washington: National Academy of Sciences.

Metcoff, Jack. "Biochemical Markers of Intrauterine Malnutrition." In *Nutrition and Fetal Development,* edited by M. Winick, vol. 2. New York: Wiley, 1974.

Miller, Herbert C., and Khatab Hassanein. "Fetal Malnutrition in White Newborn Infants: Maternal Factors." *Pediatrics* 52 (Oct. 1973): 504.

Moghissi, Kamran S. "Relationship of Maternal Amino Acids and Proteins to Fetal Growth and Mental Development." *Amer. J. Obst. & Gyn.* 123 (15 Oct. 1975): 5.

————. "Maternal Nutrition in Pregnancy." *Clin. Obst. & Gyn.* 21 (June 1978): 297.

Naeye, Richard et al. "Relation of Poverty and Race to Birth Weight and Organ and Cell Structure in the Newborn." *Pediat. Res.* 5 (1971): 17.

Pike, Ruth, and Helen Smiciklas. "A Reappraisal of Sodium Restriction During Pregnancy." *Int. J. Gyn. & Obst.* 10 (1 Jan. 1972): 1.

Pitkin, Roy M. "Nutrition During Pregnancy." In *Nutritional Disorders of American Women,* edited by M. Winick. New York: Wiley, 1977.

Rugh, Robert, and Landrum B. Shettles. *From Conception to Birth.* New York: Harper & Row, 1971.

Scott, Kenneth E., and Robert Usher. "Fetal Malnutrition: Its Incidence, Causes, and Effects." *Amer. J. Obst. & Gyn.* 94 (Apr. 1966): 951.

Stone, Martin L., and A. L. Luhby. "Folic Acid Metabolism in Pregnancy." *Amer. J. Obst. & Gyn.* 99 (Nov. 1967): 638.

Williams, Roger J. *Nutrition Against Disease.* New York: Pitman, 1971.

Worthington, Bonnie, Joyce Vermeersch, and Sue R. Williams. *Nutrition in Pregnancy and Lactation.* Saint Louis: C. V. Mosby, 1977.

The Eighth Month

Brody, Jane E. *Jane Brody's Nutrition Book.* New York: Norton, 1981.

Churchill, John A. "Factors in Intrauterine Impoverishment." In *Nutritional Impacts on Women,* edited by K. Moghissi and T. Evans. New York: Harper & Row, 1977.

Flanagan, Geraldine L. *The First Nine Months of Life.* New York: Simon & Schuster, 1962.

Food and Nutrition Board. National Research Council, 1980. *Recommended Dietary Allowances.* 9th rev. ed. Washington: National Academy of Sciences.

Liley, H. M., and Beth Day. *Modern Motherhood.* New York: Random House, 1966.

McFee, John G. "Anemia: A High Risk Complication of Pregnancy." *Clin. Obst. & Gyn.* 16 (1973): 153.

Moghissi, Kamran S. "Relationship of Maternal Amino Acids and Proteins to Fetal Growth and Mental Development." *Amer. J. Obst. & Gyn.* 123 (15 Oct. 1975): 5.

————. "Maternal Nutrition in Pregnancy." *Clin. Obst. & Gyn.* 21 (June 1978): 297.

Pitkin, Roy M. "Nutritional Support in Obstetrics and Gynecology." *Clin. Obst. & Gyn.* 19 (Sept. 1976): 489.

Rosso, Pedro. "Prenatal Nutrition and Fetal Growth Development." *Pediat. Annals* 10 (21 Nov. 1981): 21.

Rugh, Robert, and Landrum B. Shettles. *From Conception to Birth.* New York: Harper & Row, 1971.

Winick, Myron. "Cellular Growth in Intrauterine Malnutrition." *Ped. Clin. N. Amer.* 17 (Feb. 1970): 69.

————. *Malnutrition and Brain Development.* New York: Oxford University Press, 1976.

The Ninth Month

Boston Women's Health Collective. *Our Bodies, Our Selves.* New York: Simon & Schuster, 1979.

Brewer, Gail S., and Tom Brewer. *What Every Pregnant Woman Should Know: The Truth About Pregnancy.* New York: Random House, 1977.

Brody, Jane E. *Jane Brody's Nutrition Book.* New York: Norton, 1981.

Burton, Benjamin T. *Human Nutrition.* 3d ed. New York: McGraw-Hill, 1976.

Flanagan, Geraldine L. *The First Nine Months of Life.* New York: Simon & Schuster, 1962.

Food and Nutrition Board. National Research Council, 1980. *Recommended Dietary Allowances.* 9th rev. ed. Washington: National Academy of Sciences.

Pitkin, Roy M. "Maternal Nutrition: A Selective Review of Clinical Topics." *J. Obst. & Gyn.* 40 (Dec. 1972): 773.

Rosso, Pedro. "Effects of Maternal Dietary Restrictions During Pregnancy." In *Nutritional Impacts on Women,* edited by K. Moghissi and T. Evans. New York: Harper & Row, 1977.

Rugh, Robert, and Landrum B. Shettles. *From Conception to Birth.* New York: Harper & Row, 1971.

Takahashi, Yoko I., and John E. Smith. "Prenatal Biochemical Changes in Vitamin A Deficient Rats Given Retinoic Acid." *Fed. Proceed.* 32 (Mar. 1973): 910.

Williams, Roger J. *Nutrition Against Disease.* New York: Pitman, 1971.

Breast Feeding

Atkinson, P. J., and R. R. West. "Loss of Skeletal Calcium in Lactating Women." *J. Obst. & Gyn. Br. Common.* 77 (June 1970): 555.

Boston Women's Health Collective. *Our Bodies, Our Selves.* New York: Simon & Schuster, 1979.

Burton, Benjamin T. *Human Nutrition.* 3d ed. New York: McGraw-Hill, 1976.

Committee on Nutrition. American Academy of Pediatrics. "Encouraging Breast Feeding." *Pediatrics* 65 (March 1980): 657.

Filer, Lloyd J., Jr. "Maternal Nutrition in Lactation." *Clin. Perinatol.* 2 (Sept. 1975): 353.

———. "Relationship of Nutrition to Lactation and Newborn Development." In *Nutritional Impacts on Women,* edited by K. Moghissi and T. Evans. New York: Harper & Row, 1977.

Food and Nutrition Board. National Research Council, 1980. *Recommended Dietary Allowances.* 9th rev. ed. Washington: National Academy of Sciences.

Goodrich, Frederick W., Jr. *Preparing for Childbirth: A Manual for Expectant Parents.* Englewood Cliffs, N.J.: Prentice-Hall, 1966.

Hanson, L. A. "Breast Milk and Defense Against Infection in the Newborn." *Archives of Dis. in Childhood.* 47 (1972): 845.

Jelliffe, Derrick B. "Unique Properties of Human Milk." *J. Reprod. Med.* 14 (Apr. 1975): 133.

La Leche League International. *The Womanly Art of Breastfeeding.* 3d. ed. Franklin Park, Ill., 1981.

Sims, Laura S. "Dietary Status of Lactating Women." *J. Amer. Diet. Assoc.* 73 (Aug. 1978): 139.

Thompson, A. M., and A. E. Black. "Nutritional Aspects of Human Lactation." *Bulletin of the World Health Organ.* 52 (1965): 163.

Whichelow, Margaret J. "Success and Failure of Breast Feeding in Relation to Energy Intake." *Proc. Nutr. Soc.* 35 (1976): 62A.

Whitehead, R. G. "Nutrition and Lactation." *Postgrad. Med. J.* 55 (May 1979): 303.

Widdington, Elsie M. "Nutrition and Lactation." In *Nutritional Disorders of American Women,* edited by M. Winick. New York: Wiley, 1977.

Winick, Myron. *Growing Up Healthy: A Parent's Guide to Good Nutrition.* New York: Morrow, 1982.

Worthington, Bonnie S. "Nutrition During Pregnancy, Lactation, and Oral Contraception." *Nursing Cl. of N. Amer.* 14 (June 1979): 269.

What's Ahead for Future Mothers?

Crosby, Warren M. et al. "Fetal Malnutrition: An Appraisal of Correlated Factors." *Amer. J. Obst. & Gyn.* 128 (1 May 1977): 22.

"Fetal Surgery Outside Womb Called a Success." *New York Times,* 15 Nov. 1981.

Harrison, M. F. et al. "Management of the Fetus with a Urinary Tract Malformation." *J. Amer. Med. Assoc.* 246 (7 Aug. 1981): 635.

Moghissi, Kamran S., J. A. Churchill, and Dorothy Kurrie. "Relationship of Maternal Amino Acids and Proteins to Fetal Growth and Mental Development." *Amer. J. Obst. & Gyn.* 123 (15 Oct 1975): 5.

The National Foundation, March of Dimes. "Genetic Counseling." White Plains, NY.

"The New Baby Boom." *Time,* 22 Feb. 1982.: 52.

Stewart, Felicia et al. *My Body, My Health.* New York: Wiley, 1979.